PRAISE FOR
The Metabolic Approach for Cancer

"*The Metabolic Approach to Cancer* explains why medicine has failed to find a single cure for cancer. Read this important book to learn how cancer is an environmental, metabolic disease with many small causes that stack up and what you can do to prevent or even reverse it. Taking control of your environment and your food gives you control over cancer! You'll never look at sugar the same way again."

—DAVE ASPREY, *New York Times* bestselling author of
The Bulletproof Diet; creator, Bulletproof Coffee

"*The Metabolic Approach to Cancer* is a powerhouse of detailed information on how to prevent, manage, and treat cancer. How refreshing to see such a compilation of insight, structure, and sweeping scope, one that centers on the health of the entire individual, not just killing cancer cells alone. It is written in an intimate conversation style that comes from decades of deep personal experience, research, and genuine passion. It's time to welcome a new gem to the universe of books on cancer."

—TRAVIS CHRISTOFFERSON, author of *Tripping over the Truth*

"Dr. Nasha Winters and Jess Higgins Kelley have written an important book, *The Metabolic Approach to Cancer*, that can help cancer patients better manage their disease. Most cancers, regardless of cell or tissue origin, are now recognized as a single metabolic disease that feeds on fermentable fuels like the sugar glucose and the amino acid glutamine. Winters and Kelley provide cancer patients with logical, nontoxic, therapeutic strategies for starving cancer cells of their prime fuels while enhancing overall patient health. This book will be a valuable resource for all cancer patients and their oncologists."

—THOMAS N. SEYFRIED, PhD, author of *Cancer as a Metabolic Disease*

"*The Metabolic Approach to Cancer* is the book I have been yearning for since my cancer diagnosis in 1989. I have been managing my cancer with nutrition and lifestyle, but my research has led to confusing and sometimes contradictory information. This book has everything I need to know in one place. I feel empowered with knowledge about what I can do and why it will make a difference. I want everyone touched by cancer to read this book."

—JAN ADRIAN, MSW, founder and director, Healing Journeys

"In *The Metabolic Approach to Cancer*, Dr. Nasha Winters and Jess Higgins Kelley take the adage 'knowledge is power' to a new level. The book is packed with science-backed, practical, and highly relevant information that could easily overwhelm the reader. But rest assured, in a very caring way the two authors make sure you learn how to set priorities, address the main areas of concern first, and make step-by-step improvements to your well-being. This book has the power to truly transform your health!"

—PATRICIA DALY, author of *The Ketogenic Kitchen*

"*The Metabolic Approach to Cancer* is a terrific resource for anyone interested in treating cancer with natural therapies. This book is delightful and full of valuable information."

—ANN FONFA, president, Annie Appleseed Project

"In *The Metabolic Approach to Cancer*, Dr. Nasha Winters and nutritionist Jess Higgins Kelley expose the inadequacies inherent in the entrenched model of conventional cancer care. Looking beyond the manifestations of a body out of balance, they open the reader's eyes to the underlying epigenetic changes that contribute to the development and progression of this devastating disease. Also included here is a set of tools—including nutrition, lifestyle, and metabolic therapies—that address the root cause of the problem. This integrated approach offers an opportunity to bring body and mind back into balance."

—MIRIAM KALAMIAN, author of *Keto for Cancer*

The
Metabolic
Approach
to Cancer

The
Metabolic
Approach
to Cancer

Integrating Deep Nutrition, the Ketogenic Diet, and Nontoxic Bio-Individualized Therapies

Dr. Nasha Winters, ND, L.Ac., FABNO
Jess Higgins Kelley, MNT

Chelsea Green Publishing
White River Junction, Vermont

Project Manager: Patricia Stone
Developmental Editor: Makenna Goodman
Copy Editor: Jennifer Lipfert
Proofreader: Laura Jorstad
Indexer: Ruth Satterlee
Designer: Melissa Jacobson

Printed in the United States of America.
First printing May 2017.
10 9 8 7 6 5   18 19 20 21

Our Commitment to Green Publishing
Chelsea Green sees publishing as a tool for cultural change and ecological stewardship. We strive to align our book manufacturing practices with our editorial mission and to reduce the impact of our business enterprise in the environment. We print our books and catalogs on chlorine-free recycled paper, using vegetable-based inks whenever possible. This book may cost slightly more because it was printed on paper that contains recycled fiber, and we hope you'll agree that it's worth it. Chelsea Green is a member of the Green Press Initiative (www .greenpressinitiative.org), a nonprofit coalition of publishers, manufacturers, and authors working to protect the world's endangered forests and conserve natural resources. *The Metabolic Approach to Cancer* was printed on paper supplied by Thomson-Shore that contains 100% postconsumer recycled fiber.

Library of Congress Cataloging-in-Publication Data
Names: Winters, Nasha, 1971– author. | Kelley, Jess Higgins, 1978– author.
Title: The metabolic approach to cancer : integrating deep nutrition, the ketogenic diet, and nontoxic
  bio-individualized therapies / Dr. Nasha Winters, ND, LAc, FABNO, Jess Higgins Kelley, MNT.
Description: White River Junction, Vermont : Chelsea Green Publishing, [2017]
Identifiers: LCCN 2017001559 | ISBN 9781603586863 (hardback) | ISBN 9781603586870 (ebook)
Subjects: LCSH: Cancer—Diet therapy. | Integrative medicine. | BISAC: HEALTH & FITNESS /
  Diseases / Cancer. | HEALTH & FITNESS / Nutrition.
Classification: LCC RC271.D52 W56 2017 | DDC 616.99/40654—dc23
LC record available at https://lccn.loc.gov/2017001559

Chelsea Green Publishing
85 North Main Street, Suite 120
White River Junction, VT 05001
(802) 295-6300
www.chelseagreen.com

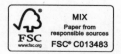

Dedicated to John "Jack" Higgins
November 27, 1954–October 19, 2016

Contents

Foreword

You only have to talk to Dr. Nasha Winters for about five minutes to realize that she's a walking encyclopedia for integrative medicine. When I first met her, I was mostly interested in studying her own radical remission, which is when someone heals from cancer against all odds. Five minutes later, I realized she was a tour-de-force naturopath with twenty-five years of clinical experience in integrative oncology and with dozens of former patients who had experienced their own radical remissions under her guidance. I knew we would have much to talk about.

To begin with, Dr. Nasha emphasized something that my radical remission research subjects had been saying for over a decade—"It's all about the underlying conditions." In *The Metabolic Approach to Cancer*, this is referred to as the "terrain," a beautiful metaphor to think about your body as a garden.

If the plants in a garden aren't thriving, a novice gardener might simply spray weed killer and hope for the best. However, a master ecological gardener will take much more into consideration: Does the soil have the proper minerals in it? Does the soil have toxins seeping into it that are harming the plants? Are the plants receiving adequate sunshine? Clean and plentiful water? Are the seeds healthy? Are environmental forces, such as high winds, causing undue stress to the plants? This is the level of in-depth analysis that this book offers for the body-mind-spirit system—and with impressive results.

If modern medicine has learned anything about cancer in the last fifty years, it's that cancer is not a simple disease. In fact, it's not even a *single* disease but rather a collection of over one hundred different diseases—each with mitochondrial dysfunction at its center. Add to this the fact that everyone's body is significantly different from their neighbor's—meaning that no two people have the same toxin exposure, immune system, metabolism, or microbiome—and you can begin to appreciate why this highly individualized approach to cancer makes sense.

For all of cancer's complexity, though, the authors and I agree on a simple (and Nobel Prize–winning) theory that boils cancer down to one idea: When the mitochondria in a cell fail, that cell will become cancerous.

This was a big "aha" moment for me during my initial years of research into radical remissions as part of my PhD at University of California, Berkeley. I had never really bought into the prevailing theory that cancer cells were simply healthy cells that—for some unknown reason—started behaving "badly." Instead, I believe that there is an explanation for *everything* in this world, including why healthy cells begin to act in a cancerous manner.

The metabolic theory of cancer—which was first introduced by Otto Warbug in the 1920's, and for which he was awarded the Nobel Prize—claims that damage to a cell's mitochondria is what causes a cell to behave cancerously. This explanation made sense to me because I knew from basic biology that the mitochondria are the "factories" of the cell, in charge of producing energy (through aerobic respiration) and of telling the cell when to reproduce and when to die. A cancerous cell does the exact opposite—it reproduces when it shouldn't, forgets to "die" when it should, and gets its energy from glucose instead of oxygen (anaerobic respiration).

If mitochondria failure leads to cancer, the next logical question is "So what caused the mitochondria to fail?" The answer: any number of things.

Cancer researchers today are often frustrated because they get conflicting results when it comes to uncovering the cause of cancer. For example, some researchers have proven that viruses can cause cancer, as is the case with the HPV virus and cervical cancer. Other researchers have proven that bacteria can cause cancer, as is the case with the *Helicobacter pylori* bacteria and stomach cancer. Still other researchers have shown that toxins can cause cancer (such as nicotine), or that radiation can cause cancer (such as Chernoybl), or that genetic mutations or traumas or chronic stress can cause cancer.

So, who is correct? All of them—assuming that any of those events can lead to mitochondrial failure.

This is where the book's individualized approach to cancer treatment fills a much-needed gap. Why specifically did *your* (or your loved one's) mitochondria fail? More importantly, how can you begin to repair your mitochondria?

As you will learn in this book, you can begin to answer those questions by first assessing your past and present lifestyle choices, and then by requesting specific blood and genetic tests from your health practitioner. In this book, Dr. Nasha and Jess Kelley teach you how to find *and correct* the root cause of cancer, as opposed to merely trying to kill off any cells that are behaving cancerously.

Once you've thoroughly assessed your terrain through the wonderful "Terrain Ten" (ten areas of your body and mind to examine and measure), the book provides an elegant solution for returning to balance: food. Yes, food, that wonderful healer of healers! As Hippocrates said, "Let food be thy medicine and medicine be thy food." I believe strongly in those words, but unfortunately modern medicine has dismissed them almost entirely. Thankfully, this book, along with the work of fellow functional and integrative medicine colleagues, is beginning to change that egregious error.

It's really quite simple: Our bodies run on food, water, and energy. If you give your body the healthy food and water it needs, while also creating emotional conditions in your life that lead to an abundant flow of energy in the body, you will be well on your way to health.

When it comes to food, this book advocates for the ketogenic diet, which strictly limits the amount of carbohydrates you eat while simultaneously increasing the amount of fat you consume in order to force your cells to receive energy from fat instead of glucose (which cancer cells love). Though many of my vegetarian and vegan colleagues may disagree with certain aspects of the ketogenic diet, I prefer to focus on the commonality of these differing points of view: namely, eating plentiful vegetables and removing sources of toxins from your life. Everyone agrees that healing begins with a sharp increase in vegetables and an equally significant decrease in toxins.

What I view as most important to the dietary approach in *The Metabolic Approach to Cancer* is the authors' belief that all people need to be on a different diet depending on their individual physiology and their particular cancer. There is no such thing as a "one-size-fits-all" diet in their eyes. I have seen the battery of tests that Dr. Nasha orders and analyzes for each one of her patients, and how those test results inform her recommendations of what that person should or should not be eating, as well as what supplements and other lifestyle changes that person needs at this moment in time—knowing full well that this person will likely need a very different set of recommendations in six months.

Some nutritional treatments are used temporarily, such as fasting, while others might work well for your body in the long-term. The point that this book makes, and with which I agree, is that every human is different, and therefore the key is to view your symptoms and lab results as messengers that are trying to tell you where and how you've gone off balance.

Once you know where you're off balance, this book will give you the tools you need to regain your health. From delicious recipes to specific exercise suggestions and stress-reducing recommendations, you will leave this book with a powerful to-do list of lifestyle changes to consider. And that's a good thing, in my opinion, since one of the biggest problems with conventional cancer treatment is that it takes all of the power away from the patient.

In this book, the authors encourage you to step into your rightful role as the head gardener of your "garden"—that is, your body-mind-spirit system—and to begin asking deeper questions: Are you giving your body the food-medicine that's right for you at this particular time? Do you have emotional or physical symptoms that are trying to tell you something? What changes can you make to reduce your stress and increase joy? What changes can you make to bring your body fully back into balance?

The answers to these questions lay in this unique, metabolic approach to cancer treatment . . . this gem of a book. Get ready to dive into a world of truly personalized medicine—this is what the future of health care should look like.

KELLY TURNER, PhD

The Cancer Crisis

As to diseases, make a habit of two things—to help, or at least, to do no harm.
                                                        —HIPPOCRATES

What we discovered, counter-intuitively, is that when you start killing a cancer cell, one of the things it does in order to survive is to spread even further.

—DR. PATRICK SOON-SHIONG, .
well-known doctor, surgeon, and scientist .

Cancer is the most elusive, cunning, adaptable, intelligent, and innovative disease in history, and it has been outsmarting us for a long time. Since the earliest cases of cancer were identified around 1.6 million years ago, humans have been invested in discovering its cause and ultimate treatment. The first written record of cancer dates back to 3000 BC, where it was declared, depressingly: "There is no cure."[1] And there still is no cure even now, thousands of years later. In fact, medical thinking has really progressed only a few paces from the antiquated idea that cancer is caused when one of the body's four humors—blood, phlegm, yellow bile, or black bile—is out of balance. The prevailing (and failing) dogma in Western medicine today is that cancer is caused and driven by genetic mutations, or just bad luck.

The somatic mutation theory (SMT) asserts that when a cell endures extensive damage to its genetic material—deoxyribonucleic acid, or DNA—it eventually reaches a point where it goes rogue from its intended function and becomes cancerous. Cancer research and treatment development have been locked within the tiny confines of this tenet since the SMT theory was cast in carbonite over seventy-five years ago. The problem is that this outdated mutation focus is not getting us any closer to preventing or curing this scary, heartbreaking, expensive, and painful disease. We simply must take a new approach because right now we're not winning the war on cancer—not even close. Today there's a better chance of surviving Russian roulette than cancer and its associated Western treatments. Something is terribly wrong with the current cancer model.

As of this writing, cancer directly affects almost half of the US population. Half. The numbers are horrifying: By today's end, approximately 1,600 cancer patients will have died. The same number will die tomorrow and the next day. In 2015 more than 1.5 million new cancer cases were diagnosed (an estimated 1,665,540), resulting in over half a million deaths (585,720, to be precise). New cancer cases have steadily increased for the last 150 years. At the beginning of the nineteenth century, only one person in twenty was diagnosed with cancer. In the 1940s that increased to one out of every sixteen people. By the 1970s it had become one in ten. In 1960, breast cancer affected one in twenty women, and by 2016, the number rose to one in eight. Today half of all men and over a third of all women in the United States will develop cancer in their lifetime.[2] For carriers of a *BRCA* mutation (a genetic mutation that can increase the risk of certain cancers including breast) who were born before 1940, the risk of developing breast cancer by age fifty was 24 percent, but among those born after 1940, when pesticides were introduced (more on this relationship later), it has almost tripled to 67 percent.[3] From 1973 to 1991 prostate cancer rates increased 126 percent. In several European countries cancer is now the leading cause of death, and in America it is expected to surpass cardiovascular disease as the number one cause of death by 2020. While cancer is not contagious, it is unquestionably the bubonic plague of our day.

It is important to know that what cancer is *not* is a disease of the aging population. From the early 1980s to the early 1990s, the incidence of cancer in American children under age ten rose by 37 percent.[4] After accidents, cancer is the next most frequent cause of death in children, and a 2016 study found that malignant brain tumors are the number one cause of cancer-related deaths in American adolescents between the ages of fifteen and nineteen.[5]

Not only is cancer affecting children at an increased rate of almost 40 percent in the past sixteen years, rates of secondary cancers, which are new cancers unrelated to a person's original cancer, are also surging like a tsunami. Nearly one in five new cancer cases in the United States involves someone who has had the disease before, a rate increase of almost 300 percent since the 1970s.

As if this is not overwhelming enough, the comorbidities resulting from cancer treatments are also increasingly alarming. A March 2016 article in the journal *Oncology* found that survivors of young adult cancers have more than twice the risk of developing cardiovascular disease than people without a cancer history.[6] A 2006 University of California, Los Angeles (UCLA), study found that chemotherapy causes changes to the brain's metabolism and blood flow that can linger at least ten years after treatment (a phenomenon many refer to as "chemo brain"). If cancer patients can survive conventional oncology's antiquated and largely ineffective treatments, they are far more likely to die earlier and with a lower quality of life.

Leading cancer treatments such as chemotherapy and radiation are, in fact, carcinogenic, meaning they actually *cause* cancer. Indeed, several cancer drugs including tamoxifen, used to treat breast cancer, are classified by the International Agency for Research on Cancer (IARC) as Group 1 carcinogens—meaning carcinogenic in humans. So is radiation. Yet when you or the person next to you is diagnosed with cancer, then surgery, radiation, or chemotherapy, or a combination of these, will be your primary treatment options. These modalities will, in words used by those in the oncology field, "slash, burn, and poison" cancer cells in hopes of killing them. (Early chemotherapies were actually derived from mustard gas, a chemical agent of war.) The trouble is that these conventional treatments also slash, burn, and poison a body's healthy cells. Not only that, but they further deplete the immune system, damage DNA, eradicate critical microbes in the gut, cause inflammation and oxidative stress—all of which are cancer-*promoting* factors (each of which we will discuss further in this book). But the sad reality at this point in time is that there are few to no other treatment options available. Until now. With this book we intend to shine a beacon of light on integrative, nontoxic diet and lifestyle approaches to cancer that *work*, without the side effects.

A new approach to cancer is sorely needed since the current model of conventional oncology is based solely on treating the tumor and cancer cells through aggressive strategies that can—and do—diminish the tumor but often with significant cost to the patient. If someone does not already have an autoimmune condition before cancer, they will usually get one after conventional treatment, as these therapies strongly override, suppress, or overstimulate the immune system (more on this in chapter 7, in "Causes of Immune System Impairment"). And while some patients bounce back after treatment, many do not. The long-term implications of these therapies can include increased gut permeability, impaired cardiovascular health, depressed cognitive health and neurological function, debilitating neuropathy, destruction of the immune system, and even death. But there is a stunningly effective cancer treatment available right at the grocery store: food.

While certainly no magic bullet or single intervention exists for treating cancer in either practice model, conventional or nonconventional, study after study shows that only 5–10 percent of cancer is caused by damaged DNA. What's more, is these inherited mutations cause cancer *only if* said mutations also alter mitochondrial function. The remaining 90–95 percent of cancer cases are caused by poor diet and unhealthy lifestyles that also damage mitochondrial function.[7] This is where we absolutely have to start focusing. Cancer is a mitochondrial disease related to a person's physiology, psychology, and ecology. Examining a damaged gene by itself is like putting on your seat belt after your car has crashed. *Cancer is not a genetic disease* but instead a metabolic disorder that occurs in response to how we are feeding and treating our bodies and therefore our genomes. Humanity's modern diets and lifestyles are in complete discordance with our evolution. Through epigenetics (which you will learn about in chapter 3) we have the ability to influence gene expression and mitochondrial function through diet, lifestyle, and thoughts. That's powerful medicine.

If a line were drawn across the bottom of every page of this whole book to represent the entire time line of human existence, the very last page would represent the era when our basic diet of wild animals and plants was changed to incorporate grains, legumes, and dairy products. On the very last inch of the very last page would be listed the following changes to humans' diet and environment that have occurred in only the last 250 years: air-conditioning, airplanes, antibiotics, artificial food color, artificial sweeteners, cars, cell phones, chronic stress, computers, electric lighting, emulsifiers, high-fructose corn syrup, genetically modified food, internet, pesticides, prescription medications, artificial preservatives, refined foods, sunscreen, synthetic chemicals, synthetic fats, television, toilets, vaccines, and much more. That's quite a list for our ancient genome to adapt to, and it's clearly not adapting very well. While we cannot go back in time and live in caves again (nor need we aspire to), we can begin to focus on resurrecting dietary and lifestyle approaches that are more in keeping with our genetics and our ancient metabolic systems, unchanged for millions of years and now disturbed by modern life. In this book you will learn how these disruptions are causing cancer and how to rectify it.

What *is* metabolism? Metabolism is the combination of physical and chemical processes that occur in the body to create the energy required to maintain life. Simply speaking, metabolism is how the body utilizes the food we eat to obtain energy. Thus, our metabolic approach to cancer is nutrition-centered. Food, air, water, and sex are what have sustained the human race for the past 2.6 million years, so clearly they are pretty important. If food is the body's gasoline, the mitochondria inside cells are the tiny engines responsible for converting that food into energy for the body to run on. It is therefore inside the mitochondria where metabolism takes place. What has been known—but largely ignored—for over a hundred years is that the root cause of cancer is actually damaged mitochondria. Think of it this way: When you pour sugar into the engine of a car, it stops running. The same concept can be applied to the human race. What we explain in this book is that while most modern diets and lifestyles are largely responsible for cancer-causing mitochondrial damage, deep nutrition, therapeutic diets (low-glycemic, fasting, and ketogenic), and nontoxic lifestyle approaches can provide the repairs.

Now more than ever it is critical to understand that cancer is about the way our bodies and our minds interact with the environment. The majority of cancers seen today are modern, man-made diseases, and a metabolic approach can prevent and halt the cancer process. Doesn't this sound simple? You may wonder why this hasn't been prescribed for the last hundred years. Indeed, it is unfathomable why a treatment so utterly obvious is not already in practice. One explanation: There is no money in food research, and the results of whatever research is done cannot be patented. Thankfully, isolated cancer-fighting phytonutrients *can* be patented (meaning there is money to be made), and there are scores of available studies proving the ability of food-derived compounds to counteract cancer's many tricks. (We cover many of these "superfoods" in this book.) In general, however, the power of nutrition as a cancer therapy—either on its own or alongside Western treatments—has been largely underestimated and ignored. Until now. But before we go into the details of the metabolic approach, let's begin at the beginning.

What Exactly *Is* Cancer?

While the American Cancer Society asserts that cancer is a collection of over a hundred different diseases and imbalances, more recent research is demonstrating that cancer is not many diseases rather a singular disease of energy metabolism. All cancers, regardless of tissue or cellular origin, use fermentation (the Warburg effect) to generate energy, which is different than how healthy cells produce energy. This energy production dysfunction is the common defect seen in all cancers, which is why targeting metabolism will target all cancers to some degree—and is the basis of this book.

More broadly, cancer is defined as the uncontrolled division of abnormal cells and the spread of those cells throughout the body. A tumor is a mass of these abnormal, or mutated, cells, each exhibiting riotous and prolific growth. Cancer cells are like teenagers hopped up on Red Bull in a mosh pit—out of control and urging others near them to join the frenzy. As cell masses grow and expand they can affect surrounding normal tissues or organs such as the liver or bowel.

It is important to know that most common cancers take months, sometimes years, to develop into a detectable mass. In fact, even healthy adults produce five hundred to a thousand new cancerous cells a day, and only one in a thousand people is truly cancer free.[8] It's scary to think about, but all of us have cancer cells in our body, no matter how healthy we are. All it takes is a hearty push from one of the ten factors we detail in this book to toss healthy cells into the mosh pit of uncontrolled growth. Then, without specific nutrition designed to repair mitochondrial dysfunction, invigorate the immune system, reduce inflammation, repopulate the microbiome, and balance hormones and blood sugar, healthy cells disappear into the chaotic realm of cancer.

The Ten Hallmarks of Cancer

1. **Sustained proliferation:** Cancer cells multiply out of control by creating proteins that encourage their explosive growth.

2. **Insensitivity to antigrowth signals:** Cancer cells disarm the processes the body uses to put the brakes on unwanted cell division.

3. **Evasion of apoptosis (also known as cell suicide):** Normal cells self-destruct when they detect an error (mutation) that cannot be repaired, but cancer cells thrive despite these errors.

4. **Limitless replicative potential:** Normal cells die after a certain number of divisions. Conversely, cancer cells are immortal.

5. **Sustained angiogenesis (development of blood supply):** Cancer cells are able to orchestrate the creation of new blood vessels to supply them with the oxygen and nutrients they need to grow.

6. **Ability to metastasize:** Cancer cells can spread to other sites in the body where space, oxygen, and nutrients are more plentiful.

7. **Reprogramming of energy metabolism (known as the Warburg effect):** Cancer cells alter their method of energy production and increase their metabolic rate in order to sustain rapid growth.

8. **Avoidance of immune destruction:** Cancer cells suppress the function of key immune cells, including natural killer (NK) cells, while also evading immune surveillance systems.

9. **Tumor-promoting inflammation:** Tumors activate an inflammatory response that can increase their access to growth factors and blood supply.

10. **Genome instability and mutation:** Almost all cancer cells have defects in their ability to repair DNA, allowing the reproduction of mutated cells.

While there exist over two hundred known types of cancers, ten specific traits have been identified that are inherent to each one. These so-called hallmarks of cancer are the anticancer defense mechanisms hardwired into all cells that must be breached in order for a cell to become cancerous. In other words, healthy cells have ten different security systems in place to keep cancer from breaking in and taking over, which is why we all don't have full-blown diagnosable cancer despite the aforementioned presence of cancer cells in our bodies. In 2000 Douglas Hanahan and Robert Weinberg published a groundbreaking review article in the journal *Cell* in which they identified the original six hallmarks, and in 2011 they updated their list by proposing four more.[9] While of course there are some critics of their assertions, in general these ten hallmarks of cancer are largely accepted by Western medicine. In this book we review several of them from a metabolic perspective. But where our approach differs is this: Western medicine identifies the genetic mutations or the pinpoint mechanisms that cause these system breaches in order to design drugs to treat them. Our approach *prevents the breaches from happening in the first place.* And if a breach does occur, we prescribe a nutritional, or metabolic, counteragent. Do be aware that each one of these biological security systems, or hallmarks, is incredibly complex; the sidebar provides only *extremely* basic synopses of their mechanisms. The main idea is to give you an idea of how truly complex cancer is.

How Conventional Medicine Uses This Information

Certainly, having an understanding of the many ways cancer works is a brilliant example of the progress made by modern science. But when it comes to the effectiveness of developing new treatments based on these hallmarks (not to mention the millions of dollars spent on research) there has, unfortunately, not been much success. Instead, we've seen or experienced the devastating physical side effects from conventional, chemical-based, and targeted treatments. Many of us have incurred significant emotional and financial costs, without success. For the last seventy-five years, the "War on Cancer" has been laser-focused on developing targeted therapies and mapping the human genome for genetic clues to cancer. But the magic bullet scientists have been searching for has remained elusive, leaving a trail of failed and highly toxic therapies. Still, 95 percent of cancer spending is allocated to genetic research while prevention accounts for only about 5 percent of spending.[10] Five percent! Truly the Western way: Treat the disease, not the cause. Even worse, our prevention model is centered on drugs (think aspirin), vaccinations, and radiation-based screening methods including mammograms, which are also a risk factor for cancer. Sadly, false-positive mammograms and overdiagnosis of breast cancer among women ages forty to fifty-nine cost $4 billion in health care spending annually, according to an April 2015 study in the journal *Health Affairs*.[11]

It probably comes as no surprise that areas of cancer research and drug development have become a big business. In 2014 alone, the global market for cancer drugs hit $100 billion.[12] Some drugs, bevacizumab (Avastin) for example, can cost the patient $8,000 per month. The average cost of a new cancer drug is over $100,000 a year, and medical costs associated with cancer cripple many families. In 2010 an estimated 40 percent of patients reported depleting their savings, almost 30 percent reported dealing with bill collectors, and 54 percent of those handling the catastrophic financial burden of cancer said it had become more difficult to afford treatment.[13] So while cancer might be spectacular for the economy, it has proven both costly and deadly for the patient.

Let's look more closely at the biological drug bevacizumab, which was developed to inhibit angiogenesis, one of the hallmarks of cancer. Bevacizumab works by blocking a protein called vascular endothelial growth factor (VEGF) that is encoded by the *VEGF* gene and promotes the formation of new blood vessels that help to feed tumor cells. Based on this mechanism, bevacizumab was approved for use with metastatic (stage IV) breast cancer in February 2008 under the "accelerated approval program" offered by the US Food and Drug Administration (FDA). This program allows a drug to be used before traditional full approval is granted, giving patients earlier access to promising new drugs that may treat serious or life-threatening conditions while the final confirmatory clinical trials are still being conducted.[14] The initial phase 3 randomized study of bevacizumab known as E2100 found that patients administered bevacizumab in combination with another drug, paclitaxel, survived a mere six months longer without their tumors progressing than those given paclitaxel alone. Six months. This is considered a huge success in the cancer world. Not only that, but VEGF is only one of twenty-six angiogenesis pathways; it just happens to be the one most stud-ied. This example illuminates the fact we have found a single drug to act on a single protein but ignore the other twenty-five pathways—something food can address simultaneously.

But in February 2011 the *Journal of the American Medical Association* pub-lished the pooled results of sixteen confirmatory studies of 5,608 patients taking bevacizumab and found that these patients in fact had a 50 percent increased risk of dying from treatment-related adverse events compared with the use of chemotherapy alone. The risk of fatal problems such as bleeding, blood clots, and bowel perforations more than tripled when bevacizumab was used with certain kinds of chemotherapy drugs, particularly platinum- and taxane-based medications.[15] With that, the FDA revoked approval for bevacizumab's use in treating breast cancer, but it remains in use for other cancers. The worst part about this story is that bevacizumab was the only hope offered to millions of women who were already dying of their cancer.

Can this really be all conventional oncology has to offer? In effect, surgery, chemotherapy, and radiation rip only the top of the weed out of the garden and leave the roots behind in the soil, only to grow back a stronger and more resilient plant. Of course, we do not discount that there may be a time and place for these treatments depending on the cancer case, but it is negligent of oncologists not to take a broader approach and look at the whole person when designing comprehensive cancer care plans. It is important to note, however, that while we are critical of the current model in conventional care, with this book we do *not* mean simply to bash Western medicine, but rather to embrace *all* existing models, while using food as the foundation for healing. Cancer treatment does not have to be "either-or"; using a metabolic approach can be effective on its own while also improving the outcome of conventional treatments when they are used in tandem.

You will learn that there is a lot more happening in and to the body that provokes cancer than we are currently told, and that you have a treatment (and prevention) option sitting right in your refrigerator or waiting to be harvested from your garden. But please remember we are up against a lot of misinformation out there, and an utter lack of support in the conventional oncology world with regard to nutrition. In fact, typically when a newly diag-nosed cancer patient asks their conventional oncologist what they should eat to help support their health, the response is: "It doesn't matter, eat what you want; just don't lose weight." Know this: Less than 25 percent of all medical schools offer a course in nutrition, and most of these are elective. Your medical doctor likely has little understanding of basic nutrition, never mind deep or integrative nutrition, and is therefore simply not qualified to offer advice on the topic. And it's not just medical doctors, either; there is a contingent of naturopathic physicians who are not up to speed in nutritional biochemistry. Throughout this book we scientifically myth-bust several diet dogmas currently prominent in the world of natural medicine. On a brighter note, more and more oncologists and other medical professionals are recognizing the role of metabolic nutrition in the health of their patients—but not nearly enough.

The nutrition recommendations of the American Cancer Society (ACS) are formulated by registered dietitians trained in the food pyramid (read: Big Agriculture) model. Their corporate sponsors are the American Dairy Association, Abbott Nutrition (maker of seasonal vaccines and ibuprofen), and PepsiCo. The "quick and easy" snacks they recommend to people undergoing cancer treatment include angel food cake, cookies, doughnuts, ice cream, and microwavable snacks.[16] (We are not kidding; visit their website and see for yourself.) These recommendations turn a blind eye to the many important studies (not to mention the suppressed work of Otto Warburg, PhD, MD, and Thomas Seyfried, PhD, in the field of the metabolic theory of cancer, which we detail in chapter 4; see "How Cancer Cells Gobble Glucose: The Warburg Effect") that have proven that sugar causes—or, at the very least, can stimulate—cancer. Even a mainstream 2016 study from the University of Texas MD Anderson Cancer Center concluded that diets high in sugar are "a major risk factor" for certain types of cancers, especially breast cancer. We simply must reverse the dismissive attitude toward the role that diet and lifestyle play in cancer prevention or progression. Because it may very well be our only hope.

A metabolic, deep nutrition, and nontoxic approach is the answer to cancer prevention and management. This book is our call to arms—we must focus on the 90–95 percent of cancers that are caused by the standard American diet and exposure to environmental toxins. We simply cannot keep shrugging our shoulders when we, or our loved ones, are diagnosed.

If a new virus began to kill one of every four people in the United States, you can bet your pink ribbon a cure would be found, and fast. While Western medicine continues to drive along the dusty, dead-end road seeking the genetic and targeted answer to cancer, it is time for us to start taking control of our own health and health care choices. We'll say it again: Cancer is a metabolic, environmental, and emotional disease. It's not just a tumor; it signifies correctable imbalances that occur inside and outside our body. Now is the time for lifelong remission. It is time for some real hope and to disarm the most deadly disease of modern times. How? With the metabolic approach to cancer.

CHAPTER 1

The Solution Is a Metabolic Approach

Illnesses do not come upon us out of the blue. They are developed from small daily sins against Nature. When enough sins have accumulated, illnesses will suddenly appear.

—HIPPOCRATES

Natural forces within us are the true healers of disease.

—HIPPOCRATES

The metabolic approach to cancer is a naturopathic nutrition program that utilizes the medicinal powers of traditional foods, therapeutic diets, and nontoxic lifestyle approaches as cancer counteragents and preventives. We developed this program during our thirty years of collective work in the fields of naturopathy, Oriental medicine, acupuncture, nutrition, and integrative oncology.

Dr. Nasha has been studying and using this very different—and very effective—approach for cancer prevention and neutralization for over twenty-five years. Her approach strays significantly from conventional oncology, and has been saving lives for many years, including her own. Dr. Nasha's personal cancer experience began over twenty years ago when a diagnosis of stage IV ovarian cancer veered her away from pursuing a conventional medical degree and toward the study of naturopathic medicine. To treat her own cancer she used an integrative approach fortified by a traditional whole food diet and environmental adaptations. Using "alternative medicine" is the reason Dr. Nasha not only remains a cancer *thriver* today, but is healthier and more vital than *before* her cancer diagnosis. This personal experience helped form the foundation of her naturopathic oncology practice, which in turn has helped thousands of other patients do what she did: not only overcome cancer but become healthier than before.

When cancer patients don't achieve the desired results from conventional treatments they come to Dr. Nasha for another option; for some, it is their last and only hope. Under Dr. Nasha's care most experience far better clinical outcomes (some cases we can truly call "miracles") and a better quality of life living *with* cancer than patients adhering strictly to the conventional medical model. Because of her emphasis on traditional, whole food, nutrient-dense, and therapeutic diets, Dr. Nasha teamed up with master nutrition therapist Jess Higgins Kelley in order to expand treatment and education options for her patients. Together we knew there had to be a better way to approach this largely preventable and debilitating disease—and we have found it.

After years of clinical practice and exhaustive research, tapping the expertise of leading and like-minded colleagues in various fields, and leaving no stone unturned in our patient assessments, we have identified ten key elements of a person's "terrain" that require optimization in order to successfully prevent and manage cancer. The term *terrain*, commonly used in the naturopathic lexicon, refers to a person's internal and external biological ecosystems. The body is a complete biosphere, a garden full of systems and networks that all communicate and interact with one another. Call it what you will—body, garden, terrain—they all mean the same thing. Every human has internal systems at work (the heart pumping blood, the lungs breathing air) that respond to outside events, including exposures to stressors or pollutants.

Comprehending the complexities of the individual's biological terrain is akin to a gardener understanding the ideal conditions for growing vegetables. A successful gardener knows it takes more than a piece of land and a packet of seeds to grow a bountiful harvest. It requires a knowledge of soil bio-chemistry, the planting requirements of all the various types of seeds, proper balance of nutrients, fertilizing agents, and the right amount of water and sunlight. It also requires insight into how pests, insects, weeds, molds, and fungi can impact the soil or plants. The ten terrain elements we've identified are like systems within that garden. Regulating a healthy human biological terrain is similar to raising a healthy, thriving garden. When the body is fed a diet that provides adequate amounts of macro- and micronutrients, vitamins, and minerals; is exposed to a variety of microbes; and has adequate amounts of exercise, sleep, fresh water, sunlight, love, and attention; then the body, like a healthy garden, will flourish. Conversely, if it is fed antinutrients and chemicals, receives insufficient sunshine, and endures too much stress, it will wither.

So the key is this: Since cancer consists of cells gone awry in response to toxic diets and environments, we must optimize the body's healing mechanisms instead of waging war on them. We need to treat the terrain, not the tumor. We must build the body up instead of attacking it. Our strategy works: The only side effect of the metabolic approach is feeling better. *Much better.* In fact, for over a decade Dr. Nasha has seen hundreds of stage IV cancer patients who have lived far beyond their "expiration date" because they have followed this model. As we will explain, each terrain element is optimized using the oldest form of medicine: *food*. It sounds simple, yet in the modern world of medicine, it's about as radical and "unfounded" as it can be.

The Terrain Ten™

The core of our approach is dedicated to the science of using therapeutic nutrition to positively impact metabolism, creating an inhospitable environment for cancer while simultaneously removing dietary and lifestyle factors that provoke it. What is astonishing to realize—yet for the most part ignored—is that dietary agents have been shown to impact each of the ten hallmarks of cancer.[1] From decreasing the spread (*metastasis*) of cancer cells to promoting cancer cell death (*apoptosis*) and inhibiting growth factors—believe it or not, *the right food* is cancer's fiercest enemy. In 2015 cancer specialist Dr. Keith Block, along with an international task force of 180 scientists, published a capstone paper titled "Designing a Broad-Spectrum Integrative Approach for Cancer Prevention and Treatment." The article identified dozens of nontoxic phytonutrients that affect the ten hallmarks of cancer and the pathways known to be significant for the genesis and spread of cancer.[2]

What this means is that eating well is not just a good idea, but that the specific phytonutrients we discuss throughout this book exert proven medicinal action against cancer. And while there are many cancer diets out there, we debunk several—vegetarian, vegan, acid-alkaline, and the Budwig Diet, to name a few—within this book. Certainly the intentions behind these diets are commendable, but each is fundamentally flawed, and we will explain how. While certain foods can act as powerful anticancer agents, other foods can be cancer's strongest ally. This book teaches you the difference between the two. By incorporating the ten terrain elements we've developed alongside the deep nutrition and nontoxic lifestyle approaches we recommend in this book, your ability to prevent or survive cancer will increase exponentially.[3] The ten terrain elements (we call them the Terrain Ten) we have identified are the physiological and emotional human elements that require balance and optimization in order to halt and prevent the cancer process.

As you read this book it will become clear that while the elements of the Terrain Ten are presented individually and in a linear fashion, in the dynamic process of health and disease they are all woven together. The ten make up the complete ecosystem that is an individual's terrain, and each one cross-pollinates the others. All systems are connected, and as throwing

The Terrain Ten™

1. Genetic, epigenetic, and nutrigenomic modifications
2. Blood sugar balance
3. Toxic burden management
4. Repopulating and balancing the microbiome
5. Immune system maximization
6. Modulating inflammation and oxidative stress
7. Enhancing blood circulation while inhibiting angiogenesis and metastasis
8. Establishing hormone balance
9. Recalibrating stress levels and biorhythms
10. Enhancing mental and emotional well-being

a rock in a still lake creates ripples over the entire surface, disrupting one terrain element negatively affects all the others. For example, high stress levels lead to hormonal and blood sugar imbalances. In turn, high blood sugar levels suppress the immune system. The point is that cancer can capitalize on imbalances found within any of the ten terrain elements. Our therapeutic model therefore addresses the *whole person*, not just the tumor. A tumor is merely a side effect that occurs when a person's terrain is out of balance, when too many big rocks are thrown into a still pond. As we've said before, cancer doesn't just show up one day at random, it doesn't just "happen" to you, and it is not bad luck. Just as the weed in the garden alerts the gardener to mineral or other deficiencies in the soil, cancer is a messenger telling you that some element within you—emotional, spiritual, or physical—is not in harmony.

Within each terrain chapter, we illustrate how elements of modern living and the American food pyramid, overconsumption of sugar, GMO foods, modern agriculture practices, processed soy, grains and gluten, pesticides, antibiotics, low-fat diets, vegan diets, processed foods, nutrient deficiencies, sedentary lifestyles, stress, and more directly contribute to imbalances in the terrain and contribute to the cancer process. There are so many insults to our terrain every day, and our objective is to educate you on how to avoid or at least minimize them. You can eat "perfectly," but if you don't clean up your external environment you won't get very far in changing your internal terrain. Even the most intelligent, well-read people don't consider the impact our day-to-day exposures to the toxins in our food, air, water, products, stressors, relationships, and attitudes have on our terrain. We aim to bring awareness to this, and we also want to acknowledge that at times what you read might feel overwhelming. It is for all of us. But knowledge is power, and you have a lot more power and control over this disease than you may realize: 95 percent of it is related to the diet and lifestyle factors we identify in this book!

Changing the Focus

Every organism on this Earth requires food to create energy in order to live and reproduce. Food is the fuel that keeps our bodies driving down the road. All of the energy, genetic instruction, and structural and regulating materials for your terrain come from nutrients. Simply put, food and the nutrients obtained from it are required to sustain life. When nutrient levels become deficient, symptoms (such as headaches, fatigue, weight gain, aches and pains) will be followed by disease. Low vitamin D causes rickets, low vitamin C causes scurvy, low folate in a mother results in spina bifida in the child. Without food, we die in approximately 40 to 180 days (this depends on a person's body weight; some obese people have survived and remained healthy without food for over five months!). With the right foods, we can heal. It's time to start giving credit where credit is due: Certain foods and dietary habits have kept us alive for 2.6 million years. Deep nutrition, a metabolic approach, is the answer to cancer. And where Western medicine is trying to isolate the active forms of food to create synthetic versions able to be patented, we recommend the whole foods and dietary practices, such as fasting, that have sustained us for millennia. Yes, *not* eating is powerful medicine. All foods contain more than one active ingredient, and we strongly believe in the therapeutic power of synergies.

When sugar, processed grains, soda, preservatives, additives, trans fats, synthetic oils, pesticides, herbicides, genetically modified corn and soy, and junk food are replaced with organic, wild, and fermented vegetables, bone marrow and organ meats, healthy fats, specific herbs, and adequate hydration, the terrain shifts in a matter of days. We've seen it happen— and tested it—hundreds of times during our multiday cancer retreats over the years. Epigenetic markers change, blood sugar levels decline, immune systems are fortified, hormones balance, digestion improves, toxins are removed, and fogs of depression are lifted. When stress, endocrine and sleep disruptors, and environmental and emotional toxins are removed and replaced with peace, purpose, nutrients, nontoxic products, rest, exercise, and healthy relationships, the body becomes incredibly resilient. All these elements are powerful enough to affect DNA, and that's good medicine. Cancer doesn't like that.

You've heard it before, but it is true: You are what you eat. But of course we take things further: "We are not just what we eat, but what our *food* eats." When it comes to deeply nutritious foods, the quality of the soil where the food was grown is also essential. When animals are fed toxic diets they become toxic to eat. If you feed animals antibiotics, hormones, and genetically modified grains and legumes, they go from being healthy to four-legged Superfund sites—not to mention propelling antibiotic resistance. Our approach dives deep into food quality and also bio-individuality. There is not, cannot, and should not be a one-size-fits-all diet all the time. What you eat needs to change with the seasons, for example, and is largely based on what your genetics can tell us. We look at many nutrigenomic factors (meaning, how our genes affect our foods and vice versa) throughout each chapter.

As you can see from the title of the book, we subscribe to the metabolic theory of cancer—the proven fact that cancer cells are fueled by sugar and that altered mitochondrial metabolism is the ultimate cause of cancer. In fact, a December 2016 meta-analysis research paper assessed more than two hundred studies conducted between 1934 and 2016 and concluded that the most important difference between normal cells and cancer cells is how they respire, or create energy.[4] Cancer cells use a primitive process of fermentation to inefficiently convert glucose from carbohydrates into energy needed to sustain their rapid growth, a process we discuss in detail in chapter 4. But the most important finding is that fatty acids (dietary fats) cannot be fermented by cancer cells, which makes a ketogenic diet the most powerful dietary approach to cancer identified to date. And thanks to more than a hundred years of research by the physicians and scientists Otto Warburg, Thomas Seyfried, Dominic D'Agostino, and Valter D. Longo, as well as a rising number of others, we know beyond a shadow of a doubt that low-glycemic, ketogenic diets and intermittent fasting should be an integral part of an effective anticancer diet program. We discuss these in relation to almost all ten terrain elements.

We realize there are many people who are drawn to what we are talking about and others who are not. Our approach aims to empower people. Sadly, many cancer patients spend more time looking at a new car than at their grocery list. Using diet to prevent and manage cancer requires engagement, and that is not always easy. Conventional medicine, on the other hand, allows the patient to be passive—the doctor performs surgery or administers chemotherapy, and the patient just waits for the test results. In the conventional model the healing, and ultimately the trust, lie with the doctor. We believe, however, and have seen over and over in our practices, that true healing occurs when the patient is an active participant in the healing process. Our process is for those who are motivated to take charge of their health and willing to make lifestyle changes. It's about getting to know yourself, and maybe changing things you never thought possible. It's about asking questions, and not shying away from answers. It's about undoing the notion that you are a victim of cancer and you have no control over the process. Because you do.

CHAPTER 2

Assessing Your Terrain

Awareness is the greatest agent for change.

—ECKHART TOLLE

Know the enemy and know yourself; in a hundred battles, you will never be defeated.

—SUN TZU

Whether you aim to prevent cancer, have recently been diagnosed with it, or are in remission, it is essential to assess the elements that could or did contribute to its development. By identifying and prioritizing the potential drivers of the cancer process, you gain the ability to put the brakes on the runaway truck that is this deadly disease. The mechanisms governing cancer development are multifaceted and interconnected—much more than a name, age, and diagnosis. Viewed in a positive light, cancer, or a concern about cancer, can act as a messenger bringing a strongly worded invitation to explore how your life may be out of balance. Then it is up to you to decide if you want to change it.

In this chapter you begin to identify where your terrain elements may be out of balance by answering ten questions that relate to each of the Terrain Ten. This questionnaire is not intended to diagnose, treat, or cure your cancer, rather simply to heighten your awareness. Often our patients have initially told us, "I was so healthy before cancer," a self-perception that can make being diagnosed that much more of a shock. Yet after completing this questionnaire and looking really carefully under the hood, the "aha" moments start to happen. This exercise will help you determine where to focus first and what the next steps are. Consider it your empowerment plan.

Begin by answering all of the questions in the ten questionnaires. Then add up the number of "yes" answers in each section and note which of the terrain areas have the highest amount. The terrain areas with the most "yes" answers will be the areas you should prioritize focusing on first. Do not be overwhelmed if you score high in *every* section; many people do. The goal is merely to draw your attention to which areas of your body or life may need support and also to recognize which of these you have control over, and which of these you do not. Do know that starting to address *any one* of these ten areas will significantly enhance your body's ability not only to respond to conventional therapies and reduce side effects from the treatments, but also to make you stronger and better able to prevent cancer from occurring in the first place.

TABLE 2.1. GENETICS AND EPIGENETICS

1. Have you tested positive for *BRCA1* and/or *BRCA2*?	Yes	No
2. Have you tested positive for any other type of gene mutation, including: *EPCAM, MLH1, MSH2, MSH6, PMS2, RB*, or *TP53*? If you don't know, circle "No"	Yes	No
3. Are you either heterozygous or homozygous for a *MTHFR* mutation?	Yes	No
4. Are you heterozygous or homozygous for a *VDR, COMT*, and/or *CYP1B1* mutation?	Yes	No
5. Do you have a family history of cancer?	Yes	No
6. Were your grandparents affected by the Great Depression, or any other type of famine, natural disaster, or major stressful period?	Yes	No
7. Were your parents exposed to large amount of stress and/or environmental toxins?	Yes	No
8. Did your mother smoke or take any types of drugs or medications while she was pregnant with you?	Yes	No
9. Did you experience any type of trauma in your childhood?	Yes	No
10. Are you on any pharmaceutical drugs, including over-the-counter medications?	Yes	No

Total number of "Yes" answers

If you scored highest in this section, please focus on chapter 3.

TABLE 2.2. BLOOD SUGAR BALANCE

1. Do you have a sweet tooth?	Yes	No
2. Do you find it difficult to fall asleep without an evening or late-night snack, and/or awaken hungry during the night?	Yes	No
3. Do you get "hangry" (irritable because of hunger) if meals are skipped or delayed?	Yes	No
4. Do you regularly skip breakfast?	Yes	No
5. Are sugar-based foods (e.g., candy, cookies, cake, soda, bread, waffles) what you crave the most, and/or consider your "comfort foods"?	Yes	No
6. Do you consume more than 25 grams of added sugar a day (more than one soda, candy bar, or flavored yogurt)?	Yes	No
7. Is your body-fat content over 25 percent?	Yes	No
8. Do you feel tired or crave sugar after a meal?	Yes	No
9. Do you or any family member have a history or diagnosis of metabolic syndrome, hypoglycemia, prediabetes, insulin resistance, polycystic ovarian syndrome (PCOS), pancreatitis, pancreatic cancer, or type 1 or 2 diabetes?	Yes	No
10. Do you consume alcoholic beverages more than 3 times a week?	Yes	No

Total number of "Yes" answers

If you scored highest in this section, please focus on chapter 4.

TABLE 2.3. TOXIC BURDEN

1. Do you currently live (or were you raised) near a toxic waste or factory site, military base, industrial complex, agricultural area, or airport?	Yes	No
2. Do you have any known environmental sensitivities, such as to odors like perfume or diesel fuel?	Yes	No
3. In total, do you use a microwave, cell phone, or laptop computer more than 3 hours a day?	Yes	No
4. Do you use pesticides or herbicides in or around your home or garden or on your pets?	Yes	No
5. Do you use any nonorganic body care or household cleaning products (e.g., shampoo or laundry detergent) and/or have your hair professionally dyed?	Yes	No
6. Do you have your clothes dry-cleaned, use nonstick cookware, drink unfiltered water, or either drink from or store food in plastic containers?	Yes	No
7. Do you have a history of first-, second-, or thirdhand cigarette smoke exposure?	Yes	No
8. Do you have any mercury fillings, work in the dental industry, eat fish more than 3 times a week, and/or have you ever been exposed to heavy metals, including lead?	Yes	No
9. Do you have an occupational history with known exposure to toxic chemicals, such as asbestos or heavy metals?	Yes	No
10. Do you find it difficult to sweat?	Yes	No
Total number of "Yes" answers		

If you scored highest in this section, please focus on chapter 5.

TABLE 2.4. MICROBIOME AND DIGESTIVE FUNCTION

1. Were you born via cesarean delivery?	Yes	No
2. Were you fed infant formula before the age of 1 year?	Yes	No
3. Have you ever, or do you now, use hand sanitizer and/or antimicrobial soap?	Yes	No
4. Have you been diagnosed with small intestine bacterial overgrowth (SIBO), ulcerative colitis, Crohn's disease, or colon cancer? Or do you have digestive symptoms such as gas, bloating, diarrhea, or constipation?	Yes	No
5. In your lifetime have you ever taken more than one course of antibiotics? Or have you ever completed the recommended prep for a colonoscopy? *(Answer yes if either is true.)*	Yes	No
6. Do you eat nonorganic meat and/or dairy products?	Yes	No
7. Have you had chemotherapy?	Yes	No
8. Do you take nonsteroidal anti-inflammatory drugs (NSAIDs)—such as acetaminophen (Tylenol), aspirin, or ibuprofen (Motrin or Advil)—or antacids more than a couple of times a year?	Yes	No
9. Do you typically eat fewer than 6 servings of different vegetables a day?	Yes	No
10. Do you eat processed, nonorganic grains such as pasta, bread, or cookies more than once a month?	Yes	No

Total number of "Yes" answers

If you scored highest in this section, please focus on chapter 6.

TABLE 2.5. IMMUNE FUNCTION

1. Have you been told that your vitamin D level is below 50 ng/mL?	Yes	No
2. Do you have a personal or family history of any autoimmune disease such as rheumatoid arthritis?	Yes	No
3. Do you use over-the-counter medications to suppress a fever?	Yes	No
4. Do you have a history of any of the following: Epstein-Barr virus (can cause infectious mononucleosis); human papillomavirus (HPV); cytomegalovirus (CMV); a sexually transmitted infection (STI or STD); herpes zoster (shingles); Lyme disease; yeast infection; or infection with a parasite?	Yes	No
5. Is either of the following true: (1) You are *never* sick, or (2) you catch every cold and flu that comes your way?	Yes	No
6. Do you have allergies (i.e., seasonal allergies, asthma, hives, and/or allergies to certain foods)?	Yes	No
7. Have you been diagnosed with celiac disease or gluten intolerance?	Yes	No
8. Have you ever received any vaccinations (including against seasonal influenza or herpes zoster, and vaccines needed for travel), or been prescribed any type of immunotherapies?	Yes	No
9. Have you ever taken steroids?	Yes	No
10. Do any children younger than 5 years live in your house? And/or do you work in a school, hospital, or medical setting?	Yes	No

Total number of "Yes" answers

If you scored highest in this section, please focus on chapter 7.

TABLE 2.6. INFLAMMATION

1. Do you have a history of eczema, psoriasis, acne, flushing, or rashes?	Yes	No
2. Have you ever been diagnosed with arthritis, or do you suspect that you have it?	Yes	No
3. Do you have any physical pain patterns, including back or hip pain, that is either constant or intermittent?	Yes	No
4. Do you have inflammatory bowel disease (i.e., Crohn's disease or ulcerative colitis)?	Yes	No
5. Do you ever eat fried or fast foods?	Yes	No
6. Do you have any known food allergies or do you experience gastric reflux?	Yes	No
7. Do you rely on NSAIDs for pain management?	Yes	No
8. Have you ever or do you now experience high amounts of stress?	Yes	No
9. Do you engage in high-intensity exercise more than 5 days a week?	Yes	No
10. Are you overweight, do you consume alcohol, and/or do you eat fewer than 6 different vegetables a day?	Yes	No

Total number of "Yes" answers

If you scored highest in this section, please focus on chapter 8.

TABLE 2.7. BLOOD CIRCULATION AND ANGIOGENESIS

1. Do you bruise easily?	Yes	No
2. Have you ever been diagnosed with a clotting disorder?	Yes	No
3. Have you ever been diagnosed with hemochromatosis or elevated ferritin level (high iron storage)?	Yes	No
4. Do you have a history of deep vein thrombosis (DVT)?	Yes	No
5. Do you have a history of pulmonary embolism (PE)?	Yes	No
6. Do you have high or low blood pressure?	Yes	No
7. Do you drink less than 2 quarts of water a day?	Yes	No
8. Do you take any pharmaceutical anticoagulants (e.g., warfarin [Coumadin] or enoxaparin [Lovenox])?	Yes	No
9. Are you on medication to control your blood pressure? And/or do you take a daily aspirin?	Yes	No
10. Do you exercise less than 30 minutes 3 times a week?	Yes	No
Total number of "Yes" answers		

If you scored highest in this section, please focus on chapter 9.

TABLE 2.8. HORMONE BALANCE

1. Do you have a history of birth control pills, bioidentical or standard hormone replacement therapy, steroid use, fertility treatments, and/or hormone blockade therapies?	Yes	No
2. (Women) Do you have a history of premenstrual syndrome (PMS), irregular cycles, fibrous breasts, and/or menopausal symptoms?	Yes	No
3. (Men) Have you had a change in sexual function and/or been diagnosed with erectile dysfunction?	Yes	No
4. Do you have a low libido (sex drive)?	Yes	No
5. Do you have a history of fertility problems, including miscarriage?	Yes	No
6. Have you ever been diagnosed with a thyroid disorder?	Yes	No
7. Have you ever been diagnosed with adrenal fatigue and/or low cortisol levels?	Yes	No
8. Do you experience weight fluctuations of more than 10 pounds on a regular basis?	Yes	No
9. Do you handle store receipts, drink out of plastic bottles, have exposure to paraben-containing products, or eat nonorganic animal protein more than once a month?	Yes	No
10. Do you now or have you ever followed a low-fat diet?	Yes	No

Total number of "Yes" answers

If you scored highest in this section, please focus on chapter 10.

TABLE 2.9. STRESS AND BIORHYTHMS

1. Did any of your symptoms or lab results worsen after a stressful period? And/or, if you have a cancer diagnosis, was the diagnosis made following a stressful period?	Yes	No
2. Are you a night owl? And/or have you ever had a job working at night or caring for a small child who kept you up late?	Yes	No
3. Do you often travel back and forth across many time zones?	Yes	No
4. Are there lights on while you sleep during the night (e.g., streetlights or a TV)?	Yes	No
5. Do you feel you are you easily fatigued?	Yes	No
6. Do you often crave salt?	Yes	No
7. Do you sleep fewer than 8 hours a night and/or go to bed after 11 p.m.?	Yes	No
8. Do you have screen time (i.e., watch TV or use an electronic device) after 5 p.m.?	Yes	No
9. Do you spend less than 15 minutes outdoors every day?	Yes	No
10. Do you feel that you experience high levels of stress every day?	Yes	No

Total number of "Yes" answers

If you scored highest in this section, please focus on chapter 11.

TABLE 2.10. MENTAL AND EMOTIONAL HEALTH

1. Do you experience irritability, mood swings, and/or unstable emotions?	Yes	No
2. Have you been diagnosed with a mental disorder (e.g., bipolar disorder, depression, anxiety)?	Yes	No
3. Are you easily offended?	Yes	No
4. Are you sensitive to other people's energy and reactions?	Yes	No
5. Do you ever experience racing, repetitive thoughts?	Yes	No
6. Do you find it difficult to speak your truth in certain situations?	Yes	No
7. Have you ever used drugs or alcohol, sex, shopping, TV, gambling, gaming, or time on the internet to self-medicate?	Yes	No
8. Do you feel that you lack a good support system (e.g., supportive spouse, friends, and/or spiritual community?)	Yes	No
9. Do you feel you lack purpose?	Yes	No
10. Do you find it difficult to feel gratitude and joy?	Yes	No
Total number of "Yes" answers		

If you scored highest in this section, please focus on chapter 12.

Ten Questions to Ask Your Oncologist

Do not be afraid to ask questions. Remember, you are paying your doctor, so they work for you. Consider yourself the CEO of your cancer care process, and your caregivers are your board of directors. Here are ten sample questions to ask when interviewing a doctor for the position of caring for your life:

1. What will you be doing to treat my cancer stem cells, since chemotherapy, radiation, and surgery do not target these and can, in fact, stimulate their proliferation?
2. How do you plan to prevent further DNA or mitochondrial damage to my healthy cells?
3. What are your expectations of and rationale for this particular treatment?
4. What is your overall expectation for this course of treatment: A cure? Palliation (meaning improving quality of life)?
5. What are the possible risks and how will the medical team address possible adverse consequences?
6. Are there treatments you cannot provide? What would you consider doing if you had my disease?
7. What would my course of disease progression be if I choose to do nothing you recommend? (What would my survival time be, for example?)
8. Are you open to integrative therapies and willing to work with my integrative oncology experts?
9. What experience and training do you have with integrative oncology, nutrition, or integrative medicine in general?
10. Are you available and willing to communicate with my entire team and be supportive of my personal choices?

Now that you have an idea about the elements of your terrain that might be promoting a cancer process, it is time to plan how you want to make a change. Remember, you are in the driver's seat of your health care plan. The real urgency of cancer lies in the shock of diagnosis; while cancer-related medical emergencies do occur, they are quite rare. In most cases (even when given a poor prognosis) you have time to explore your terrain and choose how best to approach treatment and how to support your body every step of the way.

We understand that it can be hard to trust oneself in the face of a scary diagnosis, especially since patients are often swept into their personal war against cancer at an alarming speed. Doctors can use language that makes it sound as though treatments must happen immediately and that to refuse is a death sentence. Add to that the overwhelming amount of information found on the internet and suggestions from well-meaning family and friends and it can all result in major stress and confusion. Most people diagnosed with cancer will go through the full seven stages of grief—starting with shock or disbelief, then denial, bargaining, guilt, anger, depression, finally arriving at acceptance and hope. Our best advice is to slow down, breathe, read this book, trust yourself, and hurry to hopefulness!

Cancer is most often a marathon, so you'll need to pace yourself. Maybe it's time to take that vacation you've always wanted, or spend more time doing the things you love. We've seen it hundreds of times, where cancer ends up being the best teacher and the best journey a person experiences in their lifetime. And remember, no matter what your diagnosis is, *cancer is not a death sentence*, so never believe them if a doctor gives you an expected amount of time to live. Miracles happen every day, so never lose hope.

Now it's time to go deeper into each terrain element and the specific metabolic approaches to this disease. We sincerely hope you find the same inspiration and success as our patients have.

CHAPTER 3

Genetics, Epigenetics, and Nutrigenomics
What You Inherit, What You Can Control

Genes get turned on, turned off or modified by our environment; what we eat, who we surround ourselves with, and how we lead our lives. —LYNNE MCTAGGART, *author of* The Intention Experiment

Epigenetics doesn't change the genetic code, it changes how that's read. Perfectly normal genes can result in cancer or death. Vice-versa, in the right environment, mutant genes won't be expressed. Genes are equivalent to blueprints; epigenetics is the contractor. —DR. BRUCE LIPTON, *author of* The Biology of Belief

Fortunately, the theory that our genes forecast the fate of our health has been disproven during the last two decades. This may be news to some, but suffice it to say your DNA is not your destiny. Rather, what has been learned is that genes function more like light switches. Just because a person tests positive for the *BRCA* mutation, for example, does not mean they will get breast cancer. Our genes can be flipped on or off depending on our exposure to certain environmental factors, including diet, lifestyle, and stress. Researchers in the emerging field of *epigenetics* ("upon genetics") have been studying these environmental "fingers" that are responsible for switching genes on and off and learning a lot about how our genomes actually work. You can think of your genome—your complete set of DNA—like billions of Christmas lights running through your body. Epigenetic factors such as poor diet or exposure to carcinogenic toxins are the fingers that can turn a strand of those lights from being expressed, or illuminated, to silenced, or turned off. Too much or too little exercise; trauma of any kind; chemical stressors such as infections, food allergens, and processed foods; environmental toxins such as fluoride and other metals; emotional or financial stress; issues with children, spouses, or loved ones—all of these impact genetic expression. Every thought, every bite, and every lifestyle choice affects genetic regulation. We all have mouths that can smile or frown; it is the particular environment that triggers which demeanor we choose to express.

Human evolution has transpired based on how our genes have responded to our environment for the past couple of million years; it is the reason we are all not still covered in hair. Our genes can change in response to our environment, and they always have. Just as good kids can "go bad" when exposed to a negative influence, our genes can exert harmful or helpful expressions depending on what factors they are exposed to. A poor diet can damage mitochondria, turning on cancer-promoting *oncogenes*. Yet a genetically attuned diet (similar to the one humans have eaten for over two million years) can keep these oncogenes silenced and mitochondria healthy. The genetic mutations considered by conventional medicine as the root causes of cancer are, in fact, *modifiable by epigenetic factors*.[1] Indeed, it is well established that genetics is the cause of only 5–10 percent of cancers and most of these genes encode proteins that impact mitochondrial respiration. It is mitochondrial damage that causes cancer, not the genes. If the inherited cancer gene does not damage mitochondria, cancer will not occur.[2]

What's more, genetic health is actually almost entirely contingent upon the food we eat and how it is metabolized by the body. *Nutrigenomics*, another emerging field, studies the interaction between diet and genes. So far the findings have been significant. For example, dark leafy greens can affect gene expression through epigenetic modification processes such as *methylation* (a process discussed later in this chapter). And there is a growing body of evidence that certain dietary compounds—including folate, vitamin B_{12}, tea polyphenols, cruciferous vegetables, and more—have anticarcinogenic properties because of their relationship to DNA.[3] There is now an undeniable association between diet and genetic health, and it is high time we started utilizing this knowledge.

In this chapter we will explain genetic and epigenetic concepts in an understandable way, and also present how the dietary changes that occurred as humans evolved from hunter-gatherers to farmers have negatively impacted our genome. The reason this is so important (and why genetics is the first of the Terrain Ten to be presented) is because some people choose to undergo "preventive" measures to avoid the development of cancer, such as removing breasts when they test positive for a *BRCA* gene mutation. While this has surely saved lives, and we certainly never judge people on the decisions they feel they need to make for their own health, we show in this chapter that even if an individual tests positive for a scary gene like *BRCA1* or a SNP like *MTHFR* (which we discuss in a moment), with the right diet and other terrain modifications, cancer may not be what sends them into the casket. However, those who test positive for the *BRCA1* gene but are not willing to make the diet and lifestyle changes needed to achieve an optimized terrain increase their likelihood of developing cancer by a lot—85 percent in some cases. Conversely, by focusing on prevention and on participation and engagement in our own health, the possibility of avoiding cancer decreases significantly—85 percent in the other direction. This book is all about encouraging participatory medicine through deep nutrition and nontoxic approaches. The way we live our lives determines our genetic destiny. If we expose ourselves to positive epigenetic factors like deep nutrition, exercise, good sleep, stress management, and healthy relationships, our genes will express smiles and health, not frowns and disease. Sounds simple, right? In many ways it is. But first let's try to explain DNA and genes as simply as possible so that the very complex concept of genetics becomes a touch easier to comprehend.

Meet Your Genes

Genetics is the study of genes, genetic variation, and inheritance. A gene is a segment of DNA that is inherited by a child from its parents. DNA is made of molecules arranged in a double helix, a shape that looks similar to a spiral staircase. Each step of the staircase is made of a *base pair*, a coupling of two out of the four possible nucleobases—the chemicals adenine (A), thymine (T), cytosine (C), and guanine (G). These are sometimes referred to as the *genetic alphabet*. The particular sequence of the four bases (ATCGTT versus ATCGCT, for instance) on the steps is what provides the instructions—or recipe if you will—for the cell to create the proteins the body needs to function. These proteins can become enzymes, antibodies, hormones, and so forth. The process of translating the genetic information (the recipe) from the DNA code into proteins is a technical process known as *genetic expression*. Just because a particular gene is encoded for in the DNA, its associated trait or protein will not necessarily be expressed (created). The recipe might be right there in the book, but the cook needs to be activated to make it.

Observable traits such as hair and skin color are known as *phenotypes* (from the Greek *phainein*, meaning "to show," and *typos*, meaning "type") and result from the interactions between our genes and the environment. For example, after hundreds of generational adaptations, the skin color of humans who migrated farther from the equator became lighter to enable their bodies to absorb more vitamin D, a process that took thousands of years. Today, however, with daily exposure to huge numbers of novel environmental factors and synthetic foods, our DNA does not have time to adapt; it's as if we have suddenly moved to the moon. When DNA is damaged (which can easily occur from many of the different factors we discuss throughout this book) the result can be a *mutation*. A mutation is a permanent alteration in the DNA sequence, due to either the deletion or substitution of part of the code. (You can think of it like a typo in a recipe—a tablespoon instead of a teaspoon—which creates a bad-tasting dish, or, in this case, a cancerous gene.)

There are two types of genetic mutations: *Germline*, or hereditary, mutations are inherited from a parent and are present throughout a person's life in every cell in the body. *Somatic* mutations are alterations in DNA that occur after birth. Somatic mutations can, but don't always, cause cancer. They result from numerous factors, including diet, lifestyle (stress, sleep, exercise), exposure to carcinogens such as cigarette smoke or pesticides, viruses, nutrient deficiencies, mistakes made during DNA replication or cell division, and more. Every time a cell divides its genes have a certain chance of mutating, so cells that divide more frequently—or are exposed to more mutation-causing toxins—have a greater chance of acquiring mutations. Over ten million billion cell divisions occur over the average human lifetime. And, what's wild to think about is that somatic mutations are occurring all the time—thousands of times a day—and these mutations can alter a cell's programming, sometimes in ways that convert a healthy cell to a cancerous one.

Thus, cancerous processes would develop all the time were it not for a built-in system that utilizes a system of checks and balances to repair DNA mutations as they occur. This system, called *genome surveillance*, also acts to silence oncogenes. Nearly all cancer cells have defects in their genome surveillance system. Cancer cells are basically abnormal cells with mutations that enable them to survive and reproduce better than other cells because the system of checks and balances is defective. The most commonly mutated gene found in cancers is *TP53*. When healthy, *TP53*, a tumor-suppressing gene (encoding for the protein p53), stops unwanted cells from growing and dividing. When a tumor-suppressor gene is mutated, a cell may no longer receive the instruction to stop growing and instead may begin to multiply out of control, one of the hallmark characteristics of cancer. What's more, is a mutated *TP53* also damages cellular metabolism forcing the cell to utilize the fermentation pathway in order to survive, and the dysregulated cell growth signature to cancer arises when fermentation replaces respiration.

Two of the most famous genes in cancer, *BRCA1* and *BRCA2*, also play central roles in genetic repair and mitochondrial function. When either *BRCA1* or *BRCA2* is absent as the result of a mutation, DNA repair complexes cannot form. Therefore, cells that are missing *BRCA1* or *BRCA2* become hypersensitive to damaging agents (such as various chemical carcinogens found in our food and personal care products, which are discussed in chapter 5; see "A Deeper Look at Carcinogens"). Fortunately, many food components are involved in repairing DNA and mitochondrial damage, including those found in cruciferous vegetables. But first let's look at another type of gene mutation that, in addition to the hereditary and somatic mutations already described, also alters gene function. *Single-nucleotide polymorphisms*, also known as SNPs (pronounced "snips"), are a type of genetic variation that is passed from parent to child. The analysis of an individual's SNPs is becoming a critical element in personalized medicine. SNP assessment has been a key element of our private practices for years and has made all the difference for many of Dr. Nasha's stage IV cancer cases.

Making Sense of Single-Nucleotide Polymorphisms (SNPs)

The process called *mitosis*, or cell division, is when a single cell divides to form two identical cells. The purposes of mitosis is both to grow and to replace worn-out cells. In mitosis, a cell first copies its DNA so that each new cell will have a complete set of genetic instructions. But cells sometimes make mistakes, similar to typos, during this copying process. These mistakes lead to variations in the DNA sequence at particular locations, causing a SNP (or as some like to say, a "hiccup"). There are an estimated ten million SNPs in the human genome.[4] And while some SNPs seem to have no effect on cell function, others can have profound effects, from changing an individual's response to certain drugs, to raising their susceptibility to environmental factors such as toxins, suppressing their ability to process hormones, affecting the way they metabolize food, and increasing their risk of depression and developing disease. Certain SNPs can also affect the metabolism of fats, alcohol, caffeine, vitamin D, sulfur, and lactose. We will cover many of these specific SNPs later in the book, but now we want to highlight one that has particularly far-reaching effects when it comes to cancer: *MTHFR*.

An estimated 50 percent of the population has inherited one copy of the infamous *MTHFR* SNP, which codes for the enzyme methylenetetrahydrofolate reductase (MTHFR). Similar to the *BRCA* gene, research suggests that an *MTHFR* gene mutation increases the risk of breast, colon, and other cancers and should be given equal emphasis to *BRCA* mutations during evaluation and treatment.[5] Individuals with *MTHFR* mutations can have a 40–70 percent reduction of normal MTHFR enzyme activity. This slows down methylation processes and the body's ability to create antioxidants, and impedes detoxification. Here we cover MTHFR's role in methylation, one of the body's primary epigenetic modification systems, a critical process used to silence mutated genes that also just so happens to be entirely dependent on nutrition.

The Mechanics of Methylation

DNA methylation is one of several critically important epigenetic processes the body uses to mark or *tag* genes. These epigenetic markers direct a cell's transcription machinery to either read a gene or not—to make the recipe or skip it. DNA methylation is when a structure called a *methyl group*, a unit composed of a single atom of carbon and three hydrogen atoms, binds to a stretch of DNA and either activates it or silences it—kind of like putting a sticker over its mouth. In this way methylation helps regulate the normal behavior of DNA; without methylation, the transcription of genes would occur without restraint. The process of methylation also impacts immune, neurological, and detoxification systems. From an evolutionary standpoint, methylation makes sense: For instance, it is a good way to deal with foreign DNA that has been inserted into the genome, silencing it so that it does not interfere with normal gene activity. (This is an issue we face when we eat genetically modified foods, as we discuss later.[6]) Changes in the pattern of DNA methylation have been a consistent finding in cancer cells. Reduced levels of DNA methylation, called *hypomethylation*, can result in DNA instability, while the overexpression of genes, or *hypermethylation*, has been associated with the silencing of valuable tumor-suppressor genes.[7]

One of the most important genes in the methylation process is, you guessed it, *MTHFR*. The *MTHFR* gene provides instructions for making the enzyme methylenetetrahydrofolate reductase. When foods containing folate (also called folic acid, or vitamin B_9) are consumed, the MTHFR enzyme converts the vitamin into an active, bioavailable form called methylfolate. Methylfolate has a complicated role in the DNA methylation process, but in short it is an important source of the carbon molecules needed for the creation of methyl groups, the mouth-covering stickers. When dietary consumption of folate is low or a person has an *MTHFR* mutation, the methylation process can be reduced by 40–70 percent. This hypomethylation in effect gives oncogenes the green light, which can result in the development of cancer. Fortunately, there are nutritional solutions for overcoming a *MTHFR* SNP and enhancing methylation: increasing consumption of folate-rich foods.

Folate: The Celebrity Methylation Nutrient

While by definition all nutrients are vital to overall well-being, there is one standout when it comes to genetic health: folate. Folate is a water-soluble B vitamin, B_9, and is essential for numerous genetic processes—as well as for metabolism and the production of red blood cells. Lack of the vitamin during pregnancy can cause neural tube defects in the baby, including spina bifida, which is why pregnant women are encouraged to take folate supplements. Folate is necessary for the formation of the DNA bases adenine and guanine. It is also required for DNA synthesis, cell formation, and regeneration. A lack of folate during DNA replication can increase the risk of mutations. Epidemiological studies have found that folate deficiency is also strongly associated with hypomethylation of DNA, increased risk of breast cancer, and the promotion of cancer in general.[8] Folate is the first of many examples of how important nutrition is to genetic health, and to the body's terrain in general.

Humans are not capable of synthesizing folate in the body, which means we rely on sufficient levels of it coming from our diet. The top sources of folate (from the Latin word *folium*, meaning "leaf") are spinach, endive, bok choy, romaine lettuce, asparagus, mustard and turnip greens, goose and duck liver, and the herb epazote. Epazote has a sharp flavor similar to fennel and was once widely cultivated as a medicinal herb, although many today have never heard of it. Another interesting constituent of epazote is the compound ascaridole, one of the ingredients in an essential oil that, in research studies of sarcomas in mice, has been associated with the inhibition of tumor growth by over 30 percent.[9] If you haven't ever tried this powerful herb, now is the time! It can be used much like cilantro in Mexican dishes and also makes for a savory soup topping.

When we don't eat enough folate-rich foods, fatigue sets in, and also anxiety, an increased risk of miscarriage, thyroid problems, and a condition called folate-deficiency anemia, the decreased production of red blood cells. Folate-rich foods should be incorporated on a daily basis, and supplementation needs to be in the active form methylfolate. Folic acid, the synthetic form of folate, is added to grains and supplements (such as prenatal vitamins), but individuals with a certain *MTHFR* gene mutation cannot metabolize folic acid. What's more, an elevated folic acid level has the potential to stimulate pre-existing cancer cells. In general, synthetic forms of vitamins should always be avoided.

Folate has also recently gained attention for its ability to help keep blood levels of homocysteine in check. Homocysteine, an amino acid, is a well-documented marker for cardiovascular disease and, when excessive, is also considered a risk factor for cancer. An estimated 20 percent of the population has a dietary deficiency of folate. Couple that with the 50 percent of people who have an *MTHFR* mutation and we can see why the Christmas lights of our genome are short-circuiting, oncogenes are running free, and cancer is rampant. So how has Western medicine been approaching genomic health? With lots of research and few results. Let's take a quick look.

Genetics and Cancer: The Western Approach

Sadly, we have made little progress in extending survival for patients with metastatic cancer since the "War on Cancer" was declared in 1971. When a solid-organ tumor (such as breast or pancreatic) spreads to distant sites, the likelihood of surviving today is about the same as it was fifty years ago, with rare exceptions—pretty dismal. Dismal especially when we consider that the federal government has spent well over $105 billion on genetic-focused efforts, most notably the Human Genome Project, a publicly funded, thirteen-year-long project begun in 1990 with the goal of determining the DNA sequence of the entire human genome. Based on the genetic discoveries made during this effort, new "smart" drugs were developed to target various genetic mutations. There are now over eight hundred such "targeted agents" in clinical development, including monoclonal antibodies like trastuzumab (Herceptin) that are the foundation of what is known as "precision medicine." Targeted therapy is a type of cancer treatment that literally targets the peculiarities of cancer cells that make them different from healthy cells and help them grow, divide, and spread. The targets are based largely on the ten hallmarks of cancer. While targeted therapy is certainly a step up from the "destroy-all-cells" approach of traditional cytotoxic chemotherapies, the "one mutation, one target, one drug" approach is not working. Drugs like trastuzumab not only have been found to cause heart failure, but also only increase ten-year disease-free survival rates by a mere *12 percent*—with a price tag over $60,000 a year.[10]

When you consider that the genome of a typical patient with lung cancer contains over fifty thousand mutations, you begin to understand why the "one target, one drug" approach doesn't work (and in this book we will show you additional reasons). It's like a psychologist trying to get a patient to smile without bothering to learn what is causing them to weep. Merely identifying a mutation is failing to recognize what *caused* it in the first place. Has your doctor tested your *MTHFR* gene or inquired about your folate intake? (If not, ask them to; it is important for both the prevention and management of cancer.) If we don't look at the root cause of these mutations, then conventional therapies might stall the cancer for a while, but eventually it will come roaring back. To truly overcome cancer it is the terrain, not the tumor, that requires treatment.

Cancer Is a Disease of Genes Mismatched with Modern Lifestyle

We cannot change our future without understanding our past. While it is easy to accept modern life as the norm, in reality the changes that have occurred in our diet and lifestyle within the past fifteen thousand years—especially in the last two hundred—are so significant that not only would our ancestors not recognize modern living, our genes absolutely do not. In fact, hundreds of DNA mutations first appeared during or after the emergence of agriculture, beginning about fifteen thousand years ago. The genes most strongly affected were those associated with skin color, bone structure, and the metabolism of "new" foods, including milk, meat, and grains.[11] While farming might seem like an age-old concept, it is actually relatively modern. Crop cultivation and animal domestication have existed for fewer than three hundred generations and, not surprisingly, most of our genetic mutations have also arisen within the same time frame. Unfortunately, more than 86 percent of these mutations are due to negative effects, meaning that they have occurred in response to threats to our genetic health, not because of positive selection.[12]

Our ancient diverse and nutrient-dense diet is what established the human genetic baseline, a system that is now exposed to dietary elements that are completely different from what we were eating when we evolved. Cars with gasoline engines cannot run with sugar poured into their tanks, and neither can humans. A bowl of wild greens and a bowl of Wheaties present very different messages to our genome, and our ancient engines—our mitochondria—are sputtering and stalling on standard American fare. Not only cancer, but also other noncommunicable diseases such as heart disease and diabetes, now affect more than half of all Americans. We are sadly a sick society. But why? For starters, the rise of agriculture triggered the biggest change to the human diet in all of our existence. When we learned to raise crops and keep domestic livestock, we were no longer dependent on hunting, fishing, and gathering wild plants. Our nutritional profile changed. The cultivation of cereal grains and other crops—including wheat, barley, millet, rice, corn, sorghum, beans, yams, and potatoes—enabled our Neolithic ancestors to build permanent dwellings and congregate in villages, but such progress came with massive nutritional consequences. Traditional hunting and gathering, which had been humans' way of life from the beginning, all but vanished in favor of foods that were completely foreign to our digestive systems and our genomes. The development of agriculture has been deemed by many experts as "the biggest mistake in human history."[13]

We are not being dramatic here; paleoanthropologists have also confirmed the negative impact of agriculture. Skeletons found in Greece and Turkey show an average height of hunter-gatherers toward the end of the ice ages was 5 feet, 9 inches for men, 5 feet, 5 inches for women. With the adoption of agriculture, human height averages went way down, and by 3000 BC had reached a low of only 5 feet, 3 inches for men, 5 feet for women. Studies by anthropologist George Armelagos and his colleagues at the University of Massachusetts showed that, compared with the hunter-gatherers who preceded them, early farmers had a nearly 50 percent increase in tooth enamel defects indicative of malnutrition, a fourfold increase in iron-deficiency anemia (evidenced by a bone condition called *porotic hyperostosis*), and a threefold increase in bone lesions reflecting infectious diseases and nutrient depletion.

Hunter-gatherers had a very diverse and nutrient-dense diet; they ate dozens of different species of wild plants a year. The average hunter-gatherer also ate more protein, fewer carbohydrates, ten times more fiber, substantially more phytonutrients, and double the amount of cholesterol than the average American eats today. Since our diet shifted from Paleo to agrarian, our consumption of grain-based carbohydrates has increased dramatically. The average American now obtains 52 percent of their daily calories from carbohydrates—primarily wheat, rice, and potatoes—while the average hunter-gatherer consumed closer to 35 percent of their daily calories from carbohydrates, and these were primarily vegetables.

Until very recently humans had never eaten wheat, rice, corn, barley, potatoes, or soybeans. The period of time since the Neolithic revolution—the transition from foraging and nomadism to agriculture and settlement—represents less than 1 percent of human history. Thus, the switch from a "caveman diet" consisting of fat, meat, and the occasional roots, berries, and other plant sources of carbohydrate to a diet dominated by grains has occurred too recently to allow the needed accommodations in the genes that encode our metabolic pathways. In fact, studies have shown that our current high-carbohydrate diet stresses several genes associated with the development of certain cancers.[14]

Early farmers frequently suffered such nutrient-deficiency diseases as scurvy (insufficient vitamin C), pellagra (insufficient niacin, or vitamin B₃), beriberi (insufficient thiamine, or vitamin B₁), anemia (insufficient folate, or vitamin B₉), and goiter (insufficient iodine). What's important to know is that these nutrients, notably folate and the powerful antioxidant vitamin C, have been found to have roles in reducing cellular DNA damage and to be required for mitochondrial function. Thus, a few centuries ago, when nutrient deficiencies became prominent, the door was opened to an increased probability of unrepaired genetic mutations. As consumption of new foods such as grains and sugar has persisted, cancer has affected people at younger and younger ages. Between 1973 and 1991 the diagnosis of brain cancer and soft-tissue sarcoma each increased more than 25 percent among US children.[15] We are not getting cancer because we are living longer; we are getting cancer because we are damaging our mitochondria on a daily basis with environmental toxins, poor diet, and endocrine disruptors. Most of us are not eating the foods that keep cancer at bay while simultaneously overeating the foods that encourage its riotous growth—too many cookies, too little kale.

———

Several genetic mutations caused by the dietary changes that attended the arrival of agriculture now increase our risk of developing cancer, especially those related to the increased consumption of sugar (glucose, fructose, and sucrose). The metabolism of glucose increases the creation of free radicals that can cause DNA mutations and subsequent inflammation.[16] Studies have also found that high glucose levels induce DNA damage and interfere with DNA repair capability.[17] Similarly, a study published in 2011 in the journal *Expert Opinion on Therapeutic Targets* titled "Refined Fructose and Cancer" demonstrated that the more fructose a person consumes, the greater the amount of damage done to DNA. Studies on a particular protein known as GLUT (and its relationship to glucose and fructose metabolism) show that it alters both germline and somatic DNA as well as inducing epigenetic changes and damaging mitochondria.[18] Our genes are screaming at us to stop eating sugar. And not only is the elimination of sugar good for our genes, it is at the heart of the metabolic approach to cancer. Cancer is not a disease of our genes, it is a disease caused by *what we are feeding them.*

In addition to a reduction in nutritional diversity, agricultural diets are associated with a caloric availability that exceeds growth and energetic requirements. Enter diabetes. How on earth do we expect our ancient genome to adapt to the changes of the past hundred years: high-fructose corn syrup (HFCS), processed grains, refined oils, artificial and synthetic ingredients, and Krispy Kremes! Grains, legumes, processed dairy products, and sugar were not part of the human diet until just a mere speck of time ago in the span of human existence, and since they have been introduced our health has declined. It is estimated that a third of today's children will get diabetes in their lifetime, and almost half of all adults will get cancer. We *must* start looking at the effect our modern diet is having on our health—and change it. Our nutrition has a significant impact on the health of our genes, and new discoveries in the emerging fields of nutrigenetics, nutrigenomics, and nutritional epigenetics keep proving it.

Diet and DNA

Nutrigenetics, nutrigenomics, and nutritional epigenetics are scientific fields that explore, respectively, the ways in which food affects patterns in gene regulation, the relationship between the human genome and nutrition and health, and how our grandparents' diet affects our health today, among other things. The findings have been stunning. To mention only a few:

- Macronutrients and micronutrients in the diet change the activity of enzymes that add methyl groups to DNA.
- Certain phytonutrients, such as green tea, have the ability to repair DNA.
- Molecules in food affect the kind and number of molecules attached to DNA.
- Common dietary chemicals act on the human genome either directly or indirectly and can alter gene expression or structure via several different mechanisms. (For example, intake of the element selenium is considered the major epigenetic switch regulating *BRCA* mutations.[19])
- Some diet-regulated genes play a role in the onset, incidence, progression, and/or severity of cancer.

To us the message is clear: Dietary intervention based on knowledge of nutritional requirements, nutritional status, and genotype can and should be used to help prevent or mitigate cancer. Connections among diet, DNA, and disease continue to surface; for example, a diet high in omega-6 fatty acids correlates to forty times more DNA damage than one high in anti-inflammatory omega-3 fatty acids (more on this in chapter 8; see "Prostaglandins and Essential Fatty Acids").[20] Many nutrients are considered "chemoprotective" as they can inhibit cancer growth, activate tumor-suppressor genes, and promote apoptosis. Cancer prevention studies have shown that all of the major intracellular signaling pathways, including DNA repair, deregulated in different types of cancer are protected by nutrients. Because genetic variation has not been taken into account when it comes to dietary recommendations, nutrition and health status have largely suffered. Personalized nutrition absolutely needs to be at the core of cancer treatments. Avoiding such DNA-damaging foods as grains, beans, inflammatory fats, and sugar is a surefire way to optimize your genome no matter your cancer history. You will learn more about all of these foods throughout this book, but one type of "Frankenfood"—genetically modified food—needs to be discussed straightaway.

Genetically Modified (GM) Foods and Their Impact on Human DNA

Perhaps the biggest weed in the garden of our terrains is the existence of foods that are genetically modified (also called GMOs, or GM foods). They represent the newest food source introduced into the human diet and have been wreaking havoc on our health ever since. In addition to promoting the dangerous horizontal transfer of antibiotic-resistant genes, consumption of GM foods decreases DNA methylation—and we have seen how that can allow cancerous genes to run wild.[21] Evidence of this may be found in trends in cancer incidence rates: Since GM foods entered our food supply in the 1990s, the number of new breast cancer cases has doubled.[22] Rates of other diseases have increased, too. Diagnosis of celiac disease, an immune-mediated disorder of the small intestine triggered by gluten proteins in wheat and other grains, has seen a fourfold increase in the past fifty years. This condition has been associated with mutations found in the *HLA-DQ2* and *HLA-DQ8* genes. MIT research scientists Anthony Samsel and Stephanie Seneff propose that the active ingredient in the herbicide Roundup, glyphosate, may be the most important causal factor in the celiac epidemic.[23]

Glyphosate is listed by the International Agency for Research on Cancer (IARC) as a carcinogen. Their 2015 report concluded that glyphosate exposure doubles the risk of non-Hodgkin lymphoma, while increasing the risk of a related cancer called multiple myeloma.[24] What is more, a 2013 study published in the peer-reviewed Public Library of Science journal *PLOS ONE* titled "Complete Genes May Pass from Food to Human Blood" found that meal-derived DNA fragments carrying complete genes can enter into the human circulatory system.[25] This means that altered genes enter our genome with every bite of genetically modified corn, soy, and so on. Studies have shown that the adjuvants in Roundup exert their toxic effects through interfering with mitochondrial respiration.[26] Elimination of GM foods is a critical step toward improving your metabolic terrain. Avoiding all grains (including corn), soy, canola, and nonorganic varieties of potatoes, apples, alfalfa, eggplant, tomato, sugar beet, sugarcane, plum, papaya, melons, and flax is imperative.[27]

The modern "breakthrough" in genetic modification technology came in 1973, when geneticists Herbert Boyer and Stanley Cohen developed a method of transferring a gene encoding antibiotic resistance from one strain of bacteria to another, bestowing antibiotic resistance upon the recipient. Since then foods and pharmaceuticals with interspecies DNA modifications (including Humulin, a biosynthetic insulin used to control blood sugar) have entered the public market with little to no safety testing, instead using the general public as guinea pigs. In the decades following approval, the horrendous health and environmental effects of GM foods and other substances have been enough to convince more than twenty-six countries—including Australia, Austria, China, France, Germany, Greece, Hungary, India, Italy, Mexico, Russia, and Switzerland—to ban all GMOs. As of this writing, however, GM foods are still being consumed at a rapid rate in the United States—and all without labeling. If you want to know what is causing cancer,

Testing Your Genetic SNPs

Genetic testing has come a long way. These tests used to cost thousands of dollars, but today many providers are able to perform a *MTHFR* test, and in many cases it is covered by insurance. To assess your genetic SNPs some testing options include www.23andme .com, and/or Genova Diagnostics, for a few hundred dollars or less. (Just make sure to always have genetic information interpreted by someone versed in SNP analysis, as there is a lot to it!) After you know your genetic picture, or even if you not decide to do testing, it's time to start taking a metabolic approach to encourage the health of your genes.

Getting and analyzing this data is a three-step process. Genova Diagnostics and 23andme are the tests that will give you the raw data. This data needs to then be run through companies such as StrateGene, Genetic Genie, and MTHFR Support; then analyzed by a health care provider to interpret the information and decide how to address the SNPs.

just look in your kitchen cabinets; the evidence is everywhere. Corn and soybean oils, components of practically every single processed food in the supermarket, are two examples in wide circulation. Unless a product sports an "Organic" or "Verified Non-GMO" label, then assume the food contains GMOs and has been exposed to glyphosate. One more incentive to consume whole, organic, unprocessed foods whenever possible.

The Metabolic Approach to Optimizing Genetic Health

With so many modern villains such as grains, sugar, pesticides, and GM foods capable of mutating genes, it might seem hopeless even to try to defeat them. But it absolutely is not. Several dietary approaches have been found to prevent, protect, and repair DNA damage. Practicing a ketogenic diet, fasting, balancing amino acids, increasing methyl-donor and folate-rich foods, optimizing B_{12} levels, and consuming specific plant-derived phytonutrients are the cornerstones of our genetic enhancement strategy. In the following nine chapters you will learn how the therapeutic approaches of fasting and the ketogenic diet positively affect each one of the ten terrain elements, genetic repair being no exception.

The ketogenic diet plays an integral role in the metabolic approach to cancer and in our approach. We personally have seen it work wonders with our cancer patients time and time again. It is a deeply therapeutic, high-fat, low-carbohydrate diet that enables the body to cease using glucose as its primary fuel source and to utilize ketones (the bi-product of fatty acid breakdown) instead. Ketones are a source of fuel that is more difficult for cancer cells to consume than glucose is. The ketogenic diet thus deprives cancer cells of energy targeting the fundamental cause of cancer: altered metabolism. We will go into more detail about the ketogenic diet throughout this book.

Throughout all of human evolution—until the past two hundred years or so—humans have experienced shortages of food from time to time. Existing on ketones is actually an evolutionary survival mechanism that just happens to be very genoprotective. Studies have found that intermittent fasting (that is, consuming nothing other than water or green tea) enhances the ability of nerve cells to repair their DNA, protects DNA from damage caused by chemotherapy, and switches on a number of DNA-repair genes.[28] Fasting, or subsisting on a high-fat diet (think winter months when there was little to eat besides whole animals or fat products made from them), is something humans have been doing for millions of years, and it turns out it's really good for our DNA.

Now let's take a deeper look at the foods specifically involved with maintaining the health of our genes; we'll talk more about fasting and the ketogenic diet in chapters 4, 7, and 11.

Protein Is Required for DNA Synthesis

One of the first questions a newly diagnosed cancer patient will often ask us is whether they should eat animal protein or not. This is by far one of the most confusing and controversial topics of an anticancer diet. But the answer is yes: Consumption of some amount of animal protein is an absolute requirement. In fact, estimates show that patients undergoing conventional cancer therapy may require as much as 50 percent *more* protein than usual, or in excess of 80 mg a day.[29] Further, recent research from Cornell University found that for individuals with a certain genotype, maintaining a vegetarian or vegan diet may actually increase the risk of developing cancer and other inflammatory illnesses.[30] The decision to adhere long-term to such a diet should take genetic factors into consideration. Cancer patients need complete proteins (all nine essential amino acids, found most readily in meat, fish, and dairy) for optimal functioning of the immune system, prevention and reversal of *cachexia* (that is, muscle wasting and extreme weight loss; reviewed in more detail in chapter 8), manufacture of DNA, and regulation of gene expression.

Remember those proteins that our genes know the recipes for? Wonder how they are actually made? Well, by arranging the twenty amino acids that come from our food into various distinct sequences, our DNA, with the help of ribonucleic acid (RNA), can create nearly forty thousand different proteins. Proteins have rightfully earned their title of "the building blocks of life." Without an adequate supply of these twenty amino acids, the body is more prone to developing genetic imbalances that can allow cancer to take hold and do its damage. But the devil is in the details: Healthy animal protein consumption is entirely contingent upon how the animal was raised, what it ate, how it is prepared, and how much of it is consumed. Quality and quantity are paramount. Deeply nutritive animals are either well fed or wild, such as pasture-raised (100 percent grass-fed) and organic beef, poultry, eggs, wild game, wild fish, and fowl. Conversely, caged or otherwise commercially raised animals that are fed a non-natural and highly toxic diet are downright dangerous to consume. In fact, they are carcinogenic.

It is confusing to hear on the news that "meat causes cancer." But the reason this is often said is because the majority of the population is not eating *real* meat; modern commercial animal products are basically Superfund sites on four (or two) legs. Conventionally raised animals are fed a highly toxic diet (discussed in greater detail in chapter 5) and then processed and packaged using synthetic preservatives. They are high in inflammatory omega-6 fats and low in nutrients. We don't recommend *ever* eating these animals.

Meanwhile, the popular anticancer diet that gets much attention is a plant-based diet. A vegetarian or, worse yet, vegan diet (which means no animal or animal by-products) is simply far too high in carbohydrates and lacking in complete proteins. The concept of a vegetarian diet as an anticancer diet arose from the highly flawed and since completely debunked China Study, a research collaboration between Cornell and Oxford Universities and the Chinese Academy of Preventive Medicine, which found that the tofu-eating vegetarians in Eastern countries had lower rates of cancer than in the West. The study failed to explore several other factors, however, including the population's high intake of cancer-fighting sea vegetables and fermented foods (more on these in chapter 6) and the enhanced genetic capacity of Asian populations to utilize the anticancer properties of soy, a capacity that 40 percent of Americans do not have.

The primary problem with vegetarian and vegan diets is twofold. First, as we have already noted, they are predominantly composed of carbohydrates—that is, after all, what fruits, vegetables, grains, and beans all are (one sweet potato contains roughly 26 grams of carbohydrate, more than anyone following a ketogenic diet should consume in an entire day). And second, these diets do not supply the balance of amino acids needed for optimal health.

The word *protein* is derived from the Greek word *protos*, meaning "of prime importance." Proteins control almost every biochemical reaction in the body and are one of three macronutrients (*macro* meaning we humans need it in large amounts), along with carbohydrates and fat. Every protein is made of a selection of twenty individual amino acids chained together in a particular sequence, like letters in a word. The sequence of these amino acids determines the function of the protein. For instance, some proteins are enzymes, while others are antibodies or certain types of hormones. Nine of these amino acids are considered "essential" since the body requires them but cannot make them on its own and they therefore *must* come from food. The eleven "nonessential" amino acids, while also required for health and growth, can be synthesized in the body, and are not always diet-dependent. A few of the normally nonessential amino acids can become "conditionally essential," since their creation is dependent on the presence of either another essential or nonessential amino acid as a parent substance (also called a precursor).

This system is not flawless, and errors in the production of nonessential amino acids can be caused by an imbalanced microbiome (which can occur during conventional cancer treatment—more on this in chapter 6) or depletion of certain vitamin or mineral cofactors. Also, if essential amino acids are not eaten in the diet, other conditionally essential amino acids will not be created. For example, the nonessential amino acid tyrosine is required to make thyroid hormones and neurotransmitters. Tyrosine can be made in the body from phenylalanine, an essential amino acid found in meat, fish, chicken, and eggs. If phenylalanine is not consumed in the diet, the body cannot make tyrosine, and thus it becomes conditionally essential. This illustrates an important point: When just *one* of the twenty amino acids is not readily present, the body will break down protein-rich tissues like bone and muscle in order to access them; some experts believe this begins to happen within a few hours of amino acid depletion. In other words, balance and abundance of each of the twenty amino acids is needed to form proteins. Missing one is like being down a basketball player; the team cannot compete.

A food that contains all nine essential amino acids is called a *complete protein*. If a food is missing or low in one or more essential amino acids, it is an *incomplete protein*. Animal foods such as meat, poultry, eggs, and fish

TABLE 3.1. A BREAKDOWN OF AMINO ACIDS

Nonessential	Essential
alanine	histidine
arginine*	isoleucine
asparagine	leucine
aspartic acid	lysine
cysteine*	methionine
glutamic acid	phenylalanine
glutamine*	threonine
glycine	tryptophan
proline	valine
serine*	
tyrosine*	

* Conditionally essential

are sources of complete protein. Plant foods such as vegetables, beans, and grains are incomplete proteins. Plant foods may be combined to create complete proteins in vegan and vegetarian diets, but this significantly raises both caloric and carbohydrate intake, which is contraindicated on a low-glycemic, calorie-restricted, or ketogenic diet. For example, to make a complete protein meal on a vegan diet, ½ cup of black beans combined with ½ cup of brown rice will total 420 calories, 22 grams of protein, and 80 grams of carbohydrate—more than four times the daily carbohydrate allowance for most people following a ketogenic diet. (Not only that, but as you will learn in chapter 7, grains and beans actually act as antinutrients, inhibiting the absorption of nutrients that are critical to the immune system. We recommend avoiding them.) Meanwhile, 3 ounces of wild salmon contains 177 calories, 22 grams of protein, and 0 grams of carbohydrate, not to mention the high anti-inflammatory omega-3 fat content. The fish—if it's wild—is hands down the better protein choice.

How Much Meat to Eat?

When it comes to meat consumption, we must pay attention to quantity because too much is also a problem. In the United States meat is consumed at more than three times the global average. Americans eat ten or twelve times more meat than the average person in Mozambique or Bangladesh. According to the US Department of Agriculture (USDA), in 2012 the average American consumed 71 pounds of red meat and 54 pounds of poultry. A popular steak house offers a 20-ounce porterhouse steak; 140 grams of protein all on its own. Is this too much? The right amount? While everyone is different—and recommendations vary widely—one thing is certain: That steak is *way* too much meat for anyone in modern times to eat in one meal, no matter how good the quality.

According to ketogenic diet principles, approximately 20 percent of calories consumed in a day should come from animal protein. That means that for a 150-pound woman on a 1,600-calorie/day diet, approximately 80 grams, or 320 calories, should come from animal protein (protein contains 4 calories per gram). For some people, however, even 80 grams is too much. For reference, two eggs and one fillet of trout would contain about 40 or 50 grams of protein. As a guideline, animal protein should be considered a side dish, not the main course, and some individuals should not consume red meat at all (more in chapter 9). Eating a diet too high in protein can actually inhibit ketosis in some people because protein can be converted into glucose and *increase* blood sugar levels. We recommend working with a naturopathic oncologist or nutrition therapist to customize your ideal protein intake based on your lab studies, genetics, weight, gender, age, and goals of therapy. And know that your protein requirement can vary depending on where you are in your health process; it may need to be be low or high at different times. That said, in addition to the quality and amount of protein, the way it is prepared is also very important when it comes to genetic health.

Proper Preparation of Protein

To get dinner on the table faster, meat is often cooked at high temperatures, and often over open flames. BBQ anyone? Think again. When meat is cooked above 300°F or over an open flame, carcinogenic compounds form and almost all of the powerful nutrients in the meat are destroyed. (Most restaurant grills are set to around 400°F, home grills to about 350°F.) Heterocyclic amines (HAs) and polycyclic aromatic hydrocarbons (PAHs) are two of the chemical compounds formed when meat is cooked at high temperatures. Both have been shown to induce DNA mutations and increase the risk for breast and other cancers through a variety of mechanisms. If that isn't bad enough, advanced glycation end products (AGEs)—also by-products of meat cooked at high temperatures—are compounds that contribute to the increased oxidant stress and inflammation that damages DNA. This is why nutrition nuances are so important.

Clearly, proper preparation of meat is essential. Slow cooking methods include stewing (such as in a Crock-Pot), steaming, and poaching. Braising is another great method, and involves first browning the meat in oil, then cooking it in a small amount of liquid in a tightly covered pan, either on the stovetop or in the oven (this helps add flavor and more moisture to tougher cuts). Slow roasting at low temperatures is also a good strategy. Always try to leave meat on the bone, with the skin on, as this conserves nutrients. If you do grill, the use of certain herbs, such as rosemary, has been shown to negate the carcinogenic effects of the aforementioned compounds. Adding lemon juice, black cherries, onions, garlic, and organic red wine also helps reduce the number of carcinogenic compounds formed when cooking meat at high temperatures.

Munch on Methyl-Donor Foods

In addition to the folate-rich foods we discussed earlier in the chapter, there are other compounds that help with methylation (the process that directs genes to be turned on or off). Vitamins B_6 and B_{12} are incredibly important, and we will present these two in the next section. But there are three food-derived compounds—betaine, choline, and methionine—that are key components of the methyl-making pathway. Diets high in these methyl-donating nutrients can rapidly alter gene expression, especially during an individual's early development, when the epigenome is first being established. Methylation metabolic pathways depend on choline, methionine, methyltetrahydrofolate (an active form of folate), and vitamins B_6 and B_{12}, thus all of these substances must be present at the same time, and until fifteen thousand years ago they were all well provided for by the human diet. And the importance of the relationship among these nutrients may well go beyond their role in gene methylation and epigenetic control, possibly including effects on energy metabolism and protein synthesis.[31]

Betaine is a derivative of the amino acid glycine. Humans obtain betaine from foods that contain either betaine or compounds containing choline, its precursor. Betaine has been shown to be important in protecting cell function and improving vascular risk factors, and is also an important nutrient in the prevention of cancer.[32] The best food sources of betaine are spinach, beets, and lamb's-quarter. Lamb's-quarter is a wild green with powerful anti-inflammatory actions. It is also a good source of a phytonutrient called saponin, which has been found to have an inhibitory effect on cancer cells.

Choline is a vitamin-like essential nutrient and a major methyl donor. Choline deficiency has been associated with an increased incidence of spontaneous liver cancer and increased sensitivity to carcinogenic chemicals.[33] A number of genetic mechanisms for this association have been proposed: altered expression of numerous genes regulating cell proliferation, differentiation, DNA repair, and apoptosis due to improper DNA methylation. Choline also forms betaine, so eating choline-rich foods also promotes the production of betaine. The best food sources of choline are wild shrimp, scallops, pasture-raised and organic chicken, turkey, and eggs. Do note, recent studies have implicated choline as a potential driver for prostate cancers, making it one of the few cancers that may warrant a reduced animal-protein and increased vegetable-based diet.

Eggs are the quintessential superfood. In addition to providing the essential amino acids, well-raised eggs are a great source of omega-3 fats (found in the yolk), phosphatidylcholine, selenium, vitamin D, and vitamin B_{12}. Gone are the days when it was believed that eggs contributed to high cholesterol and should be limited. That's a myth that has been debunked many times over in recent years. We now know that a high cholesterol level results from intake of sugar, not fat (more on this in the next chapter; see "How Sugar Infiltrated Human Diets"). Provided the eggs are from a good source (pasture-raised, organic chickens fed a soy-free diet), they can be enjoyed daily. Obviously the quality of eggs today is very different than it used to be. Humans have been eating eggs for millions of years, so we have to ask: Is it the egg, or the wheat toast fortified with synthetic folic acid that is eaten with it that is really the issue?

Compared with chicken eggs, duck eggs are higher in protein, calcium, iron, potassium, and pretty much every other major mineral. Quail, turkey, and goose eggs are also wonderfully nutritious egg options; think outside the chicken's egg box for more variety. The color of the eggshell is breed-dependent, and has nothing to do with nutrient content. What matters is the diet of the hen or duck that laid the egg, which is reflected in the color of the yolk. "Pasture-raised," "organic," and "certified humane" are the words you are looking for on the label. Yolks from these chickens should be a nice dark orange as compared with the light yellow yolks of commercial eggs. Poaching or soft-boiling is the most nutritious way to prepare an egg.

Organ Meat: The Genetic Superfood That Balances Methionine

The traditional diet of our ancestors paired muscle meats alongside organ meats and gelatinous bones and other connective tissues; they ate the whole animal. The combination of all parts of the animal provided the perfect balance of nutrients and amino acids: methionine from muscle meats, B vitamins from organ meats, and collagen from cartilage. Modern diets, by contrast, provide abundant quantities of methionine-rich muscle meats, while organs and connective tissue are tossed in the trash. Methionine synthesizes homocysteine, but the process is regulated by the presence of other nutrients, particularly vitamins B_{12} and folate. If these B vitamins are deficient the result is higher levels of homocysteine, which impairs methylation. It is a complicated, vicious cycle that occurs from eating only muscle meat, and it is why there are murmurings of methionine deprivation to starve cancer. Rather than avoid all the nutritious foods that contain said methionine, intermittent fasting is the answer to this when used therapeutically. There's a whole lot more to eating meat than just the muscle meats. Organ meats have been on the menu since the beginning of time and for good reason—we miss the majority of meat's complete nutritional benefits when the whole animal is not consumed.

A perfectly white chicken breast, fat and skin removed, doesn't contain much in the way of vitamins and minerals. A cup of it (over 4 ounces) contains no vitamin A, and only 8 percent of the recommended daily allowance (RDA) of vitamin B_{12}. Conversely, a mere ounce of chicken liver provides 81 percent of the RDA for vitamin A and 99 percent of the B_{12} recommendation. Organ meat is substantially higher in all vitamins and minerals than muscle meat, and is also naturally high in vitamin D and omega-3 fatty acids. Heart is (not surprisingly) a rich source of the antioxidant coenzyme Q10 (COQ10). The offal (which refers to an animal's stomach and other organs, as well as feet, bones, and tongue) is all nutritionally dense. By the way, don't worry about the misconception that the liver is the organ that "stores" toxins. It doesn't; it metabolizes and excretes them. Toxins are actually stored in fat tissue, of which grain-fed, commercial animals have a much higher amount. This is another reason you should always choose the higher-quality source no matter what. Ask your biodynamic farmer and hunter friends to save their animal organs for you and tap your elders for their favorite liver-and-onions recipe!

Vitamin B_{12}: DNA Backbone and Primary Methyl Donor

Vitamin B_{12} (or cobalamin, named for its high cobalt content) is a water-soluble vitamin absorbed in the small intestine with the help of a compound called intrinsic factor. B_{12} is required for a variety of physiological functions, including the synthesis and methylation of DNA—the genetic material that acts as the backbone of all life—red blood cell production, protein metabolism, myelin formation, and many neurological processes. A deficiency of vitamin B_{12} can damage DNA by causing single- and double-strand breaks in the double helix structure, oxidative lesions, or both, which are risk factors of cancer.[34] Therefore, this vitamin also plays a starring role in maintaining genetic health.

The bioactive form of vitamin B_{12} is found in animal but not plant foods, a biochemical fact that many in the vegetarian community seems to ignore. The richest sources are liver, kidney, eggs, and fish. Microorganisms including bacteria, algae, and fungi are the only organisms definitively known to produce their own stores of vitamin B_{12}. And even though land animals and fish cannot make vitamin B_{12} in their cells, they save up B_{12} produced by bacteria and concentrate it in their cells. Because plants do not concentrate or utilize vitamin B_{12} in the same way as animals, with the exception of fungi plant foods do not become rich in B_{12}. The B_{12} content in both fermented and fungi foods is very low—1 cup of crimini mushrooms provides only 3 percent of the RDA for B_{12}, which is 2.4 micrograms, barely enough to prevent anemia. Meanwhile, a serving of 3.5 ounces of pastured organic beef liver contains approximately 110 micrograms of B_{12}. This is why the vegan patients who come to us often display what we call "the three F's" of low B_{12} levels: They seem foggy, fatigued, and feeble.

Which brings to mind another important "F" to discuss: fortification. Both refined and whole grains can be fortified with nutrients, but the fortified forms of vitamin B_{12} and folic acid are toxic. Many vegan diets recommend the ingestion of fortified products to supply needed vitamin B_{12}. However, the form of vitamin B_{12} used in fortified cereals, bread products, milk, brewers' yeast, supplements, and other foods is cyanocobalamin, produced using the chemical form of cyanide (potassium cyanide). Cyanocobalamin is *not* a naturally occurring B_{12}, despite its ability to elevate B_{12} deficiency clinically. This artificial form of B_{12} is a mitochondrial poison! (Incidentally, potassium cyanide is not the same chemical as hydrogen cyanide, the purported anticancer ingredient found in apricot kernels. Laetrile, or amygdalin, is a nontraditional cancer therapy that uses the natural substance amygdalin commonly extracted from apricot kernels. When metabolized in the body, amygdalin becomes hydrogen cyanide.)

If there is a natural alternative that is not congregated with or produced using a known toxin, why choose the non-natural form just because it is inexpensive? An important tenet of deep nutrition is to eat naturally occurring food sources of vitamins and minerals—sources our genes recognize, not foods produced made in a lab.

Phytonutrients for DNA Repair

Phytonutrients are medically active compounds found in plants that are neither vitamin nor mineral. Many phytonutrients have shown promise in preventing DNA damage, enhancing DNA repair, and targeting deficient

DNA-repair systems.[35] We discuss many of these cancer-discouraging phytonutrients (and other food-derived vitamins and minerals) throughout this book, but two standouts when it comes to genetic health are isothiocyanates and carotenoids. There is a good reason why every single anticancer diet has a common theme: Eat lots of vegetables and fruit. This is because they are the richest sources of the phytonutrient compounds that can repair genetic damage. A gene-damaging tornado can rage through the body, similar to what one experiences during a course of chemotherapy, but phytonutrients are able to come in and repair all of the mess. Though many may wrinkle their noses at the thought of eating brussels sprouts, sometimes knowing exactly *why* a food is good for you can increase its appeal. To teach people the "whys" and "whats" of cancer—why it happens and what you can do about it—has always been one of the goals of our approach and is a main reason for writing this book. So without further ado, let's look at the colossal cruciferous vegetable family, and what it does for our DNA.

Cruciferous vegetables help prevent cancer in many ways thanks to the action of the phytonutrients they contain. From helping to eliminate potential carcinogens from the body to enhancing the action of tumor-suppressor genes, cruciferous vegetables are the most well-studied anticancer vegetable family. Food sources include brussels sprouts, broccoli sprouts, raw cabbage, cauliflower, horseradish, kohlrabi, radish, and watercress.

Isothiocyanates are one of the components derived from the hydrolysis (breakdown) of glucosinolates, the sulfur-containing compounds found in cruciferous vegetables. Sulforaphane, one of the many forms of isothiocyanate, has been found to reduce the risk of genetic damage caused by pesticide exposure.[36] Certain individual genetic SNPs in the metabolizing enzymes may lessen the protective effects of these helpful breakdown products, however—one of the reasons why nutrition studies should always take individual SNPs into account and why some studies have found no benefit from eating these vegetables! Regardless, eat your broccoli! Even better, eat your broccoli sprouts! We recommend all patients consume at least three servings (one serving is ¼ to ½ cup) of cruciferous vegetables every day.

The second gene-protecting phytonutrient we focus on is beta-cryptoxanthin, a common carotenoid found in organic red bell peppers, paprika, and persimmons (which also happen to be low-glycemic). It has been found to exert a "striking effect on DNA repair."[37] A high blood beta-cryptoxanthin level has also been associated with reduced risk of lung cancer. But buyer beware: Each year the Environmental Working Group (EWG), a nonprofit organization, publishes a list of the produce items that are found to have the highest amount of pesticide residue, and each year bell peppers make the list. Of the fifty-three pesticide residues found on red bell peppers by the USDA's Pesticide Data Program, three are known or probable carcinogens, twenty-one are suspected hormone disruptors, ten are neurotoxins, six are developmental or reproductive toxins, and eighteen are toxic to honeybees.[38]

We know that eating organically is more expensive, but so is cancer. We cannot emphasize enough the importance of food quality when it comes to the prevention of cancer. Sure, a conventionally grown bell pepper (identified by a sticker with a four-digit bar code starting with the number "4") will contain beta-cryptoxanthin, but it will also come with a whole host of cancer-causing chemicals on it. Eating organically—or better yet, biodynamically—grown produce is paramount. This can be identified at the grocery store by a five-digit bar code starting with the number "9," or purchased from your local biodynamic grower. A five-digit code starting with an "8" means the item is genetically modified (produce is one of the few genetically modified products that are labeled as such in the United States).

The Gist of Genetics

A combination of faulty genetics and bad luck—that's what Western medicine has been telling us is the cause of cancer. But this is clearly far from the truth. Genetics and epigenetics are influenced to a great extent by dietary factors—both positively and negatively. Genetic damage occurs all the time from exposure to toxins, radiation, pesticides, aging, stress, and more, but foods like eggs, duck liver, organic red bell peppers, spinach, endive, asparagus, mustard greens, turnip greens, and epazote can all help to protect and repair genes from that damage. Meanwhile, of all the foods we eat in modern America, there are two that cause the most damage to our genes: genetically modified foods and sugar. The good news is that you can change the destiny of your genetic health simply by putting different foods in your shopping cart. It's that easy, and it doesn't hurt. It might just taste a little different than what you are used to. In the next chapter we take a deeper look at how sugar infiltrated our modern diet, how it directly contributes to the cancer process, and how we can reverse that process by using the most powerful and ancient food therapy approach there is: the ketogenic diet.

CHAPTER 4

Sugar, Cancer, and the Ketogenic Diet

Sugar is celebratory. Sugar is something that we used to enjoy. Now, it basically has coated our tongues. It's turned into a diet staple, and it's killing us.

—ROBERT LUSTIG, *author of* Fat Chance

Sugar gave rise to the slave trade; now sugar has enslaved us.

—JEFF O'CONNELL, *author of* Sugar Nation

We have a major drug addiction problem in this country. Bigger than opiates, amphetamines, alcohol, heroin, and nicotine all combined. It's a legal drug, and everyone can easily get it. Even kids. You guessed it: sugar—it's in practically every modern food we eat and drink and it is fueling our cancers and other chronic illnesses. Sugar consumption is simply off the charts, and most people don't even think twice about it; it seems so innocent and so tasty. So what's the big deal? The deal is that cancer cells ingest sugar—all kinds of sugar—at a rate that's almost fifty times faster than healthy cells, and it's the main fuel that helps them to grow and spread.[1] Researchers from Harvard Medical School reported that up to 80 percent of all human cancers are driven by the effects of glucose and insulin, which stimulate the proliferation, migration, and invasiveness of all types of cancers. It is because sugar is cancer's favorite food that the positron emission tomography (PET) scans are able to detect active cancer sites. Before patients undergo a PET scan, they first must fast and then receive an injection of radioactive sugar. The sugar circulates in the bloodstream and is gobbled up by hungry cancer cells that light up the scan like a glow stick. The higher the rate of glucose consumption (that is, the more densely lit the cancer cells appear on the scan), the more aggressive the tumor.

Intermittent and chronically elevated levels of blood sugar and insulin are the foundation for all progressive and recurrent cancers. This state stimulates cancer cell growth, inhibits cell death, promotes metastasis, helps cancer cells resist radiation and chemotherapy, and increases complications from surgery and chemotherapy.[2] What's more, ingesting *any* type of sugar—glucose, fructose, sucrose, honey, even freshly squeezed orange juice—reduces the activity of certain immune cells by half for up to five hours following consumption.[3] Sugar can single-handedly paralyze the entire immune system. We now know that it is neither the type nor the location of the cancer cells but the way in which they metabolize glucose that determines their malignancy. This is one of the hallmarks inherent in all cancer cells. Named for its discoverer, Nobel laureate Otto Warburg, the Warburg effect is the foundation of the metabolic theory of cancer. We explore the effect more deeply later in this chapter, but for now the most important thing to remember is that all cancer cells have the ability to reprogram their energy metabolism in order to consume more glucose and grow faster. No conventional treatment, including the newer targeted therapies, will affect the cancerous cells if sugar consumption remains high. Period.

Yet the average American adult eats over 150 pounds of it annually—more than people in fifty other nations—and the disastrous effects on our health, even discounting cancer, may clearly be seen. In 2009 in response to escalating sugar-related illnesses including heart disease, the American Heart Association published guidelines defining the "acceptable" amount of added sugar in a healthy diet (this does not include naturally occurring sugars).[4] The guidelines advise women to limit added sugar consumption to no more than 25 grams (about 6 teaspoons; there are 4 grams per teaspoon) per day; men should have no more than 37 grams (about 9 teaspoons). Children under age eight should consume no more than 12 grams of added sugar a day (less than 3 teaspoons). Yet these guidelines—and similar recommendations made by the World Health Organization—get blown out of the water by Americans each day.

The *American Journal of Clinical Nutrition* reported that in the United States consumption of the most common sugar, high-fructose corn syrup (HFCS), increased 1,000 percent between 1970 and 1990.[5] Soda consumption has more than doubled since 1970. And consider this: One 20-ounce soda can contain 65 grams of sugar, more than five times the amount a child should have in a day. According to the USDA's Economic Research Service, the average child under age twelve consumes 49 pounds of sugar per year. Since there are 875 grams of sugar in a pound, a quick calculation reveals that kids are eating 42,875 grams of sugar a year. That's an average of 117 grams a day. In her excellent 2013 TED Talk "Debunking the Paleo Diet," archaeological geneticist Dr. Christina Warinner notes that in order to get the same amount of sugar contained in a 34-ounce soda, our Paleolithic ancestors would have had to eat around 8½ feet of sugarcane. Today we eat three times that in a single day—24 feet worth of sugarcane. A typical American kid eats more sugar in one day than one of our ancestors could eat in two years. Cancer cells like that.

How Sugar Infiltrated Human Diets

Before the Agricultural Revolution began around fifteen thousand years ago, the only sweet foods a hunter-gatherer ate were fiber-rich fruit and honey. Procuring these sweets involved a large caloric expenditure, including walking many miles to find and collect them. This is a far cry from purchasing hundreds of grams of sugary foods and drinks at the gas station and downing them in twenty minutes, while seated. The fact is that for practically all of human existence we ate neither sugar nor such foods as grains and beans that naturally convert to sugar. Sugarcane, a tall perennial grass, was domesticated on the island of New Guinea only around ten thousand years ago. At first people picked the cane and ate it raw, chewing the highly fibrous stems. *Bagasse* is the name of the soluble fiber that comprises more than half a stock of sugarcane and has been found not only to support gut microbiota (or flora) but actually improve glucose metabolism.[6]

Over the next few thousand years, sugarcane cultivation spread from tropical island to island, reaching the Asian mainland around 1000 BC. The art of transforming cane into powder then became a secret art, and the powder was used as medicine to treat headaches and other aliments. Columbus planted the New World's first sugarcane in Hispaniola around 1500, and within a few hundred more years, hundreds of thousands of slaves were imprisoned on sugarcane farms. As more cane became available, prices fell and demand increased. By the mid-seventeenth century, sugar went from being a luxury spice to a household staple. In 1700 the average adult consumed 4 pounds of sugar a year, in 1800 that number increased to 18 pounds, and in 1870, sugar consumption had nearly tripled, to 47 pounds. By 1900, adults were eating 100 pounds of sugar a year.

Today, in addition to sugarcane, sugar beets, and corn, there are over sixty different types and names for the kinds of sugar found in processed foods. Various types of natural sugars, added sugars, and starches that convert to sugar are found in whole grain cereals, bagels, donuts, waffles, pancakes, pizza, juice, iced tea, soda, coffee drinks, ketchup, pasta sauce, pasta, yogurt, granola bars, soups, salad dressing, fruit, whole grain bread, cookies, candy, and cake—the list could go on for miles. Even a "healthy" soup made at your favorite high-end, health-conscious supermarket can contain more than 18 grams of added sugar per cup.

Natural Sugar, Added Sugar, and Milk Sugar

There are many different types of sugar, and they fall into two categories: natural and added. Naturally occurring sugars are those inherently present in such foods as fruit, milk, and honey. Added sugars are those that occur in processed food and are just that: extra sugar added to a food. A processed food is any food with more than one ingredient and may have organic cane juice, table sugar, or HFCS added to it. When it comes to a cancer cell, however, whether added or natural, sugar is sugar. And as the saying goes, "You can put lipstick on a pig, but it's still a pig." So whether it's organic cane syrup, agave, barley malt, dried fruit, soda, fruit juice, HFCS, white sugar, honey, date syrup, or a banana—if it causes blood sugar levels to rise, cancer cells will eat it. (Of course, a phytonutrient and fiber-rich raspberry is a far better choice than a granola bar—processed sugars like HFCS cause a substantially higher blood sugar spike than naturally occurring sugars.)

Added sugar hides in a lot of places; it's not just in the obvious spots like candy and soda. The mistakenly "healthy" breakfast of a low-fat yogurt and granola can pack more than 55 grams of added sugar into one serving. Simply put, it is not a healthy breakfast. Meanwhile, naturally occurring sugars include fructose and glucose found in fruit and honey, galactose found in vegetables such as celery, and lactose found in breast and animal milk. One banana contains 14 grams of naturally occurring sugar, while a cup of sweet potato contains 6 grams of naturally occurring sugar. A person who eats a lot of fruit, especially on an empty stomach, is going to have spikes of cancer-promoting high blood sugar. For this reason, we suggest sticking to fruits with lower sugar values that also happen to be most nutrient-dense: berries, green apples, and persimmon.

While this might be starting to sound overwhelming, don't worry! In chapter 13 we outline ways to ease into a lower-sugar diet, but we felt it was important to first paint a picture of just how much sugar we can eat in a day. If you read nutrition labels for calorie and fat content, you are missing the bigger boat: Always read sugar and carbohydrate content as well (and, of course, the list of ingredients, which is the most important!). One of the first things Jess asks her clients to do is to track their sugar intake for three days. This exercise is often the eye-opener people need to start making changes.

The Lowdown on Dairy

Now let's look at milk and milk sugars. One cup of low-fat cow's milk contains 13 grams of sugar in the form of lactose, a natural form that 65–90 percent of the world's population cannot digest (due to a deficiency of or ineffective lactase, the enzyme needed to metabolize lactose).[7] When they are not digested, the resulting high levels of these sugars circulating in the bloodstream can cause numerous problems, including difficulties with the digestive and immune system—resulting in runny noses or ear infections—anxiety, depression, migraines, weight gain, the appearance of black eyes, and much more (more on this in chapter 12; see "Factors That Impact Emotions"). Estimates from the National Institutes of Health (NIH) are that

TABLE 4.1. SUGAR CONTENT IN COMMON FOODS

Food	Sugar Content (g)
Apple, 1 medium	11
Banana, 1 medium	14
Barbecue sauce, 2 tablespoons	15
Coca-Cola, 12 ounces	39
Cranberry juice cocktail, 8 ounces	33
Dried cranberries, ⅓ cup	26
Fat-free honey Dijon salad dressing, 2 tablespoons	8
Fruit preserves, 1 tablespoon	10
Lemonade, 8 ounces	29
Mangoes, 1 cup	24
Marinara with mushrooms sauce, 1 cup	22
Orange, 1 medium	23
Organic fruit-and-nut granola, ¾ cup	15
Organic ketchup, 2 tablespoons	8
Organic whole-milk French vanilla yogurt, 1 cup	29
Vanilla soy milk latte, 16 ounces	29

approximately 65 percent of the human population has a reduced ability to digest lactose after infancy.

Milk, cheese, yogurt, and ice cream are all new to the human diet since the Agricultural Revolution. A 2004 *American Journal of Clinical Nutrition* study linked consumption of dairy products to cancers including ovarian.[8] Low-fat dairy products are even newer to us, having existed only since the 1920s. Further, if the cow that produced the milk has been treated with growth hormones, then cancer risk increases even more (more on this in chapter 10; see "Top Three Hormone Hijackers"). Around fifteen thousand years ago, when herding began to replace hunting, humans learned how to make the once-toxic lactose content of dairy products digestible by fermenting them. In addition, the genetic adaptation called *lactase persistence* emerged about 7,500 years ago, giving some populations the ability to produce lactase and continue to drink milk after weaning age.[9]

While some people can consume dairy products without difficulty, others should avoid it, depending on tolerance and lab findings. The most important thing to know on the topic of dairy, however, is that it is always healthiest in its raw and natural state (when procured from a clean source, of course). Low-fat dairy products are absolutely not healthy at all. The golden rule when it comes to whole food nutrition is to eat foods as close to their natural source as possible. Think about it: Cows, goats, sheep, and humans do not produce low-fat milk, or products such as processed yogurts. Milk fats, especially those found in breast milk, are good for us. Sugar is not. And when fat is removed from dairy products, their sugar content increases. This concept is a major myth buster for the many people who have been brainwashed by the low-fat dogma. We are here to rewire that thought process and get you to love healthy fats like eggs, nuts, and avocado again. Your body will thank you.

Artificial Sweeteners

The FDA has approved five non-nutritive sweeteners: *aspartame, saccharin, acesulfame-K* (K for potassium), *sucralose,* and *neotame*. The most widely used is aspartame, a neurotoxic substance that accounts for over 75 percent of the adverse reactions to food additives reported to the FDA each year. Many of these reactions are very serious, including seizures and death. Among the ninety different symptoms reportedly caused by aspartame: headaches/migraines, dizziness, seizures, nausea, numbness, muscle spasms, weight gain, rashes, depression, fatigue, irritability, tachycardia, insomnia, vision problems, hearing loss, heart palpitations, breathing difficulties, anxiety attacks, slurred speech, loss of taste, tinnitus, vertigo, memory loss, and joint pain.

When aspartame is digested in the body, it breaks down into two amino acids—phenylalanine and aspartic acid—and methanol. Methanol is a wood alcohol and a known poison. Phenylalanine blocks production of serotonin, a neurotransmitter that, among other activities, helps control food cravings and mood. As you might imagine, a shortage of serotonin causes the brain and body to scream for the food that supplies more of this brain chemical—and that would be sugar.

Sucralose (known commercially as Splenda) has been linked to the development of leukemia in mouse studies, and the Sucralose Toxicity Information Center research has concluded, "It is clear from the hazards seen in pre-approval research and from its chemical structure that years or decades of use may contribute to serious chronic immunological or neurological disorders." Sucralose is produced by chlorinating cane sugar. Chlorine is toxic to the thyroid gland, which regulates metabolism.

While we discuss two of them here in detail, do note that all artificial sweeteners are highly toxic, have only been in the human food chain since the 1960s, and should be avoided at all costs.

What about Agave?

Agave nectar, beloved by many in the alternative health community, is sap derived from the agave plant. From plant to product, agave typically undergoes a chemical process that uses genetically modified enzymes, caustic acids, clarifiers, and filtration chemicals. Agave nectar, dubiously marketed as a "healthier" sugar, is actually higher in fructose content than HFCS. So high, in fact, that in 2009 the medical advisory group Glycemic Research Institute halted and banned all future clinical trials using agave, and issued warnings to the public and manufacturers about the dangers of agave because of its high fructose content and effect on blood sugar. For some reason this information has not reached mainstream media, as many agave products are still marketed as low-glycemic. Just avoid it.

Caution with Sugar Alcohols

The sugar alcohols commonly found in foods, gum, and toothpaste are *sorbitol, mannitol, xylitol, isomalt,* and *hydrogenated starch hydrolysates.* Sugar alcohols do not contain the ethanol found in alcoholic beverages, and occur naturally in plant products such as berries. However, the majority of the store-bought granulated versions (including xylitol) are commonly derived from genetically modified corn that is altered through a highly toxic chemical process. They can stimulate diarrhea and exacerbate existing irritable bowel syndrome (IBS)–related symptoms. Common side effects of sugar alcohol consumption include bloating, gas, and abdominal pain. We do not recommend these mainstream types of sugar alcohols.

When it comes to the best types of sweetener, raw honey, monk fruit, chicory root, and fresh stevia leaf in small amounts are the optimal choices. (We outline how to get started on a low-sugar diet in chapter 13; see "A Tiered Approach to Starting a Low-Glycemic Diet.")

All Carbohydrates Turn to Sugar

All types of carbohydrates—including vegetables, fruit, grains, legumes, and all sugars—are naturally converted into glucose by the digestive system. In general, as we learned in the last chapter, proteins are broken down into amino acids, and fats become fatty acids. All sugars, carbohydrates, and starches are converted to glucose via the action of a very important group of pancreatic enzymes called *amylases*. Research has found that low serum amylase levels cause abnormal glucose metabolism and impaired insulin action.[10] Symptoms of low amylase can include allergies, eczema, and asthma. One of the leading causes of amylase deficiency is a high-carbohydrate diet, and since Americans eat an estimated 200 pounds of grain products a year each, widespread amylase deficiency in the United States is not far-fetched. Plants store their glucose supply in the form of starch, long chains of thousands of glucose molecules linked together. Plants with the highest concentrations of starch include grains, corn, rice, yams, potatoes, beans, and peas. When these plants are consumed, the body breaks down the starch and converts it to glucose.[11] When whole plants, such as wheat, are refined and the fiber removed, what is left is a powdery white flour that converts to sugar in an instant. If you have ever held a soda cracker in your mouth for longer than a minute, you know how rapidly the taste changes from salty to sweet. By contrast, a wheat berry won't taste sugary in your mouth for quite some time.

The difference between a refined or simple carbohydrate (the soda cracker) and a complex carbohydrate (the wheat berry) is the fiber content. Fiber is basically plant material that cannot be digested. The more fiber, the less sugar—think sugarcane versus granulated white sugar. (Read more about fiber in chapter 6; see "The Metabolic Microbiome Reboot Plan.") What is scary to consider is that when it comes to carbohydrate intake, the current US Dietary Guidelines, published every five years by the Office of Disease Prevention and Health Promotion, provide the perfect recipe for diabetes and are a main driver behind today's obesity epidemic. Currently the US government suggests that carbohydrates make up 45 to 65 percent (approximately 225 to 325 grams of carbohydrates) of a person's total daily calories. They suggest consuming low-fat dairy, grains, and beans in addition to fruit and vegetables. The genetically tuned human diet of our ancestors was closer to 35 percent of calories from carbohydrates a day, and these were primarily from fiber-rich vegetables. A piece of white bread contains 15 grams of carbohydrates and less than a gram of fiber. It converts to sugar fast, just like that cracker. However, a cup of broccoli has 6 grams of carbs and almost 2.5 grams of fiber, not to mention far more phytonutrients.

When half our plate is full of carbohydrates—especially in refined forms— the result is high blood sugar levels. When carbohydrate-derived glucose enters the bloodstream and blood sugar levels begin to rise, the pancreas produces a very important hormone called *insulin*. Insulin allows glucose to enter cells, unlocking the gate like a key. The mitochondria inside cells convert the glucose into energy molecules. When there is too much glucose, cells get full and the leftover glucose is converted into fat. A meal of a soda and a candy bar packs upward of 70 grams of sugar, far more than our bodies are able to process. It's like trying to drink water from a fire hose. *This* is why people gain weight. It's not because of eating fat, it's because of all the extra sugar that gets converted into fat.

This connection between sugar and weight gain has been shown hundreds of times over in more studies than we can count. In the thirty or so years since the ludicrous low-fat movement began, estimates now show that more than two-thirds (68.8 percent) of American adults are considered overweight or obese. The US Department of Health and Human Services has concluded that almost three in four men (74 percent) are considered to be overweight or obese.[12] Approximately 40 percent of women are now considered obese, and about a third of children and adolescents ages six to nineteen are considered to be overweight or obese. That's simply out of control, and heartbreaking. We are devastating our children's immune systems and increasing their risk of cancer with holidays like Halloween, when over 600 grams of sugary candy can be collected by one child. Now, *that* is scary.

Sadly, along with these dramatic, sugar-rich dietary changes has come the increase in cancer. Cancer, as it turns out, likes sugar just as much as the next kid, and the effects of sugar on the body create a very hospitable environment in which cancer cells can thrive. All the extra body fat that Americans carry around produces *estrogen*, a hormone that is a major promoter of cancer growth (more on this in chapter 10; see "The Basics of Hormones and Cancer"). The rates of individuals in the United States with blood sugar imbalances, including type 2 diabetes, are reaching pandemic proportions, just like cancer. One in every ten adults has diabetes, and one of three adults has prediabetes. Rates of type 2 diabetes in ten- to nineteen-year-olds increased 21 percent between 2001 and 2009. Evidence from large cohort studies shows a higher cancer incidence in people with type 2 diabetes, with the highest mortality observed in those using insulin.[13] As we will see, insulin, too, has an extremely potent effect on cancer.

Alas, it is not easy to stop eating sugar, even when we know it's bad. Sugar stimulates the same pleasure centers of the brain that respond to heroin and cocaine; naturally, we want more of it. Sugar is a powerful drug and is really just as dangerous as the illegal drugs we hear about on the news. When people can't or don't stop eating it, they get sick.

Glucose and Insulin: The Evil Twins of Cancer

There are a number of ways elevated glucose and insulin can cause metabolic imbalances throughout the body and increase cancer risk. An increased metabolism of glucose promotes several hallmarks of cancer, including excessive proliferation of cancer cells, antiapoptotic signaling (helps cancer cells remain immortal), cell cycle progression, and angiogenesis.[14] In addition to feeding the cancer beast and helping it grow, high levels of glucose and insulin stimulate cancer-promoting pathways. In a study published in 2013 in the *Journal of Clinical Investigation*, researchers reported that high glucose levels trigger the expression of several growth factors.[15] Additional research has found that high glucose levels inhibit the functioning of the p53 protein.[16] (As we mentioned in chapter 2, p53 is a tumor-suppressing protein. It has been described as "the

Weight-Gain Shake Smackdown

Below is the information copied from an ingredient label from a commonly recommended "weight-gain shake" that contains only 240 calories, 10 grams of protein, 4 grams of fat, 20 grams of sugar, and 41 grams of carbohydrate. The first five ingredients (after water) are GMO and the forms of vitamins are synthetic!

INGREDIENTS: WATER, CORN SYRUP, SUGAR, MILK PROTEIN CONCENTRATE AND LESS THAN 2% OF VEGETABLE OIL (CANOLA, HIGH OLEIC SUNFLOWER, CORN), SOY PROTEIN ISOLATE, ACACIA GUM, FRUCTOOLIGOSACCHARIDES, MAGNESIUM PHOSPHATE, POTASSIUM CITRATE, INULIN (FROM CHICORY), POTASSIUM CHLORIDE, CELLULOSE GEL AND GUM, SALT, CALCIUM CARBONATE, SOY LECITHIN, SODIUM ASCORBATE, CHOLINE BITARTRATE, NATURAL AND ARTIFICIAL FLAVOR, ALPHA-TOCOPHERYL ACETATE, CALCIUM PHOSPHATE, ASCORBIC ACID, CARRAGEENAN, FERROUS SULFATE, ZINC SULFATE, PURIFIED STEVIA LEAF EXTRACT (SWEETENER), VITAMIN A PALMITATE, NIACINAMIDE, VITAMIN D_3, CALCIUM PANTOTHENATE, MANGANESE SULFATE, COPPER SULFATE, PYRIDOXINE HYDROCHLORIDE, THIAMINE HYDROCHLORIDE, BETA-CAROTENE, RIBOFLAVIN, CHROMIUM CHLORIDE, FOLIC ACID, BIOTIN, POTASSIUM IODIDE, PHYTONADIONE, SODIUM SELENITE, SODIUM MOLYBDATE, VITAMIN B_{12}.

guardian of the genome" because of its role in preventing genome mutation.) What that means is that high-sugar diets take p53 off the job, leaving cells more prone to unchecked DNA damage and the formation of cancer.

There's more. Insulin also stimulates the release of pro-inflammatory chemicals called *cytokines* from human fat cells. Therefore, a diet that

Optimal Terrain Metabolic Rescue Shake

Here is our version of a weight-gain shake recipe. It contains 20 grams of protein, 25 grams of fat, 18 grams of carbohydrate, and no sugar. Plus, it is made from whole foods and has ingredients you can actually recognize and pronounce!

2 tablespoons whey
   or egg protein powder
   or collagen powder
   (15 grams protein)
2 teaspoons whole flaxseeds
   (not oil)
1 tablespoon medium-chain
   triglyceride (MCT) oil

1 teaspoon modified citrus pectin
1½ cups filtered water, or
   cooled green or Tulsi tea
½ avocado
2 tablespoons raw cocoa powder
2 teaspoons cinnamon
1 tablespoon vanilla extract
Ice

Blend in a high-powered blender until all ingredients are completely mixed and enjoy!

repeatedly elevates blood glucose levels (such as a banana for breakfast, a sandwich for lunch, pasta for dinner) promotes a pro-inflammatory environment that is considered the match that lights the fire of cancer. High insulin levels also increase other inflammatory molecules that inhibit immune cells, such as natural killer (NK) cells, while also causing the production of insulin-like growth factor, type 1 (IGF-1). IGF-1 is a hormone that promotes tissue growth, and it exerts very powerful effects at several key stages of cancer development including cellular proliferation, apoptosis, angiogenesis, metastasis, and the development of resistance to chemotherapeutic agents.[17]

Insulin resistance (which occurs after prolonged periods of high glucose levels) is a lowering of cells' ability to respond to insulin and resultant difficulty allowing glucose to enter cells. Insulin resistance is also a hallmark of cachexia, the "wasting from within" syndrome that kills 50–80 percent of all cancer patients. (This is reiewed in more detail in chapter 8, but simply note here that consuming a high-carbohydrate diet that includes sugar will only worsen cachexia.) Drinking the often recommended sugar-laden meal-replacement drinks (Boost or Ensure, for example) is like throwing gas on the fire. A study in the September 2014 issue of the journal *Cancer and Metabolism* concluded that cachexia is partly due to "metabolic alterations in tumor cells, which can be reverted by a ketogenic diet, causing reduced tumor growth and inhibition of muscle and body weight loss."[18] That's right, the ketogenic diet, consisting of approximately 20 grams of carbohydrates a day, can reverse cachexia, and we've been doing it with patients for years.

What you will discover as you continue reading is that everything we talk about for cancer also applies to other modern diseases. We can't say it enough: It is crucial to limit your intake of glucose if you want to stop cancer and other diseases like diabetes, heart disease, and nearly every other noncommunicable disease there is. But cancer in particular has a very strong sugar addiction, and it has figured out a very clever way to use it.

How Cancer Cells Gobble Glucose: The Warburg Effect

We are not the first to assert that cancer loves glucose. Otto Warburg, a medical doctor and Nobel laureate, first described a theory for the metabolism of cancer cells, now known as the Warburg effect, in the 1920s. Thankfully, Warburg's early work has more recently been carried forward by several researchers and scholars, notably Dr. Thomas Seyfried from Boston College and Dr. Dominic D'Agostino at the University of South Florida, as well as many others. What they have found (and what has been largely ignored by Western medicine—just read the excellent book *Tripping over the Truth*, by Travis Christofferson) is that cancer cells use glucose to create the energy they need to sustained their frenzied growth. But they do not use glucose the way normal cells do; they use it faster. One of the widely accepted hallmarks of cancer is exactly this ability of cancer cells to reprogram energy metabolism, allowing them to create energy at a very rapid rate. Let's explain how.

First, we know that uncontrolled growth defines cancer. Growth requires a cancer cell to replicate its DNA, RNA, and other cellular components in order to divide into two offspring cells. All this doubling and dividing requires energy. Just as climbers on Mount Everest burn an average of 10,000 calories a day, cancer cells require a lot of energy to sustain their vigorous activity. In order for any cell, not only a cancer cell, to remain alive and to perform its genetically programmed functions, it must produce energy. Cancer cells devised a way to do this much more rapidly. For starters, they consume blood sugar fifty times faster than normal cells, a feat they accomplish in a number of ways. One is by creating more insulin receptors on their surfaces than healthy cells have, allowing more glucose to enter. Breast cancer cells have been found to have three times the number of insulin receptors on their surfaces compared with healthy cells, and colon cancer cells can have almost twice as many.[19]

The energy required by cancer cells is created by breaking down glucose through a process called *respiration*. Respiration occurs when glucose is converted into energy storage molecules called *adenosine triphosphate*, or ATP. All cells need ATP molecules (picture tiny batteries) for energy, and when the body runs out of ATP it burns first carbohydrates then fats, typically not protein, to make more. This respiration process can happen in two different ways, either *aerobically*, which requires oxygen (the method normal cells under normal conditions typically use), or *anaerobically*, which does not require oxygen.

Aerobic respiration is a multistep process during which healthy cells, using oxygen, convert a molecule of glucose into two pyruvate molecules (a process called *glycolysis*, literally meaning "splitting glucose"), ultimately forming over thirty molecules of ATP and releasing carbon dioxide as a waste product. Conversely, cancer cells use a metabolic pathway called anaerobic respiration to break down glucose into pyruvate and form ATP, but instead of carbon dioxide, lactic acid is produced as a by-product. While aerobic respiration can provide over thirty molecules of ATP per molecule of glucose, anaerobic respiration produces only two.

Because of mitochondrial damage, cancer cells have no choice but to use anaerobic respiration (also called fermentation) to produce energy, even when oxygen is available. How do cancer cells use this inefficient metabolic pathway? The answer is twofold. By using what Warburg termed the "aerobic glycolysis" energy production method, cancer cells produce *less* ATP per molecule

Acid-Alkaline Diet Myth Buster

Proponents of the acid-alkaline diet believe that cancer cells thrive in acidic (low pH) environments but not in alkaline (high pH) environments. Therefore, they assert that a diet high in alkaline foods (such as fruits and vegetables) that also limits acidic foods (animal products) will raise blood pH levels and create an environment in the body that discourages cancer growth. However, as we explain, cancer cells are able to create their own acidic microenvironment by performing anaerobic glycolysis, which creates lactic acid as a by-product. Tumor acidification occurs because of how cancer cells reprogram energy metabolism. Basically it is the cancer itself that creates the acidic environment, not the acidic environment that creates the cancer.

Tumors are also surrounded by pH buffers, so alkalinizing a tumor through diet is neither realistic nor useful.[20] In fact, the acid-alkaline diet is very pro-inflammatory, and a diet high in fruits and legumes increases insulin, glycolysis, growth factors, and other tumor promoters. Of course, anyone who starts eating more of the plant foods that are rich in powerful cancer-suppressing compounds will experience benefits, but the assertion that an acid-alkaline diet will work against cancer is, unfortunately, incorrect and misguided.

of glucose but they produce it *faster*. Much faster. In fact, cancer cells produce ATP almost a hundred times faster than normal cells. This is possible because cancer cells have damaged mitochondria. Remember those tiny engines inside each cell where metabolism takes place? Each cell contains hundreds to thousands of mitochondria, and these engines are responsible for supplying energy and also for controlling genetic signaling and regulating apoptosis.[21] In cancer cells, the mitochondria are damaged and dysregulated—like little

Learning from Your Labs

Blood sugar (glucose) markers such as those described below are a way to assess and monitor how the body is handling glucose.

HbA1C: Glycated hemoglobin is a form of hemoglobin used to identify the average blood glucose concentration over the preceding three months.

Fasting glucose: Detects the amount of glucose circulating in the blood when no food has been consumed for at least eight hours.

IGF-1: Detects levels of this growth hormone, whose activity is similar to that of insulin, in the blood.

Fasting insulin: Detects the amount of insulin circulating in the blood when no glucose has been consumed for at least eight hours. This can be helpful in diagnosing insulin resistance.

We strongly recommend that our patients have these blood sugar markers tested. In general, Dr. Nasha likes levels to be below "normal" lab reference values. Do speak to your primary care provider about ordering these tests if you would like to see whether high blood sugar may be contributing to your cancer or other disease process. Knowing what your baseline levels are can also help you gauge your response to following a reduced-sugar and -carbohydrate diet.

runaway trains without conductors. What damages mitochondria? Many elements of modern living, including toxins, drugs, and—yes—sugar.[22]

But for the cancer cell, it's not just about faster ATP production. By using this form of altered energy production, cancer cells are able to secrete large amounts of the resulting lactic acid into their extracellular microenvironment, which in turn lowers extracellular pH to between 6.0 and 6.5 (normal pH is around 7.4). The lactic acid (or lactate) contributes to acidosis, which turns on signals for angiogenesis (new blood supply) and acts as a cancer cell metabolic fuel, while also inducing immunosuppression.[23] (There are several excellent books that look much more deeply at this process. *Cancer as a Metabolic Disease* by Dr. Thomas Seyfried is a must-read.)

For the layperson, the take-home point is that cancer requires metabolic therapies—including the ketogenic diet and balancing the other terrain elements as outlined in this book—for effective management and prevention. So now let's look more closely at the ketogenic diet and its incredible ability to reverse and prevent the cancer process.

The Ketogenic Diet and the Metabolic Approach to Cancer

(Note: We suggest that you consult with a professional and be monitored on a ketogenic diet before starting it on your own. There are many clinical considerations, and it may not be right for everyone. It may also induce side effects that should be monitored by a ketogenic-savvy practitioner.)

We have been using low-glycemic (meaning blood-sugar-lowering), calorie-restricted, fasting, and ketogenic dietary approaches with our patients for several years with incredible results. We know (and have witnessed) that reducing intake of sugar and high-glycemic foods is the most important dietary step patients can take to prevent and manage their cancer. This is the ultimate key to exploiting the metabolic weakness of cancer. No other dietary therapy exerts such powerful protective and anticancer effects. But to be clear, the ketogenic diet is not a *cure* for cancer, per se. As you will discover, there are nine other terrain factors that contribute to the cancer process, but sugar affects each one of them negatively. Therefore, a metabolic dietary approach is a highly effective tool that benefits all of the terrain areas, and is a powerful tool to have in your toolbox alongside the other approaches we detail throughout this book. The ketogenic diet *is* emerging as a stand-alone treatment far superior to what Western medicine has to offer for many cancers, including brain cancer, and is also beneficial for the treatment of neurological conditions such as epilepsy and Alzheimer's and Parkinson's diseases. This is why we refer back to the ketogenic diet and fasting over and over again. Fasting, calorie restriction, and following a ketogenic diet are hardly new or novel therapies; rather, they are "diets" that humans have followed since the beginning of time with unintentionally therapeutic results.

Until a very recent moment in human existence, we often experienced times when food was scarce to absent. Being hungry and going long periods without eating—also known as fasting—was really quite commonplace. Not so today. Being hungry is a very uncomfortable feeling for many Americans. When was the last time you let yourself be hungry for more than an hour? How ketosis ultimately works is this: When the body is deprived of dietary carbohydrates (which generally means below 50 grams a day), the liver becomes the sole provider of stored glucose, in the form of *glycogen*, which it uses to feed hungry organs like the brain, a particularly high-needs organ that utilizes about 20 percent of total energy expenditure. But the liver stores only enough glucose to last the body somewhere around twenty-four to forty-eight hours. If we didn't have a backup energy source, humans would have disappeared a long time ago. But luckily we do: ketones. Once it is depleted of glycogen, the liver can make ketones either from fatty acids in the diet or from body fat. These compounds are released into the bloodstream and taken up by cells in the brain and other organs. Ketones are shuttled into the mitochondria's energy factories just like glucose and used to create ATP. But here's the kicker: Healthy cells have the metabolic flexibility to switch from using glucose to using ketones for energy; we've been doing this for millions of years. However, initial research has suggested that cancer cells may *lack* this metabolic flexibility. The elimination of glucose and being in a state of nutritional ketosis effectively cuts off cancer cells' main fuel supply and puts them in a state of metabolic stress.[24] In addition, ketosis provides several other anticancer benefits, including:

- Reducing angiogenesis (development of new blood vessels needed to fuel tumor growth)
- Restoring normal apoptosis (cell suicide) in cancer cells
- Destabilizing tumor tissue DNA, causing effects that damage cancer cells
- Reducing tumor size over time
- Reducing levels of insulin and IGF-1

- Enhancing the action of standard treatments, including chemotherapy and radiation, while reducing common side effects[25]

Yes, it's true and has been shown several times over—the presence or absence of sugar can make or break conventional cancer treatments, therefore we are proponents of its absence! It is a myth that the ketogenic diet only helps brain cancers. *All* cancers except prostate, mucinous adenoma of colon, bronchoalveolar lung cancer, and thyroid cancer are highly glucose dependent.

Nuts and Bolts of the Ketogenic Diet

By now you are probably wondering just how to achieve ketosis, the state where your body is burning ketones for fuel as opposed to glucose. Here's how it works in a nutshell: According to the ketogenic diets that we generally prescribe, an individual's daily nutrient intake works out to be approximately 70–75 percent of calories from healthy, anti-inflammatory fats, 20–25 percent from quality proteins, and 5–10 percent from carbohydrates, which should consist of low-carbohydrate, phytonutrient-dense vegetables. You may recall that the Atkins diet promoted high protein and moderate fat. Why does the ketogenic diet suggest instead a high-fat, moderate-protein ratio? First, it's because fats have no effect on blood sugar and insulin levels. Protein, however, can affect both of these if large quantities are consumed. If too much protein is consumed, more than 50 percent of any excess protein will be converted to glucose in the body, and that extra glucose can increase insulin levels and put the brakes on the body's ability to release and burn fatty acids and get into ketosis. Caloric intake and macronutrient ratios need to be assessed—and reassessed—on an individual basis; however, here is an approximate example of what a 2,000-calorie/day ketogenic diet looks like:

Fat (9 calories per gram) = 165 grams or 1,500 calories
Protein (4 calories per gram) = 100 grams or 400 calories
Carbohydrate (4 calories per gram) = 25 grams or 100 calories

Carbohydrates have the biggest impact on glucose levels, which is why they are consumed in the smallest amounts and should come from the most nutrient-dense and low-glycemic vegetables possible. These include dark greens, fresh herbs, cruciferous vegetables, mushrooms, garlic, and onions. A legitimate criticism of the ketogenic diet is its low amounts of phytonutrient-rich vegetables. However, it *is* possible to eat a good amount of lemon, lime, basil, broccoli, cilantro, spinach, garlic, and more every day and still remain in ketosis. Our goal is always to infuse the most nutrient-dense foods into the ketogenic diet plan. Over the years we have found that most people can achieve a ten-vegetable-a-day goal while following a ketogenic diet. However, each individual responds differently to the diet: Some achieve ketosis easily with a larger amount of carbohydrate (30 grams or so per day), while others must lower their daily carbohydrate intake to below 20 grams. When first starting out, the most helpful thing to do is track the carbohydrate intake. Try to keep the total below 20 grams a day.

Table 4.2 shows a formula that Jess created and recommends in order to maximize the amount of anticancer phytonutrients while on a ketogenic

TABLE 4.2. THE KELLEY KETOGENIC PHYTONUTRIENT FORMULA

Food	Serving Size	Carb Content (g)	Phytonutrient
Arugula	½ cup	0.4	glucosinolate
Asparagus	1 spear	0.6	saponin
Basil	¼ cup	0.2	orientin, vicenin
Black raspberry	10 berries	2	ellagitannin
Broccoli, raw	½ cup	2.9	kaempferol
Garlic	1 clove	1	allicin
Nori (seaweed)	1 sheet	1	sulfated polysaccharide
Shallot	1 tablespoon	1.7	thiosulfinate, quercetin
Shiitake mushroom	2 mushrooms	2	glucan
Swiss chard, raw	1 cup	1.4	betalain
Total Carbohydrates		13.2 grams	

diet. As you will see from tables 4.3 through 4.5, most foods contain some carbohydrate. The priority is to "spend" as much of your daily carbohydrate allowance on the most powerful vegetables and herbs possible. (Also, do strive to select organic vegetables whenever they are available.)

Foods to Focus On

Since healthy, anti-inflammatory fats and quality protein constitute the majority of the ketogenic diet, let's take a closer look at these.

Healthy Fats (75%)

Good, healthy fats include nuts and seeds, which should be raw (soaked and sprouted if possible), as well as their fresh milks, butters, oils, and flours. Varieties include almond, Brazil, chia, flax, hazelnut, macadamia, pecan, pine nut, pistachio, pumpkin, sesame, sunflower, and walnut (notice no peanuts or cashews; these are technically legumes). Coconut products are wonderful, including fresh and shredded coconut, coconut oil, coconut cream, coconut milk (canned and full fat), coconut flour, and coconut aminos. Other oils that we recommend are cold-pressed extra-virgin olive oil, avocado oil, sesame oil, walnut oil, lard (from a clean source), and duck fat. Medium-chain triglyceride (MCT) oil is often derived from coconut oil and can increase the production of ketones. Organic, full-fat, pasture-raised, and fermented dairy products (if no allergies or sensitivities) are also good, including full-fat cheeses, pastured butter, ghee, organic sour cream, cream cheese, ricotta cheese, plain full-fat yogurt from grass-fed cows, and whey protein powder. We also recommend olives, avocado, and lamb as great sources of healthy fat.

Quality Protein (20%)

Animal proteins tend to be lower in carbohydrates. When it comes to selecting animal foods, we can't say it enough times: Quality is paramount. Focus on grass-fed and finished beef and lamb; wild-caught salmon, halibut, mackerel, cod, haddock, and sardines; organic and pasture-raised chickens and their eggs; organic turkey; and fresh shellfish, such as shrimp, lobster, and scallops. (Note: The consumption of red meat may be assessed on an individual basis based on the results of certain lab tests; we discuss red meat in more detail later.)

Testing for Ketosis

The presence and amount of ketones can be assessed using either urine, blood, or the breath. Most people find that urine test strips are the easiest and most affordable home testing option; however, blood and breath tests are slightly more accurate. While the body is technically "in ketosis" when blood ketones reach a level of 0.5 mmol/L, for individuals with active cancer, ketone levels are optimally kept at or above 3.0 mmol/L and glucose levels at 70 mmol/L or lower. There are home testing options that can read both ketones and glucose, such as the Precision Xtra Blood Glucose Monitoring System. Another tool used in clinical settings is the Glucose Ketone Index Calculator, designed by Dr. Thomas Seyfried, which monitors therapeutic levels of ketosis.

Calorie Restriction

When humans eat, the body metabolizes the food to produce energy and assist in the building of proteins to make immune cells, DNA, and so forth. When fewer calories are consumed, the amount of nutrients available to the body's cells is lower. This inherently slows metabolic processes, reduces the production of free radicals, and limits the function and expression of some of the proteins involved in the cancer process.[26] We will talk more about fasting in future chapters, but the key point is that when the body doesn't have to work as hard to metabolize food, genetic damage decreases. Calorie restriction is therefore a very powerful metabolic approach to the prevention and treatment of cancer.

Following a calorie-restricted ketogenic diet (often shortened to CRKD) means reducing caloric intake anywhere from 30 to 75 percent of baseline. Before beginning this deeper metabolic process, you should first consult with your primary care provider.

Tables 4.3 through 4.5 provide the macronutrient content of over a hundred foods so that when you are ready you can start playing with diet combinations. There are also many wonderful books to look at, including

(continued on page 80)

**TABLE 4.3. MACRONUTRIENT CONTENT IN
COMMON KETOGENIC DIET–FRIENDLY FOODS: VEGETABLES**

Vegetables	Amount	Calories	Fat (g)	Protein (g)	Carbs (g)	Sugars (g)
Artichoke	1 whole	60	0.2	4.2	13	1.3
Arugula	½ cup	3	0.1	0.3	0.4	0.2
Asparagus	1 cup	27	0.2	3	5	2.5
Basil	¼ cup	1	0	0.2	0.2	0
Beet	1 cup	59	0.2	2.2	13	9
Bell pepper	1 medium	24	0.2	1	6	3
Broccoli	½ cup	15	0.2	1.2	2.9	0.8
Brussels sprouts	1 cup	38	0.3	3	8	1.9
Cabbage	1 cup	17	0.1	0.9	4.1	2.2
Carrot	1 medium	25	0.2	0.6	6	3
Cauliflower	1 cup	27	0.3	2	5	2
Celery	1 cup	16	0.2	0.7	3	1.8
Cilantro	9 sprigs	5	0.1	0.4	0.7	0.2
Chard	1 cup	7	0.1	0.6	1.4	0.4
Chive	1 tablespoon	1	0	0.1	0.1	0.1
Collard greens	1 cup	11	0.2	1.1	2	0.2
Cucumber	½ cup	8	0.1	0.3	1.9	1
Eggplant	1 cup	20	0.2	0.8	4.8	2.9
Fennel	1 cup	27	0.2	1.1	6	0
Garlic	1 clove	0	0.2	0	1	0
Green bean	1 cup	31	0.2	1.8	7	3.3
Kale	1 cup	33	0.6	2.9	6	0
Leek	1 cup	54	0.3	1.3	13	3.5
Mint	½ cup	20	0	0	4	0
Mushroom (crimini)	½ cup	8	0.1	1.1	1.1	0.7
Nori	1 sheet	10	0	1	1	0

Portobello mushroom	1 medium	22	0	2	4	2
Pumpkin	½ cup	42	0	1	10	4
Radish	½ cup	9	0.1	0.4	2	1.1
Red leaf lettuce	1 cup	5	0.1	0.1	0.6	0.1
Red onion	1 medium	44	0.1	1.2	10	4.7
Spaghetti squash	1 cup	31	0.6	0.6	7	2.8
Spinach	1 cup	7	0.1	0.9	1.1	0.1
Tomato	1 medium	22	0.2	1.1	4.8	3.2
Zucchini	1 medium	33	0.6	2.4	6	4.9

Sources: The US Department of Agriculture and individual food manufacturer labels

TABLE 4.4. MACRONUTRIENT CONTENT IN COMMON KETOGENIC DIET–FRIENDLY FOODS: NUT AND SEED MILKS/BUTTERS/FLOURS/OILS

Nut & Seed Milks/ Butters/Flours/Oils	Amount	Calories	Fat (g)	Protein (g)	Carbs (g)	Sugars (g)
Almond butter (Artisana)	2 tablespoons	180	16	7	7	1
Almond meal	3 tablespoons	90	8	3	3	1
Almond (whole)	1 ounce (23 nuts)	162	14	6	6	1
Almond (slivers)	¼ cup	180	15	6	6	1
Brazil nut	1 ounce (6 nuts)	185	4	4	3	1
Cacao butter (SunFoods, SuperFoods)	1 tablespoon	126	14	0	0	0
Chia seed	2 tablespoons	137	9	4	12	0
Cocoa powder (Equal Exchange)	1 tablespoon	20	0.5	1	2	0
Coconut cream (Nutiva manna)	1 tablespoon	100	9	1	3	1

Coconut flour (Bob's Red Mill)	2 tablespoons	60	2	2	8	1
Coconut oil (Nutiva)	1 tablespoon	130	14	0	0	0
Coconut milk (canned, Native Forest)	¼ cup	100	10	0	3	1
Flaxseed meal	1 tablespoon	37	3	1	2	0
Hazelnut	½ ounce (10 nuts)	88	9	2	2	1
Macadamia butter (Artisana)	2 tablespoons	210	20	4	6	2
Macadamia nut	1 ounce (10–12 nuts)	203	21	2	4	1
MCT oil (NOW)	1 tablespoon	100	14	0	0	0
Olive oil (Spectrum)	1 tablespoon	120	14	0	0	0
Pecan	1 ounce (19 halves)	196	20	2.6	4	1
Pecan butter (Artisana)	2 tablespoons	210	20	4	6	1
Pine nut	1 ounce (167 kernels)	191	19	3.9	3.7	1
Pistachio	1 ounce (49 nuts)	159	13	6	8	2
Pumpkin seed	1 cup	285	12	12	34	0
Sesame oil (Kevala Organic Extra Virgin)	1 tablespoon	130	14	0	0	0
Sesame seed	1 tablespoon	50	5	2	1	0
Shredded coconut (Let's Do Organic)	¼ cup	147	13	1.3	5.3	1.3
Sunflower butter (Sunbutter)	2 tablespoons	220	20	6	5	1
Sunflower seed	1 cup	830	76	23	28	0
Walnut	1 ounce (14 halves)	185	18	4	4	1

Sources: The US Department of Agriculture and individual food manufacturer labels

**TABLE 4.5. MACRONUTRIENT CONTENT IN COMMON
KETOGENIC DIET–FRIENDLY FOODS: ANIMAL PROTEINS**

Animal Proteins	Amount	Calories	Fat (g)	Protein (g)	Carbs (g)	Sugars (g)
Bacon, pork (Applegate Farms)	2 pan-fried slices	60	5	4	0	0
Beef (grass-fed)	3 ounces	123	4	21	0	0
Beef brisket	2 ounces	156	6	5	0	0
Beef hot dog (Applegate Farms Organic)	1 dog	90	7	6	0	0
Bison	3 ounces	202	13	20	0	0
Chicken	1 cup	306	18	35	0	0
Clam	20 small	281	4	49	10	0
Cod	3 ounces	70	0.6	15	0	0
Crab (Crown Prince)	½ can (2 ounces)	40	0	9	0	0
Egg	1 large	78	5	6	0.5	0.5
Gelatin (Great Lakes)	1 tablespoon	25	0	6	0	0
Haddock	1 fillet	136	0.8	30	0	0
Halibut	3 ounces	94	1.4	19	0	0
Lamb	3 ounces	250	18	21	0	0
Lobster	3 ounces	76	0.7	16	0	0
Mackerel	3 ounces	174	12	16	0	0
Mussels	3 ounces	146	3.8	20	6	0
Oysters	6 medium	175	11	8	10	0
Pork chop	1 chop	505	31	52	0	0
Salmon	3 ounces	177	11	17	0	0
Sardine	2 sardines	50	3	6	0	0
Shrimp	3 ounces	85	1	18	0	0
Trout	1 fillet	215	8	33	0	0
Tuna	3 ounces	99	1	22	0	0

Animal Proteins	Amount	Calories	Fat (g)	Protein (g)	Carbs (g)	Sugars (g)
Turkey bacon (Applegate Farms)	1 slice	35	1.5	6	0	0
Turkey breast	1 slice	22	0	4	1	1
Turkey hot dog	1 dog	60	3.5	7	1	0

Sources: The US Department of Agriculture and individual food manufacturer labels

The Ketogenic Kitchen, by Domini Kemp and Patricia Daly, and a forthcoming guide to the diet *Keto for Cancer*, by Miriam Kalamian, a keto-nutrition specialist, which we highly recommend to help you get started with recipes.

Making Sense of Sugars

Our modern diet provides our bodies with more sugar than our genes, mitochondria, and hormones have experienced in all of human history. It is a poison to us and the elixir of life to cancer cells. Reducing the amount of sugar and carbohydrates we eat to those consumed by our pre-agricultural ancestors is clearly a very powerful step in reducing the threat of cancer. Sugar lurks in many places, so immediately limiting sugar consumption to natural sugars, such as those found in low-sugar fruit like berries, is a simple way to start.

In the next chapter we shift focus to another primary cause of cancer: exposure to toxic chemicals and environmental carcinogens. We explain how to avoid them and how to rid them from the body. You may be surprised to learn where some of these cancer-causing agents are found.

CHAPTER 5

Carcinogens, Cancer, and Detoxification

All substances are poisons; there is none which is not a poison. The right dose differentiates a poison and a remedy.

> —An early observation concerning the toxicity of chemicals made by PARACELSUS (1493–1541)

You can't live a healthy life on a sick planet.

> —JOHN REPLOGLE, *president and CEO of Seventh Generation Inc.*

Our exposure to cancer-causing chemicals often happens on a completely unconscious level. While toxic chemicals are everywhere, most of them are invisible. Since the Second World War, more than eighty thousand new synthetic chemicals have entered commercial use. In all, more than twenty million chemicals have been created; most are not in direct commercial use, but the by-products of their manufacture contaminate the air, the earth, and the water. Globally a new chemical is synthesized on average every twenty-seven seconds.[1] Unbelievably, less than 5 percent of these chemicals have been tested for their safety, and none have been tested for their synergistic effects (meaning how they interact with one another, important because in some cases inert chemicals can become carcinogenic when combined). Meanwhile, we ingest, inhale, inject, absorb, and endure ambient exposure to them.

As you've probably gleaned by now, the term *carcinogen* refers to any substance that can contribute to the process of cancer formation, including causing mutations and promoting tumor growth. Exposure to carcinogenic toxins causes mitochondrial damage, inflammation, and oxidation, disrupts hormone balance, and suppresses the immune system. Sadly, our exposure to them is chronic and daily.

Cancer rates have soared since the Industrial Revolution approximately three hundred years ago, with scores of studies linking toxin exposures to the development of cancers, including breast cancer, childhood leukemias, and brain cancer. For example, there is a positive correlation between exposure to domestic use of weed killer and garden pesticides and the development of leukemias and brain tumors.[2] In fact, it is estimated that almost 90 percent of all cancers are due to the exposure to environmental carcinogens. Not only that, but exposure to high levels of carcinogens in tandem with suboptimal functioning of the body's detoxification system significantly increases the risk of cancer.[3] You will learn later in this chapter about a few SNPs that can greatly affect how well your liver is able to neutralize and excrete toxic chemicals, making genetic analysis a key consideration before embarking on any detoxification program.

The role played by exposure to carcinogens is not to be underestimated when it comes to cancer. In our clinical practices we have developed and integrated environmental toxin assessments that are part of all new patient intakes. Often this area is the highest priority. Even if patients are eating a very clean and ketogenic diet, if they are exposed to carcinogens on a daily basis, cancer cells will have access to agents that encourage their proliferation, regardless of good nutrition. After years of seeing a cancer recur or a new cancer arise on the heels of a toxic exposure (a common one being home renovations), we knew that this area of the terrain needed our focused attention.

A Deeper Look at Carcinogens

Carcinogens can be found in new cars, couches, lawn care products, baby pajamas, baby powder, air fresheners, laundry detergent, pesticides, dry-cleaning chemicals, cookware, certain foods, food wrappers, arts and crafts supplies, kids' toys, building supplies, hair coloring, drinking water, perfume, prescription medications, and more. They have names like *aflatoxins*, found in stored grains; *arsenic*, used in vegetable pesticides and animal feed; and *formaldehyde*, used in cosmetics, house paint, and vaccinations. Many of the treatments conventionally used to *treat* cancer are also known carcinogens. Nine different chemotherapy agents are designated as known IARC Group 1 carcinogens (meaning cancerous to humans). These include *chlorambucil*, used to treat leukemia, and *melphalan* used to treat ovarian cancer. Why do we wonder that rates of secondary cancers are on the rise? Our Western model's best practice is to treat cancer with agents known to cause cancer. How is this considered good science? It is time we started poking holes in our flawed cancer model.

Some carcinogens are eliminated by the body's detoxification systems within a matter of days or months. Others toxic chemicals can persist in the body for a lifetime, circulating between organs and storage in fat cells. These are called persistent organic pollutants (POPs), and are compounds that are resistant to environmental degradation through chemical, biological, or photolytic processes. Because of their persistence, POPs accumulate in the body, significantly affecting human health as well. The pesticide dichlorodiphenyltrichloroethane (more commonly referred to as DDT) is probably the most well-known POP. Its devastating effects on health were illuminated by the 1962 bestseller *Silent Spring*, written by biologist Rachel Carson.

In their "Fourth National Report on Human Exposure to Environmental Chemicals" (2009) the Centers for Disease Control and Prevention (CDC) declared that the average person living in the United States had at least 212 synthetic chemicals in their system. At birth, many newborns in the United States already have over 200 toxic chemicals in their bodies that entered via the mother's placenta. The types of chemicals detected in humans include toxic metals, polycyclic aromatic hydrocarbons, volatile organic compounds, dioxins, organophosphate pesticides, herbicides, and pest repellents.

Many people assume that toxic chemicals are regulated, and therefore don't think about reading the list of ingredients on their sunscreens, bug sprays, or art supplies. Sadly, however, the only watchdog we have in the United States is the outdated and toothless Toxic Substances Control Act, adopted by Congress in 1976. Until June 2016, the core provisions of this law that supposedly actively regulates household and industrial compounds had not been amended since its adoption. It has proven ineffective at outlawing the use of agents known to cause cancer, such as asbestos, which is still legal in the United States yet has been banned in fifty other countries. Pre-market testing and safety provisions were also not incorporated into the law, nor does it require safety testing for the roughly sixty thousand "grandfathered" chemicals that were already in use prior to its passage.[4] This has allowed thousands of chemicals to remain on the market without any review of their safety. Chemical companies have since added hundreds of new chemicals to products in daily use without any required safety demonstration. In fact, the government had to have evidence that a chemical posed a risk *before* it could require testing. Our chemical regulations have been about as safe as letting a wolf guard sheep.

Cigarettes are a perfect example. Smoking is known to cause cancer, even second- and thirdhand smoke is known to cause cancer, and yet still cigarettes are legal. The warning label on the box is supposedly sufficient to deter potential smokers. But warning labels do not exist for many other products. In early 2016 Johnson & Johnson's baby powder and other talc-containing products used for feminine hygiene were determined by a Missouri state court to cause ovarian cancer. In 2013 the manufacturer Banana Boat recalled twenty-three different spray-on sunscreens because users' skin was literally catching on fire in the sun's heat. Sadly, cosmetics and body care products are the least regulated arm of the FDA.

Meanwhile, concerns over commonly used chemicals have been at the fore for many political and public-interest groups for decades. The IARC, the official cancer agency of the World Health Organization, was first convened in France in 1965. The agency conducts studies to identify factors that can increase the risk of cancer in humans, including chemicals, occupational exposures, physical agents, biological agents, and lifestyle habits. The results of the studies are grouped according to the item's carcinogenic potential:

Group 1: carcinogenic to humans
Group 2A: probably carcinogenic to humans
Group 2B: possibly carcinogenic to humans
Group 3: not classifiable as to its carcinogenicity to humans
Group 4: probably not carcinogenic to humans

Since 1971, the IARC has evaluated nine hundred chemical agents, of which more than four hundred have been identified as carcinogenic, probably carcinogenic, or possibly carcinogenic to humans. To say that another way, when chemicals are actually assessed in scientific trials, almost 50 percent of them are found to contribute to cancer. *Almost half.*

This is a very troubling statistic, and it begs the question of why we are not erring on the side of precaution. Why do we not *resist* the introduction of a new chemical whose ultimate effects are disputed or unknown? Instead, chemical production and subsequent use is being approached with reckless abandon. And while our daily dosage of carcinogens has reached lethal limits, the bigger problem is—as toxicologists explain—that the timing, pattern, and duration of toxic exposure are just as important as the dose. That is, carcinogenic agents have varying levels of cancer-causing potential. Some may cause cancer only after prolonged, high levels of exposure, while others have a more acute effect. The risk of developing cancer from exposure to a carcinogenic agent is contingent upon factors including the dosage, method, length, and intensity of exposure, but also individual genetics and the body's detoxification capabilities. The more cigarettes smoked, the higher the risk of cancer.

With all the carcinogens we are exposed to, it is critical to learn not only how to identify and avoid them, but also how to actively support the body's elimination of them through deep nutrition and lifestyle approaches. As you will learn a bit further on in this chapter, there are many foods that have been found helpful in the removal of toxins and reduction of radiation exposure risk. But first let's look at how carcinogens actually cause cancer.

How Carcinogens Cause Cancer

Cancer develops in stages, and carcinogens disrupt multiple biological pathways in a manner that facilitates the cancer process. Some carcinogens may cause direct DNA damage, or genetic mutations, while others may disrupt the liver's detoxification system. Some carcinogens do not affect DNA directly, but rather lead to cancer by stimulating cells to divide at a faster-than-normal rate, similar to sugar. In a review published in the June 2016 issue of the peer-reviewed journal *Environmental Health Perspectives*, the IARC completed a review of all Group 1 human carcinogens and identified their mechanisms of carcinogenesis. They presented a novel new categorical method that identifies the ten key characteristics of human carcinogens. These are similar to the ten hallmarks of cancer we presented in chapter 1 and help to illustrate the varied mechanisms by which carcinogens cause cancer. The cancer-causing characteristics of toxins are that they:

1. Initiate metabolic activation, which means the chemical conversion of a benign substance into a more hazardous one via the normal biochemical processes of cells
2. Induce DNA damage and/or mutation
3. Alter DNA repair or cause genomic instability
4. Induce epigenetic changes, including DNA methylation
5. Induce oxidative stress
6. Induce chronic inflammation
7. Suppress immune system function
8. Activate or deactivate cellular receptor sites
9. Cause cell immortalization
10. Alter a cell's proliferation, death, or nutrient supply

What researchers concluded is that any given carcinogen will exhibit at least one, perhaps more, of these characteristics.[5] For example, heavy metals—to which we are exposed through our drinking water, food supply, and occupational exposures—can cause genomic instability. Perfluorooctanesulfonic acid (PFOS), a chemical used as a stain repellent on fabrics, can facilitate angiogenesis, a cancer cell's ability to create its own blood supply. The metabolism of ethanol from alcoholic drinks forms acetaldehyde, a compound that can damage DNA.

Now that it has been established how these agents cause cancer, let's discuss our exposure to them. To address all the toxic compounds humans are exposed to would deserve an entire book of its own. So the following listings are simply a gentle reminder to help raise your awareness around products of daily living that have toxic potential. We recognize that the content of this next section can feel extremely overwhelming; we are all living on a very toxic planet. If you have been using any of the products or have had exposure to the substances we outline, please do not beat yourself up about it.

Just employ the detoxification strategies detailed at the end of this chapter, replace your products, and start questioning chemical regulations!

A Carcinogen's Route of Entry

The manner in which a harmful substance or carcinogen enters the body is called the route of entry, and there are five such routes:

1. Absorption (through the skin)
2. Inhalation (through the lung)
3. Ingestion (through the digestive tract)
4. Injection (into the bloodstream)
5. Ambient exposures (through the immediate surroundings)

When a carcinogenic substance enters the body by any of these routes, acute or chronic effects can ensue. Before cancer develops, symptoms of toxicity can surface, from an immediate reaction, such as a rash or difficulty breathing, to more delayed and chronic symptoms including fatigue, skin eruptions, constipation, autoimmune conditions, fibromyalgia, chemical sensitivities, and depression. By now most people are aware that cigarette smoking and overconsumption of alcohol can cause cancer. But what many do not realize is that seemingly benign products such as bubble bath, cell phones, clothes, lettuce, chicken, nail polish, hair dye, tattoos, tampons, and tanning beds all either contain or expose us to carcinogens. The average American is exposed to at least five known carcinogens a day.

The first route of entry we will examine is absorption. Our skin is really like a million little mouths, and it can absorb 60 to 100 percent of the agents it comes into contact with.

Absorption

Many carcinogens are able to cross through the skin and enter the bloodstream, damaging cells and organs along the way. Because skin thickness varies in different parts of the body—it is thinner on the eyelids and thicker on the soles of the feet—the body absorbs chemicals at differing rates depending on the location of exposure. For example, when compared with the bottom of the feet, the skin of the scalp and forehead can absorb forty times as fast, while the delicate skin surrounding the scrotum has a three-hundredfold greater rate of absorption. Our skin is exposed to carcinogens in various ways, and while we do not list them all in this book, we do want to highlight those commonly found in personal care products including hair dye, tampons, and textiles.

Cosmetics and Personal Care Products

Of the 113 agents listed by IARC as Group 1 human carcinogens, the Campaign for Safe Cosmetics reports that at least 11 of these have been, or are currently used in personal care products: formaldehyde, phenacetin, coal tar, benzene, mineral oils, methylene glycol, ethylene oxide, chromium, cadmium, arsenic, and crystalline silica or quartz. Coal tar is found in hair dye, shampoo, dandruff or scalp treatments, and rosacea ointment. (Interestingly, in reviewing our patients' toxin assessments, we found that many of our patients with ovarian cancer used black hair dye at one point or another.) Methylene glycol is used in nail polish and hair straighteners, and phenacetin is an ingredient commonly found in bubble bath, hair conditioner, shampoo, wave sets, moisturizer, and other bath and hair care products. Unfortunately, rather than being a rejuvenating experience, a trip to the beauty salon can actually be carcinogenic. The pink hair dye used by many in solidarity with those who have breast cancer may not be such a good idea after all.

Because health and beauty products are poorly regulated by the FDA, it becomes critically important for the consumer to read labels on all products applied to the hair or skin. Especially when the product is being used on children. The subsidiary website run by the EWG, Skin Deep (www.ewg .org/skindeep), provides an exhaustive searchable database of toxic ingredients in cosmetic and personal care products. Meanwhile, our golden rule for body care and beauty products is: If you can't eat it, don't use it. Thankfully, there are many organic and natural body care products on the market, and simple solutions like using coconut oil for body lotion not only reduce toxic exposure, but improve the health of your skin. And yes, there are many organically focused beauty salons!

Many commonly used, cotton-based feminine-hygiene products are also highly toxic. First, in 2015 researchers from the University of La Plata in

Argentina found that almost 85 percent of tampons are contaminated with glyphosate, the Group 2A chemical used in the herbicide Roundup. Second, not only is cotton one of the most common GM crops in the United States, cotton's bleaching process makes use of another Group 1 carcinogen and POP, *dioxins*. And third, some tampons contain synthetic fragrance, which can also be carcinogenic. Vaginal wall tissues are highly permeable, allowing carcinogens to be freely absorbed and enter the bloodstream. From 1973 to 2004 the incidence of vulvar tumors increased an average of 3.5 percent each year, and while this has been largely attributed to human papillomavirus (HPV), the role of toxic tampons should not be underestimated. Organic tampons are the best way to go.

Clothing

Carcinogens are present in many of the fabrics found in everyday textiles such as clothes, bed linens, and towels. These agents can diffuse into the skin and lead to systemic exposure. Skin cancer is one of the most common cancers in the world, and squamous cell carcinoma—which begins in the top layer of the epidermis—accounts for about 20 percent. While sun exposure is often blamed for skin cancer development, cancers also arise in areas not commonly exposed to the sun, rather covered in clothing. Turns out, the production of textiles can involve the use of a large number of carcinogenic compounds, including azo dyes, flame retardants, formaldehyde, dioxins, solvents, biocides, and heavy metals.

The chemicals used to make fabrics remain, even after the clothes have been produced. Pentachlorophenol, for example, an organochlorine pesticide and Group 1 carcinogen, has been detected in many fabrics. In one study, volunteers wore shorts and T-shirts during five minutes of sweat-inducing exercise. Subsequent skin analysis revealed the presence of benzothiazole (a carcinogen) on areas covered by the clothes but not on uncovered areas. Another study proved the transfer of another carcinogen, polychlorinated dibenzo-p-dioxin, from textile to skin. When pajamas treated with this flame retardant were worn by children while they slept, a fiftyfold increase in the metabolite 2,3-dibromopropanol was detected in children's urine the following morning. After the children wore flame-retardant-free pajamas, the urine concentration of the metabolite slowly decreased, but even after five days it was still twenty times higher than the baseline concentration. Findings like this are why many states, including Washington and California, have attempted to ban the use of flame retardants in all clothing and furniture. Clothing, bed linens, and the upholstery used to cover furniture should be made from naturally grown fibers free of flame retardants. It is important to check with individual manufacturers about how their fabrics are produced and treated. (To learn more about the toxic dangers of clothing, we recommend the book *Killer Clothes* by Drs. Brian and Anna Maria Clement.)

We also must not overlook the use of highly toxic detergents and fabric softeners common in many households. Clorox bleach is a highly toxic solvent known to cause thyroid disorders. The synthetic petrochemical and likely human carcinogen 1,4-dioxane is a by-product formed when ethylene oxide, used to create laundry detergent, reacts with other ingredients. A study done by the Green Patriot Working Group (GPWG) and the Organic Consumers Association (OCA) found 1,4-dioxane in most laundry detergents, including even natural brands. If you think laundry detergent doesn't seem like that big a deal, consider this: We have had excellent results in children with asthma and other respiratory ailments when we suggest discontinuing the use of highly toxic laundry and dryer sheets.

We recommend switching to clothing brands that use sustainable production practices and nontoxic fibers. We also recommend making your own laundry detergent with borax and other natural soaps.

Inhalation

Breathe in, breathe out. On average, humans take twelve breaths per minute, or approximately twenty thousand a day. Without oxygen, we can live for only about three minutes. With every breath, nitrogen, oxygen, water, carbon dioxide, ozone, vapors, smoke, dust, acid droplets, pollen, and, in some cases, *hazardous air pollutants* (HAPS) enter our lungs. HAPS are defined by the Clean Air Act as substances known or suspected of causing cancer, birth defects, or other adverse health problems. Currently 188 HAPS have been identified, including dioxins, benzene, arsenic, beryllium, mercury, and vinyl chloride. Sources that emit these carcinogenic chemicals include tobacco smoke, engine exhaust, cleaning products, solvents found in paint, arts and crafts supplies, building materials, synthetic and fragranced products, and coal combustion. *Volatile organic contaminants* (VOCs) are toxic off-gassed by-products in homes that come from paint, varnishes, cleaning solutions, solvents, insulation, wood, furniture, carpeting, and other products. Inhaled HAPS and VOCs are caught either in the nose or by the hairlike cilia that line the airways and are either exhaled or deposited into the lungs, where they are free to enter the bloodstream. When HAPS or VOCs enter the lungs, damage occurs through direct contact with lung tissues, and when they are absorbed into the blood, they damage the organs involved in toxin metabolism, including the kidney, liver, colon, and bladder.

Unfortunately, there has been a steady increase in air pollution over the last decade. More than 3.5 billion people—half the world's population—breathe air deemed unsafe by World Health Organization standards. It's not surprising that lung cancer is currently one of the most common cancers in the world. An IARC evaluation showed increased risk of lung cancer as exposure to outdoor air pollution increased. Because there are so many toxic inhaled carcinogens, part of the toxin assessment in our clinics investigates patients' exposure to common products, especially those that are somewhat easier to control, such as cleaning products and synthetic fragrances.

In many cases these seemingly benign products are in fact highly malignant. For example, in a study published in *The FASEB Journal*, the journal of the Federation of American Societies for Experimental Biology, scientists concluded that *phthalates*, a class of plasticizing chemicals often used in synthetically fragranced products (perfumes, scented candles, and plug-in air fresheners), help fuel the growth of some of the most hard-to-treat types of breast cancer. Plainly put, we cannot trust store-bought products to be safe. But there's more to be concerned about than the products we make: The two most prevalent, deadly airborne carcinogens are the naturally occurring and odorless radon and benzene.

After smoking, exposure to radon, a Group 1 carcinogen, is the second leading cause of lung cancer in the United States and the leading cause of lung cancer in nonsmokers. Radon is a radioactive gas created by the breakdown of uranium, a heavy metal found in rock and soil. Exposure can occur inside homes, offices, or schools, especially in basements. Radon enters through cracks in floors, walls, and foundations, and accumulates inside the building. Radon levels can be higher in homes that are well insulated, tightly sealed, or built on top of soil rich in uranium or radium. Houses right next door to each other can have different levels of radon, and the US Environmental Protection Agency (EPA) estimates that approximately one in fifteen homes in the United States has an unsafe level. This odorless gas is also released from building materials or from well water containing radon. When radon decays, it emits tiny radioactive particles that damage lung cells. We cannot emphasize enough the importance of testing your home for radon and making sure to open windows daily all year long to allow fresh air to circulate through your home, office, or school building. (When buying a new home, a radon test is a mandatory part of the inspection process. For good reason.)

The other naturally occurring airborne Group 1 carcinogen, benzene, is a colorless or light yellow liquid chemical, and exposure has been linked with leukemias, multiple myeloma, and non-Hodgkin lymphoma. Benzene is found in crude petroleum, and any activity involving petroleum can lead to exposure. It is used primarily as a solvent in the chemical and pharmaceutical industries and is found in plastics, resins, synthetic fibers, dyes, detergents, drugs, pesticides, and vehicle exhaust. Benzene is just about everywhere. Levels of benzene are higher in homes with attached garages, in homes close to gas stations and airports, and in homes located near fracking sites.

Automobile and airplane exhaust accounts for the largest source of benzene in the environment. The poison circle from a single runway can extend six miles from its hub and run twenty miles downwind. In fact, according to a study by the Citizens Aviation Watch Association (CAWA), cancer rates for people living on the perimeter of Chicago's O'Hare airport are 70 percent higher than for the average Chicagoan. The Earth Island Institute, a nonprofit environmental public interest organization, compared health data from 1991 to 1995 of people living near Seattle's Sea-Tac airport with that of Seattle residents overall and found infant mortality near the airport was 50 percent greater, while cancer deaths were 36 percent greater. For those living near the airport, overall life expectancy was more than five years shorter. And a 1993 EPA health-risk assessment concluded that aircraft engines are responsible for approximately 10.5 percent of the cancer cases within a sixteen-square-mile area surrounding Chicago's Midway airport.[6]

When it comes to air quality in your home, we highly suggest use of a HEPA or charcoal air filter to help reduce the amount of benzene inhalation.

Additionally, NASA has found that some species of houseplants can eliminate up to 87 percent of toxins from the air, including formaldehyde, benzene, toluene, trichloroethylene, carbon monoxide, and even dust. These plants include English ivy, spider plants, and Boston fern. A single plant won't make much difference, however. You'll need to fill your entire house with plants. But it's worth it; they're also beautiful to look at! Lastly, we highly recommend clearing the air with burning sage, a practice called *smudging* that has been used for thousands of years. A study published in the *Journal of Ethnopharmacology* determined that smudging reduces a variety of airborne pathological microbes. Burning essential oils is also purported to clear the air of toxins and is the best alternative to synthetically fragranced products if your home is in need of some pleasant aromas. Burning scented candles—unless they are made naturally with 100 percent essential oils—should be completely avoided.

If you live near an airport, oil and gas activity, or fracking area, you may not be able to pack up and move to the mountains, but you can begin implementing these air-purification practices and actively pursuing the detoxification steps we outline at the end of this chapter.

Ingestion

Ingested carcinogens—from food, water, and medications—harm the gastrointestinal tract on their way down and, if not destroyed by gastrointestinal fluids (including the stomach's highly acidic hydrochloric acid), are absorbed and transported by the blood to internal organs where they wreak havoc. Worldwide, the rates of digestive tract cancers have exploded. In 2010 the organization Cancer Research UK reported that esophageal cancer rates in men rose 50 percent over the previous twenty-five years in the United Kingdom, and high rates are also prevalent in China and Iran, where these cancers have been directly linked to the preservation of food using synthetic nitrosamines (more about these to come).

There is currently pervasive use of carcinogenic pesticides and heavy metals in modern conventional agricultural practices. Far too often our clients tell us that it's too expensive to eat organically. And yes, thanks to farming subsidies, it is cheaper to drink soda and eat chips than it is to eat vegetables. But the carcinogens found in our modern food and water supplies—in produce and meat items, in addition to artificial preservatives and colors—are very dangerous to our health. In the previous chapter we discussed the use of carcinogenic glyphosate in GM foods, but heavy metals such as cadmium, arsenic, and nickel—all Group 1 carcinogens—are also frequently used in pesticides. Heavy metal exposure can contribute to genetic damage as well as disabling various DNA repair pathways.[7] The USDA's Pesticide Data Program documented more than fifty different pesticide residues found on conventional lettuce, three of which are known or probable carcinogens. You can't really wash these chemicals off, either. If only it were that easy. Sorry, but if it's not organic, there are cancer-causing pesticides on your "healthy" salad.

We cannot overemphasize the importance of eating organic foods—and growing your own—whenever possible to avoid exposure to carcinogenic pesticides and the heavy metals they contain. If you are just learning about eating organically, we recommend taking a look at the EWG's annual "Dirty Dozen" report. This is a listing of the produce items found to have the highest amount of pesticide residues, and it has included strawberries, apples, celery, and grapes. You should try to eat only organic versions of the foods on this list. The EWG also publishes a "Clean 15" list of produce items with the lowest pesticide residues. These foods have less need to be organically grown and includes avocados, cabbage, and onions.

Finally, because adequate hydration is so important to the body's detoxification process, the quality of the water you drink becomes paramount. Many of our cities add "treatments" like fluoride to water and do not filter it. Highly toxic substances have also been detected in public drinking water supplies, including chemotherapy agents, antidepressants, birth control hormones, pesticides, herbicides, flame retardants, and more. But refrigerator filters, plastic water bottles, and other types of water filtration systems offer false peace of mind, unfortunately. It is very difficult to find a filter that can remove all of these toxic substances. (Reverse osmosis is the best, and companies such as Pure Effect, Inc., offer other excellent filtration options.)

Toxic Meat vs. Nutritious Meat

The red meat and processed meat controversies are widely misunderstood and misinterpreted. In 2015 the IARC classified processed meat as a Group 1 carcinogen, and red meat as Group 2A, probably carcinogenic to humans.

Processed meats, which include hot dogs, ham, bacon, sausage, and deli meats, are defined as animal products that have been treated in some way to preserve or flavor them, either by salting, curing, fermenting, or smoking. Experts from ten countries reviewed hundreds of studies and came to the conclusion that eating 50 grams of processed meat a day (the equivalent of about four strips of bacon or one hot dog) increased the risk of colorectal cancer by 18 percent.

To start the myth-busting process here, it is important to know that the origins of these preservation practices are not new. Meat preservation techniques have been used for thousands of years in every culture. As early as 3000 BC in Mesopotamia, cooked meats and fish were preserved in sesame oil and dried. But industrial man has significantly manipulated these preservation techniques, rendering certain animal products totally toxic. For starters, the casings used for many types of sausages and hot dogs are made from synthetic thermoplastic materials, including polyester and polypropylene.[8] The meat inside these casings could also be called synthetic. Conventionally raised cows, pigs, and chickens are fed a specifically formulated growth-promoting diet comprising animal by-products (including crab guts and recycled animal manure), antibiotics, hormones, dioxin residues, genetically modified grains, and organoarsenicals, pesticides and herbicides made of metals that are carcinogenic to humans when metabolized in the body. These animals are sick and unhappy. In addition to a non-natural diet, they spend their entire lives trapped inside, some not even able to move. Imagine living your whole life on an airplane—without the bathroom. Eating meat that comes from sick animals will make us sick.

Processed meats are also treated with synthetic nitrates, a highly misunderstood concept. Nitrites (NO_2) are naturally occurring chemical compounds found in soil, water, and plants, and made naturally by our own bodies. They can also be formed synthetically. In 2010 the WHO listed ingested nitrites as probable human carcinogens. Cured meats account for only about 5 percent of our dietary nitrate consumption, however, while about 20 percent comes from drinking water, and 75–80 percent from vegetables (celery, leafy greens, beets, parsley, leeks, endive, cabbage, and fennel are the most potent sources). Vegetables pick up nitrates from the soil, nitrogen-based fertilizer, animal manure, water, and nitrogen in the atmosphere.

The naturally occurring salt sodium nitrate ($NaNO_3$) is exceptionally effective in preserving meats and has been used for this purpose since ancient times to inhibit growth of the harmful bacterium *Clostridium botulinum*, the origin of botulism, a severe paralyzing illness. It also keeps meat looking pink as opposed to a less appetizing gray. On the flip side, however, synthetic sodium nitrite is made by passing "nitrous fumes" into an aqueous sodium hydroxide or sodium carbonate solution, which is a far cry from a simple coating of sea salt. The bottom line here is, know where your food comes from, and if you're not making it yourself, make sure you understand every step of how it's being made. Sea salt versus chemical cocktails present very different messages to our mitochondria.

Another issue with modern processed meats is the addition of synthetic vitamin C. In the 1970s researchers discovered that when meat containing sodium nitrite is heated above 266°F, it creates *nitrosamines*, which are carcinogenic. This triggered the USDA to limit the amount of nitrites that may be added to cured meats and require that all products containing nitrites also include vitamin C, which they believed would prevent the formation of nitrosamines. The ascorbic acid added to processed meats is generally derived from genetically modified corn syrup and does not confer the same benefits as the naturally occurring vitamin C found in a bell pepper, for example. In summary, modern processed meats contain loads of added carcinogens, and they are often cooked at high temperatures on nonstick pans coated with toxic materials to boot!

It is not natural for humans to consume overprocessed meat, regardless of how much our children might love the taste. In fact, people used to take wild fish or meat and rub it down with salt that they found near the ocean to preserve it, and that has sustained us for millions of years. Today, we eat conventionally raised animals that are highly processed with GMOs, fumes, and chlorine, and then packaged in plastic. Think simple: When the meat you eat is pasture-raised, naturally processed, and cooked at low temperatures, and you consume plenty of vitamin C–containing foods, there is little cause for concern.

Medications: Not Always Worth It

Lastly, another form of ingested carcinogen is our medications. We drastically underestimate the role over-the-counter and prescription medications play in the development of cancer. Several links have already been documented, and if you listen to the fast talkers on the commercials for most prescription medications, you will hear many that acknowledge an increased risk of certain types of cancer with their use. In particular:

- Sulindac (Clinoril), a nonsteroidal anti-inflammatory drug (NSAID) used to treat pain and inflammation, can increase the risk of gallbladder cancer and leukemia.
- Hyoscyamine (Levsin), an antispasmodic used to treat gastrointestinal problems, can increase the risk of non-Hodgkin lymphoma.
- Nortriptyline (Pamelor), a tricyclic antidepressant, can increase the risk of esophageal and hepatic cancer.
- Oxazepam (Serax), a benzodiazepine used to treat anxiety and insomnia, can increase the risk of lung cancer.
- Fluoxetine (Prozac) and paroxetine (Paxil), both antidepressants, are associated with an increased risk of testicular cancer.
- Microzide (hydrochlorothiazide), used to treat high blood pressure, is associated with increased risk of renal and lip cancer.[9]

Long-term use of proton pump inhibitors including omeprazole (Prilosec) to control stomach acid was found to cause esophageal cancer in a study published in 2012 in *Archives of Surgery*. This class of medications has been identified as a primary contributor to mitochondrial damage.[10]

And while synthetic medications are a problem, even all-natural supplements can present toxicity issues. Ingestion of nutrient toxins such as copper, iodine (especially if one suffers from Hashimoto's autoimmune thyroiditis), iron, boron, calcium, and synthetic folic acid (often overprescribed for pregnant women) can accelerate the cancer process. Dr. Nasha is hesitant to recommend any multivitamin or supplement without further laboratory investigation. It is better to focus on deep nutrition than to take a supplement to remedy a deficiency. It rarely works.

In short, you should carefully consider anything you want to put in your mouth; the more synthetic it is, the worse it is for you. And many of the conditions we are prescribed medications for are directly related to nutrition and can be either prevented or mitigated simply and nontoxically by following the recommendations outlined in this book.

Injection

Toxic substances can easily enter the body when the skin is penetrated or punctured by needles. Negative effects then occur as the substance circulates in the blood and is deposited in target organs. This route of exposure can include tattoos, vaccinations, and intravenous drugs or nutrition. In 2011 a report published in *The British Journal of Dermatology* revealed that carcinogenic nanoparticles are present in tattoo inks. Red tattoo ink contains mercury, and most other colors of standard tattoo ink are also derived from such heavy metals as lead, antimony, beryllium, chromium, cobalt, nickel, and arsenic, a known carcinogen. Therefore, whether you or a loved one are fighting cancer or simply wanting to prevent it, getting a tattoo to commemorate your journey or your loved one—or anything else—may do more harm than good.

Two common vaccination adjuvants (substances added to a vaccine to increase the body's immune response) include formaldehyde, a Group 1 carcinogen, and aluminum, a neurotoxin. Particularly dangerous is the amount of these two substances that are injected into infants and small children over the course of multiple vaccinations. While the amount of formaldehyde and aluminum in each vaccine dose is low, the cumulative amount can become substantial when you consider the current recommended vaccine schedule includes thirty-three doses of ten different vaccines before age six. In addition to vaccines, several chemotherapy drugs administered intravenously are in fact known carcinogens, so it is important to discuss the ratio of risk versus benefit with your doctors if they are recommending a carcinogen to treat your cancer.

Ambient Exposures

Ambient exposures are carcinogenic factors present in immediate surroundings, which are sometimes also referred to as a person's microenvironment. Two common ambient exposures that are known to be related to the development of cancer are radiation and artificial lighting. Radiation is energy that travels in the form of waves or high-speed particles and is a known carcinogen; it interacts with DNA to produce a range of mutations. Radiation occurs naturally with exposure to sunlight and also occurs with exposure to x-rays, mammograms, nuclear weapons, nuclear power plants, some cancer treatments, and cellular devices. Another common exposure is through food irradiation, the application of ionizing radiation to foods to prevent the growth of pathogens. According to the Organic Consumers Association, an advocacy group, irradiation damages food by splitting molecules that create free radicals. These free radicals kill *some* bacteria, but also destroy essential fatty acids, vitamins, and enzymes, and combine with existing chemicals (like pesticides) in the food, forming new chemicals, called *unique radiolytic products* (URPs). Some URPs are known carcinogens, such as benzene, which has been found in irradiated beef. When fat-containing food is treated with ionizing radiation, 2-alkylcyclobutanone compounds are formed. When these compounds are exposed to human colon cancer cells, they have been found to cause DNA strand breaks.[11] Despite the known risks, food irradiation is a widely used practice in the United States. Irradiated foods can be identified by a very misleading label: a two-leafed plant surrounded by a circle.

Ultraviolet (UV) radiation is a form of electromagnetic radiation. The main source of UV rays is the sun, although it can also come from manufactured sources such as tanning beds and welding torches. Basal cell and squamous cell cancers tend to be found on sun-exposed parts of the body, and their occurrence is typically related to lifetime sun exposure. People who first use a tanning bed before age thirty-five increase their risk of developing melanoma by 75 percent.[12] Tanning beds were classified by the IARC as Group 1 carcinogens in 2009.

While the sun and its rays are often blamed for causing cancer, we also have to remember that humans lived for over two million years without sunscreen, hats, or umbrellas. We also had higher levels of vitamin D and consumed more sun-protective antioxidants like astaxanthin, a terpene that acts as a natural sunscreen. The toxins contained in most sunscreens (synthetic vitamin A and oxybenzone) can actually cause and promote the spread of cancer, according to a 2011 report issued by the EWG. Lucky for us, the EWG issues an annual list of nonhazardous sunscreens. Coating our children in toxic sunscreen—recall the one that was setting people's skin on fire—not only depletes them of needed vitamin D, but also exposes them to unhealthy chemicals. As the ozone layer decreases, avoiding the midday sun becomes more and more important; UV rays are most potent during that time. But let's not be afraid of the sun—we need the vitamin it offers (more on this in chapter 7; see "Causes of Immune System Impairment").

The Dangers of Cancer Screening

Ironically, radiation is used in two cancer screening methods, and it is one of the most common cancer treatment modalities. All involve exposing targeted sites on the human body to high doses of a known Group 1 carcinogen. Radiation can kill cancer cells, but it can also contribute to gene mutations. Mammograms use doses of ionizing radiation in order to obtain x-ray pictures of breast tissue that can reveal tumor growths undetectable by physical exam. The Institute of Medicine, the nonprofit health arm of the National Academy of Sciences, reviewed possible causes of breast cancer among women in the United States in 2012 and concluded that about 2,800 breast cancer cases a year directly stem from medical radiation. A 2015 Danish study concluded that mammography is simply too harmful to continue using. The National Cancer Institute (NCI) has released evidence that, among women under age thirty-five, mammography may cause seventy-five cases of breast cancer for every fifteen it identifies. And another study found a 52 percent increase in breast cancer mortality in Canada among young women who received annual mammograms. In fact, since mammographic screening was introduced, the incidence of a form of breast cancer called ductal carcinoma in situ (DCIS) has increased by 328 percent.[13]

In addition to the harmful effects of radiation, mammography may also help existing cancer cells to disseminate due to the considerable pressure that is placed on the woman's breast during the procedure. According to some health practitioners, this compression may cause any existing cancer cells to metastasize from the breast tissue.

And lastly, cancer researchers have identified a gene present in a significant percentage of women in the United States that is extremely sensitive to even small doses of radiation. Possessors of this gene may have an even further increased risk of developing mammography-induced cancer.

But despite these findings, the American Cancer Society recommends that women ages forty to forty-four should have the choice to start annual breast cancer screening with mammograms if they want to, women ages forty-five to fifty-four should have annual mammograms, and women fifty-five and older should have a mammograms every two years. Another source of practice guidelines, however, the US Preventive Services Task Force (USPSTF), suggests that most women can wait until age fifty and then have a mammogram biennially. Mammogram screening for breast cancer in the United States costs $8 billion per year, and false-positive mammograms contribute to a 20 percent overdiagnosis of breast cancer among women ages forty to fifty-nine.

A radiation-free mammogram alternative that Dr. Nasha has been using with her patients for years is thermography, which uses digital infrared imaging to detect masses. Additional cancer screening and detection options include Biocept (a liquid biopsy) and circulating tumor cells enumeration. These can help determine best treatment options, response to therapy, and early detection of recurrence or progression. These may be options you would like to discuss with your provider.

Electromagnetic Fields

Electromagnetic fields (EMFs), which result from the motion of an electric charge, are produced by mobile phones, computers, wireless networks, and other ubiquitous devices. EMFs are classified by the IARC as Group 2B, possibly carcinogenic to humans. Independent research shows a 540 percent increased risk of brain cancer with more than two thousand hours of cell phone use, and a Swedish study concluded that an individual's risk of brain cancer is increased more than five times if cell phone use begins in the teenage years rather than as an adult. In 2016 researchers at the National Toxicology Program, a federal interagency group under the National Institutes of Health, chronically exposed rodents to radio frequency (RF) radiation levels designed to roughly simulate what humans with heavy cell phone use or exposure might experience in their daily lives. What they found was that many of the thousands of rats that were exposed to greater intensities of RF radiation developed rare forms of brain and heart cancers, while none of the control group rats did.

With escalating rates of wireless device usage (including laptop computers, e-readers, electronic exercise trackers, TVs, cell phones, and meters that wirelessly track home electricity usage), our ambient exposure to radiation is constantly increasing. In her book *Zapped*, author Ann Louise Gittleman, PhD, provides excellent evidence for the health hazards of electronic pollution. We have seen many patients over the years who have presented with nonspecific, seemingly unidentifiable complaints, including fatigue, whose symptoms resolved once we identified their electromagnetic sensitivity and cut back on their usage of electronic devices. Over the years we've also noted that nearly all of our prostate cancer patients carry their cell phones in their pant pocket. We recommend using EMF-reducing cases and earphones for cell phones and shields for laptops.

The good news is that there are many foods that have been shown to help neutralize radiation. For example, there is some evidence that bee pollen may significantly lower the adverse effects of radiation exposure, making this sweet little superfood a wonderful addition to smoothies. But bee pollen notwithstanding, we absolutely must reduce our use and exposure to electronic devices.

Assessing Your Toxic Load

By now you may be feeling overwhelmed by the realization of how toxic our world and the products we live with every day are. It is hard not to be, given all this information. But knowledge is power, and assessing exactly how "toxic" you are is extremely important. If you already experience symptoms of toxicity—fatigue, allergies, chemical sensitivity, brain fog, constipation, chronic fatigue syndrome, and so forth—or if you scored high in the assessment quiz in chapter 2, then you may want to forgo laboratory assessments. The answer is already known. As environmental medicine expert Dr. Walter Crinnion once explained,

Taking It Further: Testing

Several companies offer testing for toxins: US Biotek offers an environmental pollutants profile; Genova offers a toxic effects panel; and Quicksilver Scientific offers a heavy metals test that includes potential nutrient toxins. We suggest talking to your health care provider about testing options.

You may obtain a detoxification profile by making a donation and plugging your 23andme test results that we discussed in chapter 3 into geneticgenie. Genova Diagnostics also offers a Detoxigenomic profile that shows detox-related SNPs.

"It is never a question of 'if' someone is burdened with toxicants. It is a question of is their toxicant burden a causative factor in their illness or if it is an obstacle to cure."[14] Starting with a realistic idea of how toxic their world is and what types of toxins are present has been paramount to the success of our patients.

Another critical piece of information to know about when it comes to detoxification is genetics. When there are SNPs in an individual's detox genes, there may be a significant impact on which drugs or medications should be used. Certain SNPs can affect the rate at which the body metabolizes and excretes certain compounds. It is critical to have your detox-pathway SNPs assessed by a professional. As you will learn in the next section, certain detox processes can be completely inhibited by variations in your genes and will therefore need to be circumvented through natural medicine.

How Detoxification Works in the Body, and the Impact of SNPs

Detoxification of the body is a multistep process whereby multiple organs mobilize, neutralize, transform, and eliminate toxins. Environmental toxins as well as toxins produced by the body as by-products of normal metabolism are processed the same way. The kidneys, intestines, gut microbiota, skin, gallbladder, and lungs all play a role. The liver, however, is the primary waste-treatment organ. It's the dump, so to speak. Toxins are sent to the liver, sorted, and processed according to type. Envision the recycling area of the dump: Plastics go in one spot, cans and bottles in another. Similarly, the liver sorts and processes toxic material by type, and the end products are added to the bile produced by the gallbladder. Toxin-infused bile then binds to fiber and is excreted through feces. Because bile is so critical in the removal of toxins, anyone who has a sluggish gallbladder (symptoms include intolerance to fatty foods, burping, and flatulence) or whose gallbladder has been removed should optimize the body's natural production of bile through the use of bile salts and bitter herbs (see below).

The process of transforming toxins into substances that can be safely eliminated from the body takes place in two main stages, usually referred to as phase 1 and phase 2 detoxification. Proper detoxification is an incredibly vital terrain process, and if either of these complex phases isn't working properly, it's as if the refuse collector went on vacation without a sub; the body's waste continues to accumulate, taking up more and more space, and becoming more and more rancid. This is where deep nutrition comes in—specific nutrients are absolutely required for the proper functioning of both phases of detox. When these nutrients (including protein and vitamin C) are not present, the refuse collector goes on permanent vacation, and carcinogenic compounds accumulate and circulate throughout the body, causing mutations and cellular damage.

Successful detoxification also hinges on the synchronization of the two phases. If phase 2 can't keep up with phase 1, the harmful intermediate toxins produced in phase 1 are reabsorbed by the intestines and circulated throughout the body, causing damage to the liver, brain, and immune system. It is very similar to an assembly line: If one person is working faster or slower than the next person, the entire process goes awry. People with active phase 1 detox systems but slow or inactive phase 2 systems are referred to as pathological detoxifiers. These are the folks who will have severe reactions to medications or supplements, or experience other extreme chemical sensitivities. A too-fast phase 1 can be caused by enzymatic and nutrient deficiencies as well as by certain SNPs, paint fumes, alcohol, cigarette smoke, alcohol, and steroids, all of which hasten the activity of phase 1 without a concomitant increase in the speed of phase 2. Let's look at these two phases and the nutrients required for their function.

During phase 1 detoxification, carcinogens, prescription and recreational drugs, hormones, endotoxins, pesticides, food additives, and other toxic chemicals are either directly neutralized or transformed into intermediate, often more toxic, compounds. Phase 1 detox is carried out by approximately fifty enzymes, collectively called the *cytochrome P450* or *CYP system*. (There are several enzymes commonly used in phase 1, including CYP1A1 and CYP1B1, whose function should be assessed in every person before starting any type of detox.)

During phase 1, for every toxin that is metabolized, one free radical molecule, or reactive oxygen species (ROS), is generated, therefore antioxidants are paramount for the entire detox process (we learn more about antioxidants in chapter 8). From a nutrition standpoint, in order for all these phase 1 enzymes to work, it has been clinically shown that a person must be consuming high-quality and bioavailable proteins, phytonutrients, vitamins, and minerals.

Detoxifcation depends on nutrition. In fact, the metabolism of toxic chemicals and drugs has been shown to be impaired when protein intake is low.[15]

In addition to the presence of all amino acids—and why vegan and vegetarian diets can be contraindicated during detoxification—the key nutrients involved in phase 1 detox include folate, vitamin B_2, vitamin B_3, vitamin B_6, vitamin B_{12}, and the antioxidant glutathione. Without the presence of these nutrients, cytochrome P450 enzymes cannot function, slowing phase 1 detox and pushing the assembly line out of balance.

Certain foods and nutritional supplements can influence both phase 1 and phase 2 by either overactivating, supporting, or inhibiting enzyme activity. These are called either *activators* or *inhibitors*. Compounds that can debilitate cytochrome P450 enzymes include a diet low in protein, or a diet high in carbohydrates, antihistamines, and grapefruit. The CYP3A4 enzymes reduce the amount of drug entering the bloodstream, and grapefruit juice contains compounds that inhibit CYP3A4, thus allowing too much of the drug to enter the circulation. Both caffeine and alcohol can overactivate phase 1 detoxification, and for some coffee is contraindicated. Conversely, cruciferous vegetables are needed for proper activation of phase 1 to avoid sluggish activity.

After phase 1, toxins that have undergone biotransformation are then sent to one of six phase 2 conjugation pathways for further transformation into forms that are safe for excretion. These six pathways involve *acetylation, glucuronidation, glutathione conjugation, sulfation, amino acid conjugation,* and *methylation.* Not surprisingly, the function of each of these six pathways is also entirely dependent on good nutrition and genetic function. For example, glutathione conjugation, which accounts for 60 percent of the toxins excreted in the bile, including industrial carcinogens, requires certain amino acids to be formed. And the sulfation pathway, which transforms toxins, neurotransmitters, steroid hormones, drugs, industrial chemicals, and the phenolics in plastics and disinfectants, requires adequate amounts of sulfur, which can be obtained only through the diet (through consumption of foods such as garlic, eggs, and cruciferous vegetables). We already know how important the nutrients folate and vitamin B_{12} are for methylation, a process that is critical not only to our genome but also for detoxification. Because various nutrients and amino acids are required for all six of the conjugation processes, they can become depleted over time; thus the importance of consistent, deep nutrition cannot be overemphasized.

Genes also regulate both phase 1 and 2 activity, and people who have SNPs in their sulfur detox pathway, for example (suggested by an intolerance to foods such as onions and asparagus), may need to follow a low-sulfur diet. Additionally, genetic SNPs in the cytochrome P450 system can either slow or speed the metabolism of toxins. Meanwhile, cruciferous vegetables (such as cabbage and broccoli), glycine, folic acid, vitamin B_{12}, fish oils, betaine, dill weed, caraway seeds, nicotine, birth control pills, and compounds from the Japanese horseradish wasabi have all been shown to stimulate phase 2 enzyme activity. Phase 2 pathways can be inhibited by a number of dietary deficiencies, including selenium, magnesium, vitamin B_2, glutathione, zinc, protein, and vitamin C. Aspirin and yellow food dye can also inhibit phase 2 activity.

In summary, the process the body uses to properly deactivate and remove carcinogenic compounds is a complex dance requiring nutrients every step of the way. Further complicating these steps is individual genetic variability. You can see why executing successful toxin removal is a whole lot more involved than simply drinking juice for a few days and picking up a cleanse kit from the local health food store. In fact, the number of people we have seen who have become horribly sick as a result of a poorly thought-out detox plan is in the hundreds. There are many considerations to approaching the successful elimination of toxic carcinogens, and next we will tell you all about them.

The Metabolic Approach to Reducing Toxic Burden

Due to how toxic our modern world is, implementing detoxification measures is not a question, it is mandatory. And it should happen frequently, in fact. Adopting a completely nontoxic lifestyle for the rest of your life is paramount. There is little point to eating a clean, organic, and wild diet if you continue to use highly toxic products. Therefore, the first step to implementing a nontoxic lifestyle is to purge your kitchen, bathroom, laundry room, and garage of all toxic products and replace them with natural ones. Take every action you can to avoid plastics, perfumes, new furniture, exhaust fumes, toxic cleaning products, paints, and solvents. While it might sound like adopting the lifestyle of a monk, it's actually not that difficult. You may be surprised by how many nontoxic products there are on the market. And yes, it can be expensive, so if you can't do everything at once, as you run out of a certain product, replace it with a new nontoxic one. Or make your own!

Once you have removed the toxic and carcinogenic items from your daily living spaces, foods, and beverages, then it's time to look at how to successfully and safely promote detoxification within the body itself. Our detox approach integrates therapeutic fasting, which has the ability to not only reduce toxic burden, including toxic side effects of chemotherapy, but also activate the immune system. We also infuse detox-promoting foods into the daily diet, along with proper hydration. We also strongly advocate saunas and regular exercise to promote sweating. Much consideration goes into the specific foods we recommend to the individuals in our practices, but those outlined in the following pages can be recommended to the general population.

We always let our patients know that detoxification can elicit uncomfortable systems as toxins become released into the system. Fatigue, diarrhea, headaches, joint pain, cold and flu symptoms, emotional symptoms, and more can all arise as a result of detoxification. This is sometimes referred to as a healing crisis or a Herxheimer reaction. These reactions can occur when the body tries to eliminate various toxins at a faster rate than they can be properly disposed of. The more toxic one's bodily systems are, the more severe the detoxification, or healing crisis, may be, so gentle approaches are needed in those circumstances. Detox symptoms can last from a few days to a few weeks, so it is important to be in close contact with a professional who can help you manage any uncomfortable symptoms. Throughout the entire detox process, proper bowel movements are essential, and therefore we advocate for enemas or colonic irrigation. By gently rinsing the colon with warm water, coffee, or oils, bowel movements and the removal of toxic materials from the liver are promoted. Do consult with a professional hydrotherapist or your primary care provider about the best type of enema or colonic program for you.

Top Detox Foods

Here we discuss the top foods for detoxification and, in general, recommend that at least two or three of these foods be consumed on a daily basis. Bear in mind that for any of the detox foods outlined below to work, a high-fiber diet is essential. Fiber acts like the car that drives toxins out of the body. (We discuss fiber in greater detail in chapter 6; see "The Metabolic Microbiome Reboot Plan.")

High-Quality Animal Protein

Foods to focus on here are pastured eggs, wild Alaskan salmon, and high-quality organic and pastured whey protein powder. Both phase 1 and 2 detox pathways are dependent on the presence of all amino acids, and these are found only in animal foods. Eggs are an excellent source of sulfur, a critical component of a phase 2 pathway; salmon is a great source of both vitamin B_{12} and the selenium that is needed for the formation of glutathione; and whey protein is one of the best foods to encourage production of the powerful antioxidant glutathione. It is important to eat these animal-based foods once you complete your fasts to properly eliminate the toxins that will be released. (We discuss fasting later in this chapter.)

Dandelion Greens and Roots

All parts of the dandelion (yes, the weed in your yard!) are edible and have both medicinal and culinary uses. They are an excellent addition to salads and smoothies. Dandelion has long been used as a liver tonic, and is one of the first greens to appear in the springtime, signaling the traditional time of year for the body to detox. The dandelion roots contain *inulin* and *levulin*, starchlike substances that support microbiome health. In fact, dandelions stimulate mucosal membranes all along the intestinal tract, which helps remove toxins from the bowel and also aids in their removal through the urine.[16] Dandelions also contain *taraxacin*, a substance that stimulates bile production. Dandelion greens are commonly used in the production of bitters. Why are bitters good? Because when the tongue recognizes the bitter flavor it sets off a series of reactions in the neuroendocrine system called the bitter reflex, which supports both digestion and detoxification. In Chinese medicine dandelions are thought to clear "liver wind," and in Ayurvedic medicine they are also used to clear heat. Energetically, people who have congested livers are often angry and "hotheaded," so foods like dandelion greens can help cool them down. Frequently drinking a bitter herb formula before meals is highly recommended.

Beets and Beet Greens

Beetroots are rich sources of betalain (red or yellow pigments) and betaine, also called lipotropic factor, which help the liver process fat. Several different betalains have been shown to exert antioxidant, anticancer, and detoxification effects.[17] Beets also happen to be an excellent source of folate, needed for the methylation detox pathway. It is important to note, however, that beets are on the high end of the glycemic spectrum. If you are following a ketogenic diet, large amounts of beets are not optimal. (One cup of beets contains 13 grams of carbohydrates and 9 grams of sugar.) However, small amounts (around 2 tablespoons) of grated raw beets make a great addition to a salad. Beet greens, which contain far less sugar than the root, are an excellent source of vitamin A, which is fundamental to immune functioning and becomes depleted with exposure to pesticides. Lastly, beet greens are a great source of vitamin C, which prevents the formation of carcinogenic nitrosamine from nitrates.

Lemon Zest, Rind, and Juice

The outer part of a lemon contains a *limonene*, a terpene that has been investigated for its anticancer and chemopreventive activity. Limonene can activate both phase 1 and phase 2 detoxification pathways. Terpenes such as limonene have been found to prevent carcinogenesis at both the initiation and progression stages and have been shown to prevent mammary, liver, lung, and other cancers.[18] Thus, adding lemon zest and eating the nutrient-dense rind is highly recommended. Lemon juice is high in vitamin C, which is helpful in the detoxification of heavy metals. In fact, vitamin C flushes where the dose of vitamin C is increased to bowel tolerance are an excellent way to promote detox. The zest of lemon can be added to just about everything!

Be aware that conventionally grown lemons can be coated with a petroleum-based wax to protect them during shipping. So be sure to always buy organic lemons. Starting the day with a glass of warm water with lemon helps to kick-start the liver and gallbladder and is another practice we highly recommend. This is also helpful because so many people are dehydrated. You should be drinking at least half your body weight in ounces of clean, filtered water a day (a 135-pound woman needs roughly 70 ounces of water daily).

Chlorella

Chlorella is green algae that has been found to inhibit the absorption of heavy metals including mercury, arsenic, and lead into the bloodstream. It contains what are called *phytochelating peptides* that work like natural chelating agents. By the way, chelation therapy is a process where EDTA (ethylenediaminetetraacetic acid) is injected into the bloodstream to remove heavy metals and/or minerals from the body and is sometimes used—and largely misused—in natural medicine. When a patient has leaky gut syndrome (more in chapter 8) they also have a permeable blood-brain barrier. Pushing chelation in people with compromised barrier function (and with detox SNPs) causes major neurological issues, and we don't advise it while someone has active cancer. However, foods like chlorella have shown evidence of having gentle metal chelation actions. Chlorella is very chemoprotective to the liver and has been found to induce cell death in liver cancer.[19]

Chlorella grows in fresh water, and there are also ways to grow your own. It is available in powdered forms, too, and makes a nice addition to a green drink or taken in water in lieu of wheatgrass shots (which we do not recommend due to the toxicity of cereal grains in any form) and when more powerful benefits can come from sea vegetables. Lastly, chlorella has also been found to naturally detox radiation. The one caveat with chlorella, and also with chlorophyll discussed below, is that they are both high in copper, so for folks who have angiogenesis and/or high copper levels these two should be avoided.

Chlorophyll

Chlorophyll is the green pigment found in plants and algae that absorbs sunlight and uses its energy to synthesize carbohydrates from carbon dioxide and water in order to grow. In a similar way, it is able bind and "trap" toxins in the gut, preventing their absorption and encouraging elimination. In animal models, chlorophyll was found to lower the bioavailability and accelerate the excretion of several environmental carcinogens, including benzene, and also offered protection from radiation. The toxin-trapping abilities of chlorophyll were also demonstrated in a human trial of residents of Qidong, China, an area with high rates of aflatoxin-induced liver cancer. Among the

180 people who took 100 milligrams of chlorophyll three times daily, urinary levels of DNA-aflatoxin conjugates (a marker for DNA mutation) went down 55 percent when compared with untreated people.[20] The best food sources of chlorophyll include all leafy vegetables, but organic spinach, parsley, and watercress in particular. Some practitioners recommend wheatgrass shots for their chlorophyll content; however, again, we do not recommend cereal grains or grasses because they are not part of a genetically supportive human diet.

Broccoli Sprouts

Broccoli sprouts are members of the cruciferous vegetable family, long hailed for their ability to promote detox on several levels, including enhancing the body's ability to remove pollutants. We also recommend other cruciferous vegetables including broccoli itself, cauliflower, and brussels sprouts, all of which are highly supportive of liver detoxification. Broccoli sprouts, though, get the gold star. In a randomized-controlled trial of approximately three hundred Chinese adults, those consuming a beverage made with broccoli sprouts every day for three months had increased excretion rates of two known carcinogens: benzene and acrolein. The rate of excretion of benzene increased as much as 61 percent over the twelve-week period. We strongly support adding broccoli sprouts to your daily diet, especially if you live near an airport or gasoline station. (Hint: These are easy to grow at home with a sprouting kit.)

Milk Thistle

This sharply spiked edible plant with bright pink flowers may be poisonous to the touch, but is powerful medicine for the liver. After careful harvest and spike removal, the roots can actually be eaten fresh. Its potent antioxidant activity has supportive effects on phase 1 detox by protecting the liver from chemical damage. Additionally, because it inhibits depletion of the liver's stores of glutathione, it is highly beneficial for phase 2 detox as well. Milk thistle has over a dozen powerful anticancer effects beyond liver support, including reducing cancer cell growth and inhibiting inflammation. Because milk thistle extracts exert such powerful effects on both phases of liver detox, there is conflicting thought about their use during chemotherapy, yet many oncology nutrition experts state that milk thistle will not increase liver clearance of chemotherapeutic drugs and does not blunt their effectiveness. It can be taken fresh or as a tea and grows throughout the United States.

Globe Artichokes

These vegetables are the edible flower bud of a plant from the thistle family, *Cynara scolymus*. They have a folk-medicine history of successfully treating liver diseases. More scientifically, artichokes contain caffeoylquinic acids, shown to have both regenerative and protective effects on the liver. Artichokes also promote the flow of bile and fat to and from the liver, facilitating a decongesting response. The powerful polyphenol-type antioxidants found in artichokes can contribute to the prevention and management of prostate cancer, breast cancer, and leukemia. Studies have found that the antioxidants rutin, quercetin, and gallic acid, all found in the edible portions of the artichoke leaf, are able to induce apoptosis of cancer cells and reduce their proliferation.[21] They make an excellent stand-alone low-carbohydrate, high-fat dinner if the leaves are dipped into mayonnaiase, oils, pestos, or organ-meat-based sauces.

Reduce Toxic Burden and Cancer Growth with Fasting and Calorie Restriction

To eat when you are sick is to feed your sickness.

—HIPPOCRATES

Instead of using medicine, rather, fast a day.

—PLUTARCH, *Greek historian*

The modern definition of fasting is abstaining from all food and drink, except water, for a specific period of time for a therapeutic or religious purpose. Throughout most of human evolution there have been times when food was scarce, and as a result fasting was a normal part of human existence up until the Agricultural Revolution when food became more abundant.

Periodic fasting is absolutely critical to human health and disease avoidance. There is not a person alive who can't start by fasting at least six hours a day. Perhaps in regard for its powerful, multilevel benefits, fasting is integrated into every major religion around the world. It is the primary published and research-supported approach to detoxification, and offers several other well-documented benefits, including immune system regeneration.

The body is resilient; it can survive for approximately forty days without food, as proven by spiritual leader Mahatma Gandhi (although we are not necessarily recommending long-term fasts, and certainly they should be done alongside a practitioner who can monitor your progress). During a fast, insulin decreases, growth hormones increase, and adipose tissue is eliminated, thus releasing stored toxins. Fasting has been found to reduce levels of polychlorinated biphenyls (PCBs) and DDT and also to reduce the toxic effects of chemotherapy agents. It makes instinctive sense: When wild animals get sick, they stop eating. Similarly, when people undergo chemotherapy, their appetite declines. They are being exposed to cytotoxic agents, and the body sends natural signals to stop eating.

Fasting is one of the best and most innate ways the body can heal itself. Those who assert that detox cannot be achieved by fasting may not have taken an anatomy and physiology course. The migrating motor complex (MMC), also known as the housecleaning wave, is a recurring motility pattern that occurs in the stomach and small bowel during fasting and is interrupted by feeding. During periods of fasting the MMC is activated approximately every 90 to 120 minutes and sweeps residual debris and bacteria through the gastrointestinal tract. When these bacteria remain stagnant, they overgrow and can lead to a condition called small intestine bacterial overgrowth (SIBO), a gut ailment that is becoming more and more common. Overgrowth of bacteria results in release of compounds that can damage DNA and also inhibit the absorption of nutrients, including amino acids and vitamin B_{12}, both critical factors in phase 1 and 2 detox. In general, Americans eat too much and too often. Eating right before bed inhibits the MMC and, in fact, research has found that it is optimal to limit eating to eight hours of the day during daylight.

Fasting is a form of short-term starvation that causes cells to switch into a protective mode known as *differential stress resistance* (DSR). During DSR remarkable changes in the levels of glucose, IGF-1, and many other proteins and molecules happen, and these changes are capable of protecting healthy mammalian cells and mice from various toxins. Cancer cells, however, do not make this switch, which makes them more vulnerable to chemotherapy drugs and other anticancer agents. In one study, ten patients who fasted in combination with receiving chemotherapy reported that fasting was not only feasible but also reduced a wide range of side effects, including nausea. This study, and the continuing work of Dr. Valter Longo at UCLA on the role of starvation and nutrient response genes on cellular protection, has opened up an incredible body of evidence to support of the many benefits of fasting. In mice, short-term starvation provided total protection to the animal, but not to the injected neuroblastoma cells against a high dose of the chemotherapy drug etoposide. These starvation-based strategies increase the efficacy of chemotherapy.[22]

We have seen it over the years in our practices as well. Our patients who opt to fast before, during, and into the day following chemotherapy seem to almost breeze right through the cytotoxic effects. Nausea is reduced, energy is retained, and even hair loss is reduced (hair loss is a common side effect of chemotherapy). Chronic calorie restriction has been known for decades to prevent or retard cancer growth, but its weight-loss effect has prevented its clinical application despite clinical evidence. Further, in human studies, those who did lose weight during a fast regained their normal weight once they started eating again. In summary, fasting helps healthy cells survive chemotheapy and reduces the toxic effects, while cancer cells take the brunt of it. Therefore, fasting should absolutely be considered as an adjunct chemotherapy approach, in direct contrast with the typical advice to eat as much as you can during treatment.

In addition, fasting and calorie restriction (lowering caloric intake by 30–70 percent) both have incredibly powerful effects on the immune system, including increasing macrophage and NK cell activity. In 2003, an article in the *Annual Review of Medicine* reported that fasting and calorie restriction is the most potent, broadly acting cancer prevention regimen in experimental carcinogenesis models.[23] Furthermore, dietary energy restriction specifically targets the IGF-1/PI3K/Akt/HIF-1 signaling pathways, which underlie several cancer hallmarks (cell proliferation, evasion of apoptosis, and angiogenesis), according to Dr. Thomas Seyfried, the current leading scientist behind the metabolic theory of cancer and author of *Cancer as a Metabolic Disease*. Amazing the healing power of "nothing"!

Reducing toxic load through fasting can be accomplished in a number of different ways. We recommend, and over the years have implemented with many patients receiving chemotherapy, fasting for twenty-four to seventy-two hours just prior to chemotherapy, and breaking the fast the day after treatment with a high-fat meal to further promote the ketogenic effects. For cancer prevention, fasting with water or green tea for three to five days once a month is excellent. By no means drink juice or consider the Master Cleanse (water, cayenne pepper, lemon, and maple syrup) during the fast; both are extremely high in sugar and will exert growth rather than inhibitory effects on cancer cells. One cup of carrot juice contains 9 grams of sugar and 22 grams of carbohydrate. Instead we recommend our "keto clean green drink": green tea, lemon juice, and melted coconut oil. Intermittent fasting is also an excellent approach. This involves either fasting or restricting calories to 400–600 a day for two days a week. In 2007, the *American Journal of Clinical Nutrition* found that alternate-day fasting—in which every other day the "fast" consisted of a single 400-calorie meal for women or a single 600-calorie meal for men—was associated with reduced blood levels of glucose, insulin, and IGF-1. The regimen was also associated with a long-term reduced risk of cancer. At the end of the day, in addition to reducing toxic load and stimulating the immune system, fasting promotes a healthy weight. And because toxins are stored in fat cells, reducing the amount of body fat means a person has reduced toxic storage space!

The Power of Sauna

It is interesting to note that the second-best proven method for removing toxins is sweating in a sauna. Interesting because the practice of taking saunas and steam baths has been a part of several cultures for thousands of years, just as fasting has. *Sauna* (a Finnish word pronounced "sow nah") means "bathhouse." Sauna has been a way of life in Finland, where it was invented, for over two thousand years. From a detox perspective, there is published evidence that using high-temperature saunas or baths in tandem with exercise, increasing doses of niacin (a B vitamin that makes you sweat when taken on an empty stomach), and electrolyte replacement reduces levels of chemicals including polychlorinated biphenyl (PCB) and hexachlorobenzene (HCBs).

This protocol, designed by L. Ron Hubbard, founder of Scientology, was originally dubbed the "Hubbard purification rundown." Today variations on the niacin, sauna, and/or charcoal flush are used in various clinical settings across the globe, achieving substantially reduced levels of toxins. Saunas and raising body temperature can reduce levels of BPA, phthalates, and other toxins. We always worry when our patients don't sweat. It can be a sign of impaired detoxification, and this is one approach to really encourage sweating.

One way to do this at home is to plan on three, thirty-minute sauna sessions (infrared saunas are great) a week. Just before each sauna session, take approximately 100 milligrams of niacin on an empty stomach and spend twenty minutes dry-brushing (to remove dead skin and stimulate the lymphatic system) and twenty minutes doing high-intensity exercise to stimulate the circulation. (Be aware that niacin, a vasodilator, can make you feel very flushed and hot, which can be uncomfortable but is not a cause for concern.) If you don't have access to a sauna, simply drinking yarrow or ginger tea in a hot shower or taking an Epsom salt bath can also encourage detoxification and is far more gentle.

Concluding Remarks on Coming Clean

The prevalence of so many new and untested chemicals in our environment and products of daily living—and the ways in which they cause cancer—is a prime example of how living so far removed from our natural environment promotes disease. Toxic burden can cause imbalances in so many terrain areas, including immune suppression, hormone imbalance, oxidative stress, and inflammation. Along with eating the clean and low-glycemic diet we advocate throughout this book, actively working to avoid or detox environmental carcinogens and toxins is of equal importance when it comes to creating a terrain that is inhospitable to cancer. Fasting exerts a powerful metabolic effect on many areas of the cancer process. Sweating exerts a powerful detoxification effect, as do foods such as broccoli sprouts, artichokes, and dandelion greens.

In the next chapter we explore the most exciting, evolutionary, revolutionary, and emerging terrain area when it comes to cancer: the microbiome. As it turns out, the health of the microbiome is also dependent on the metabolic effects of food.

CHAPTER 6

The Mighty Microbiome

Guts of Our Terrain

All disease begins in the gut. —Hippocrates

The microbiome is our newest ally in understanding how to prevent and manage cancer, one dirty Jerusalem artichoke at a time. The trillions of microbes that live within and on you make up this delicate body-wide organ that can work to either increase or decrease cancer susceptibility and progression. The role that these supportive microbes, also called beneficial bacteria, play in cancer came into medical consciousness only in the late 1990s. The *oncobiome*, in fact, is the term for an emerging area of investigation into the role specific microbes play in carcinogenesis. New information is emerging about the microbiome all the time. Since researchers began to peek at the relationship between microbes and cancer in the past few decades, the findings have been astounding. We've learned that bacteria are involved in regulating tumor cell proliferation, inducing cancer cell apoptosis, modulating inflammation, training our entire immune system, and influencing the metabolism of foods and pharmaceuticals; they also have a profound effect on genomic stability.[1] These invisible microbes have a larger-than-life impact on the terrain—as big as if not bigger than our genome.

In fact, since microbes have their own DNA, the microbiome is actually considered humans' "second genome." That's right: A complete additional set of nonhuman DNA lives inside each one of us, within each microbe.

Human microbial populations were much more diverse and prolific in pre-agricultural times, when dirt covered us like a brown blanket and before we adopted our modern daily hygiene habits. For millions of years humans wore no shoes; had no running water, no antibacterial soap, no bleached vegetables, no antibiotics; and ate a very high-fiber and microbe-rich diet. Modern improvements in hygiene and sanitation, along with the overuse of antibiotics and the standard American diet, have resulted in the killing off of our cancer-fighting microbial ecosystems, while giving rise to a set of noncommunicable, human-made diseases—like cancer. Food and lifestyle choices have everything to do with preserving the presence of beneficial bugs while keeping pathogenic or cancer-causing microbes regulated. So skip the shower, grab a dirty asparagus from the garden, and keep reading.

What Exactly Is the Microbiome?

Again, we go back in time. Humans coevolved with these *commensal* (from the Latin, meaning "sharing a table") microbes. Coevolution is the process of reciprocal and adaptive change in two or more interacting populations— think prey and predator, plant and herbivore—or, in this case, microbe and human host. Both organisms live together and benefit from each other's existence. In fact, according to the widely accepted endosymbiotic theory, human mitochondria are actually organelles descended from bacteria! *Symbiosis* happens when two different species benefit from living and working together. When one organism lives *inside* the other it's called *endosymbiosis*. The endosymbiotic theory asserts that if a large host cell ingests bacteria they can become dependent on one another for survival, resulting in a permanent relationship. According to the theory of human evolution—humans were first microbes. Over millions of years of evolution, the mitochondrion, which has striking similarities to a bacterial cell *and* has its own DNA, has become more specialized and cannot live outside the cell. Remember, mitochondria are responsible for creating more than 90 percent of the energy needed by the body to sustain life and support growth. Mitochondria drive metabolism, and supporting the health of mitochondria is at the heart of a metabolism-centric approach to cancer. Since there is increasing evidence that mutations in mitochondrial DNA–encoded genes contribute to the development of cancer, we cannot ignore their structure, function, and origin—which is microbial.

Individual microbes outnumber human cells ten to one and collectively weigh approximately 3 pounds, about the same as the human brain. In other words, approximately 90 percent of all the cells in your body are technically nonhuman. Rather, they are microbial cells—bacteria, viruses, protozoa, fungi, and archea—that perform a vast array of metabolic and protective functions for us, their "host." Entire ecosystems of microbes are resident at every location on the inner and outer surfaces of the human body. Hair follicles have their own set of microbes, as do the armpits, nasal cavity, skin, and groin. The miraculous tube that runs through your body from mouth to anus, the gastrointestinal tract, is home to the vast majority of microbes. In the mouth, the richest zone of microbes live between the teeth and gums. (We advise our patients to avoid dental work—especially root canals—when they have active cancer or are receiving treatment. It can release potentially pathogenic bacteria into the bloodstream, and we've seen many cancers recur on the heels of major dental work!) Downhill from the oral cavity, the bacterial capital of the body is the colon. One milliliter of colonic contents contains more bacteria than there are people on the planet.

Within each colony, there are different types of microbes that are grouped according to their type of relationship with us. Commensal microbes, also called microflora, derive benefit from us, but we do not benefit from them. Most of the commensal bacteria are *symbiotic* (meaning good) where they are, but if they relocate to an unintended location they can cause pathology. Specific microbes are supposed to live in specific areas of the body to carry out specific functions. For example, the bacterium *Streptococcus pyogenes* is part of the commensal flora of the nose of a healthy person, but can cause tonsillitis and strep throat if it migrates into the throat.

A *symbiont*, or beneficial microorganism, has a mutually beneficial "you pat my back, I'll pat yours" relationship with humans. A great example of a symbiont is *Bacteroides thetaiotaomicron*. Its "glycobiome" contains the largest collection of genes capable of metabolizing carbohydrates. These microbes, along with many others, are *required* for the metabolism and synthesis of macro- and micronutrients. This is the basis of much of the research that has discovered links among obesity, diabetes, and microbes.[2]

The last group is *pathogenic* microorganisms. These benefit from us, but can cause disease if their populations get too big. An infection of the stomach with *Helicobacter pylori* (*H. pylori*) can cause inflammation and damage the inner layer of the stomach, causing lymphomas. It is a leading cause of stomach cancer. And while *H. pylori* has been named a Group 1 carcinogen, it may also have a role in inhibiting development of gastroesophageal reflux disease (GERD) and esophageal cancer.[3]

Having a balance of all these bacteria is critical for maintaining homeostasis, and beneficial bacteria help keep the pathogenic microbes and fungi in check. The composition of microbial communities varies across different anatomical sites, and imbalances in the composition of the bacterial microbiota, also known as *dysbiosis*, are a major factor in human illness. Illnesses such as cancer, autoimmune conditions, obesity, asthma, autism, colitis, and mental disorders—as well as reduced vaccine response—have all been linked to the microbiome. In reality, our microbes are running the show.

But poor diet, antibiotics, sterile environments, and other threats to microbiome health can lead to the overgrowth of harmful bacteria and depletion of good bacteria. Too many pathogenic thieves leads to cancerous crimes in the terrain. For example, a 2013 study published in the *Journal of the National Cancer Institute* found that colon cancer patients tended to have higher levels of fusobacteria (a type of bacteria that promotes inflammation in the gut and fuels cancer growth) and lower levels of clostridia (a bacterial class that prevents the development of colon cancer by helping to break down dietary fiber and carbohydrates). Similarly, significant differences in the breast tissue microbiome have been identified in women with cancer versus women without cancer.[4]

Each person has a unique microbiome, just like a fingerprint or a face, which varies with gender, diet, climate, age, occupation, hygiene, exposure to animals, and other environmental factors. A baby's first bacterial inoculation happens at birth. Vaginally born babies are colonized by bacterial communities similar to their mother's vaginal microbiota, mainly *Lactobacillus*.[5] Following birth, colonization of the baby microbiota continues through contact with the environment and breastfeeding. Microbes are collected from what babies eat, touch, and put in their mouths—an evolutionary way that babies self-populate their individual immune-regulating microbiomes. Children who grow up around dogs have different microbiomes than those who do not. From age six months to three years, the number of species continues to increase, numbering about a hundred species in the gut of young infants to about a thousand in adults, and their functions also change. Babies have folate-producing microbes (needed for methylation!), while adults have more folate-harvesting microbes. By age three years, a child's microbiome looks a lot like an adult's, and it becomes much more stable.

Natural life events such as puberty, pregnancy, and menopause can cause expected shifts in the microbiome, after which they return to baseline. Puberty affects skin microbes by causing changes in skin oils, while pregnancy elicits changes in the vaginal microbiome resulting in the growth of species that will colonize and benefit the baby when it's born. Non-natural events, such as cesarean deliveries, antibiotic treatment, chemotherapy, chronic stress, diet changes, and many other factors, also cause shifts, or imbalances—dysbiosis—in the microbiome. But do not fear: Even if your microbiome has been damaged from chemotherapy or antibiotics, it can be repaired. (Take a look at the "reboot" plan at the end of this chapter.)

The Microbiome's Role in Health and Cancer

The mighty microbiome plays an entire orchestra of critical terrain roles in human health: immunologic, digestive, and metabolic, just to name a few. Specific microbes have specific roles, like a violinist or drummer, and can act to harmonize bodily functions, but can also play out of tune. For example, *Bacteroides fragilis* is largely considered useful for fighting off bacteria and fungi; however, it can also turn against the body, causing cancer in the colon when it is not kept in check by other microbes. All microbes must play together for a well-tuned terrain.

Here are just a few more examples of the roles various microbes play:

- More than 50 percent of xenobiotic, hormone, and toxin detoxification is facilitated by beneficial gut bacteria. On the flip side, pathogenic bacteria can directly secrete toxic substances while also promoting inflammatory pathways.
- Bacteria can actually change the DNA of human cells, which can lead to the onset of cancer. Scientists from the University

of Maryland School of Medicine found that a bacterial genetic transfer is linked to over-proliferation and the transformation of healthy cells into cancerous ones.

- Microbes are needed for the digestion, absorption, and synthesis of many vitamins and foods including vitamin B_{12}, vitamin K, fiber, and protein. They are also responsible for the synthesis of folate, which is produced by a number of *Lactobacillus* species.[6] As noted earlier, folate is critical for the epigenetic process of methylation, or gene silencing, to occur.

- Gut microbes—or a lack thereof—can significantly affect the efficacy of certain cancer therapies. Multiple studies confirmed that certain chemotherapy agents including cisplatin and also radiation rely on gut microbiota for successful eradication of the tumors. Germ-free mice were untreatable with these agents.

- Recent studies found that the composition of the gut microbiota is affected by the presence of tumor cells and involved in the development of cancer-related cachexia. However, a mix of good bacteria, including *Lactobacillus reuteri* and *Lactobacillus gasseri*, can reduce inflammation, anorexia, and muscle atrophy.[7]

We are continually astonished by what these invisible microbes can do. You will learn that it is our microbes that render soy and its metabolites as having an anticancer benefit—or not—and are also quite involved in estrogen metabolism. And while research continues to uncover the many different roles microbes play in cancer, one of the most compelling arguments for eating and living with our microbes in mind is their critical role in immune system function.

Microbes: Our Immune System's Personal Trainers

By virtue of its amazing capacity and responsibility to recognize, respond, and react to foreign and self-molecules, the immune system is central to the processes of health and disease. And microbes basically train the immune system how to do this. In the absence of effective microbiome-based training, the immune system does not learn to distinguish between what is safe to allow into the body and what to mount a response to. This results in haphazard, inappropriate reactions to such harmless environmental factors as allergens—pollen, mold, cat dander, and peanuts. And as we are witnessing in modern times, allergies of all kinds are on the rise. In 2013 the CDC reported that food allergies among children had increased approximately 50 percent between 1997 and 2011. Our missing microbes are largely to blame. A powerful example of this came in January 2015 when Australian researchers cured 80 percent of their study population of peanut allergies with courses of the *Lactobacillus rhamnosus* probiotic, while gradually increasing doses of peanuts themselves. Kids with peanut allergies were able to eat them again with help from their missing microbes!

Without a balanced microbiome, the immune system also fails to properly recognize and ignore harmless healthy human cells and tissues. This can lead to misdirected and unwanted autoimmune and inflammatory responses. Because we are lacking so many necessary microbes as a result of the hygiene practices enforced by modern living, our immune systems have started fighting things that do not pose a threat, like our thyroids and joints. Our intestinal and colonic mucosa hosts the body's largest proportion of immune cells—more than 80 percent! Without the presence of beneficial gut microbes to run a tight ship, the immune system is easily overtaken by pirates. In fact, research has found that forms of certain pathogenic bacteria are able to block and switch off a vitamin D receptor that is intricately involved in the immune response (more about this in the next chapter).[8] The examples go on and on, but the point is, the microbiome is literally the guts of our terrain. So why are our terrains are being overrun by thieving pirate bacteria while the good guys are jumping ship? Let's take a look.

Threats to the Microbiome

Many things can impact the health of our microbial populations, either positively or negatively. But many threats to the microbiome are also avoidable, preventable, and fixable! For those you cannot avoid, remember that the body has an incredible ability to heal. However, we cannot ignore the alarmingly increased rates of cancer that seem to grow in parallel to these modern assaults to the microbiome. It is time to become empowered and put a stop to many of the factors that are wreaking havoc with our microbes.

Cesarean Delivery

Invented during the Roman times, this procedure removes a baby from its mother by means of an abdominal incision and is necessary in some cases to save the life of the baby, mother, or both. And thank goodness we have this option for the people who really need it! However, as this procedure has become more and more safe and routine, it has become the preferred choice of some mothers to avoid the pain of vaginal delivery, accommodate work schedules, and for many other reasons. It is also the preferred option for some doctors—it's faster, more lucrative, and more easily scheduled. In 2013 payment for cesarean delivery is about 50 percent higher than average payments with vaginal births ($27,866 versus $18,329).[9] It's no wonder rates of cesarean births increased in the United States by 50 percent between 1996 and 2011.[10]

So what's the problem? It's simple: Babies are being introduced at birth to the wrong kind of bacteria. Infants born by cesarean delivery are colonized by bacteria found on the maternal skin surface, including the *Staphylococcus* species, while babies born vaginally are populated by their mothers' vaginal microbes. There is a reason human babies were designed to pass through the vaginal canal. The specific bacteria transferred from mom to baby are what train the baby's immune system to distinguish between what is "friend" and what is "foe." This process kick-starts the baby's immune system and is designed to help protect the infant from disease for its entire lifetime. New research has found that infants born by cesarean delivery have an increased risk of developing asthma, allergies, and autoimmune disease in later childhood.[11] Compared with babies delivered vaginally, those delivered by cesarean were 26 percent more likely to be overweight and 22 percent more likely to be obese.

Again, there are times when a cesarean delivery is imperative. When this is the case, there is the opportunity to "seed" the baby manually by rubbing the mother's vaginal secretions onto the baby (for more information about this, check out *Your Baby's Microbiome*, a book by Toni Harman and Alex Wakeford).

Diet: Breastfeeding, GMOs, and Low-Fiber Diets

The nutritional factor with the greatest impact on the development of a child's gut flora and long-term immunity is whether or not it is breastfed. "Breast is best," as the saying goes. In scores of studies, breastfeeding has been associated with a host of positive health outcomes ranging from fewer ear infections to a lower risk of leukemia. In fact, because breast milk is the most incredible superfood on the planet, some adults have begun using it in their fight against cancer. (Researchers in Sweden discovered that a substance found in human breast milk called HAMLET [human alpha-lactalbumin made lethal to tumor cells] has selective ability to kill cancer cells.)

Breast milk is rich in living white blood cells, immunoglobulins, and oligosaccharides that feed a particular strain of beneficial bacteria from the genus *Bifidobacterium*. Not surprisingly, the female breast contains a unique population of microbes relative to the rest of the body. *Proteobacteria* is the dominant type found in healthy breast tissue, and it is found only in small proportions at other sites in the body. Conversely, *Escherichia* and *Bacillus* have been found to dominate in cancerous breasts. Breast tissue produces high concentrations of fatty acids, and these bacteria are fatty acid metabolizers. *Proteobacteria* is also the predominant phylum in human milk. Studies have revealed that differences in the bacterial colonization pattern between formula-fed and breastfed babies lead to changes in the infants' expression of genes involved in the immune system and in defense against pathogens. Sadly, formula-fed children have been found to be eight times more likely to develop cancer than children who are nursed for more than six months.[12]

The World Health Organization recommends breastfeeding until a child is two years of age, with exclusive breastfeeding until six months. In ancient times, children were breastfed until age four or five, and in some cultures until age seven. Unfortunately, trends in the United States now show that less than 50 percent of moms were breastfeeding at six months, and only 27 percent were at twelve months. This means that approximately 70 percent of American infants are receiving formula before they are a year old, according to the CDC. Unfortunately formulas—even organic brands—can be harmful to the body's terrain and specifically the microbiome as they contain high amounts of inflammatory oils, cow's milk protein, soy proteins, and sugar, and are devoid of immune complexes and microbes. Commercial infant formulas can also contain genetically modified corn and soy ingredients. Research has shown that glyphosate disrupts gut bacteria, leading to an overgrowth of *Clostridium difficile* bacteria, which in turn create a toxic compound called p-cresol. This by-product has been identified as one of a multitude of factors that may be associated with autism.[13]

Recent data has shown that 26 percent of children hospitalized with *C. difficile* infections were infants younger than one year, and overall incidence of the infection among children has been rapidly increasing across the United States since 1997.[14] In addition, glyphosate has been shown to preferentially kill the beneficial bacteria strains *Lactobacilli* and *Bifidobacteria* while causing an overgrowth of pathogens. It has been proposed in several papers that the high consumption of GM foods by children is the reason behind the increased incidence of celiac disease, which has more than quadrupled since 1950.[15]

First foods are usually introduced into babies' diets around the age of six months. A March 2015 survey of 8,900 children ages two to eleven found that fewer than 10 percent ate the recommended four to five servings of fruits and vegetables a day, while more than 50 percent consumed more than the recommended daily amount of sugar. Fiber from plant foods is the preferred food of the microbiome, but sadly many kids are not getting any. Refined and processed foods, boxed cereals for one, are like bulldozers to the microbiome and contribute to the overgrowth of bad bacteria. Our preferred foods to first feed a baby are liver, egg yolks, avocado, and pureed greens.

The diet of American adults is no better. In 2014 the average daily dietary fiber intake was 16 grams per day, despite the recommended 38 grams. In 2009 the USDA's Economic Research Service found that in American adults a mere 3 percent of calories a day came from fruits and 5 percent of calories from vegetables (the majority of which were potatoes). This is a very far cry from the fiber-rich and plant-centered diet humans ate up until the Industrial Revolution in the late 1800s. Dietary fiber is the one food that beneficial bacteria require to survive; too little fiber starves them, and they die. Our microbes evolved eating hundreds of different kinds of fibrous plants and roots, not Cheerios.

Unfortunately, our modern diets are filled with microbiome-altering foods. Sugar and artificial sweeteners such as aspartame and saccharin have been found to alter microbial communities in such a way that the body's usual blood sugar controls are disrupted. Refined flours and cereal grains feed the harmful, abnormal bacteria and microbes in our gut. Consumption of gluten-containing grains like wheat and barley triggers the release of zonulin, a protein that leads to leaky gut, intestinal wall damage, and autoimmune reactions (see chapter 7, "Causes of Immune System Impairment," for more about this). Researchers have also discovered that overconsumption of alcohol directly damages cells along the digestive tract, driving inflammation in the gut. Last but not least, emulsifiers, detergent-like food additives, alter the composition of the gut's microbiota leading to increases in inflammation and other various health conditions including metabolic syndrome and colitis.[16] All of these factors and more can contribute to what's known as small intestine bacterial overgrowth (SIBO), a condition that has increased rapidly in the past few decades. The evidence against a high-sugar, grain-based diet is unquestionable. But what we really need to start working on is the rampant overuse of antibiotics.

Overuse of Antibiotics

The discovery of antibiotics occurred in 1943. Penicillin changed medicine forever by giving us the ability to successfully treat bacterial diseases such as pneumonia and many others; it was a medical miracle. In 1945, approximately sixty-five people *in total* were treated with antibiotics. In 2010, over *258 million* courses of antibiotics were prescribed. We've gone completely ballistic with them. Current estimates are that US kids have had an average of seventeen courses of antibiotics by age twenty, with an average of three courses even before age two. To treat anything from the common cold to ear infections to upper respiratory infections (at best 20 percent of which are caused by bacteria; most are viral), many doctors hand out antibiotics to kids as readily as grandmas hand out candy. For all of humankind's existence, we've lived with bacteria. (*Antibiotic* literally means "anti-life;" *probiotic* means "pro-life.") The outcome of many broad-spectrum antibiotics is analogous to clear-cutting an entire rain forest to harvest one tree. This is a huge problem, since antibiotics not only cause oxidative damage to DNA but also directly target and damage mitochondria.[17] Since damage to mitochondria is one of the root causes of cancer from a metabolic perspective, we really need to pay attention here.

Current wisdom asserts that antibiotics be taken only in life-or-death situations. In reality, many bacterial infections can be cured with probiotics and herbal antibiotics—or cure themselves. We have seen this hundreds of times with our patients and with our own children. If prophylactic antibiotics are recommended as part of your cancer treatment—which they often are because of immunosuppression—do consult with your naturopathic oncologist or nutrition therapist first. A side effect of antibiotic use is deep fatigue, not to mention the mitochondrial damage. And, in fact, many cancer treatments do not respond *unless* the gut microbiota is intact, but more on that in a minute.

Sadly, even if you are not knowingly taking prescription antibiotics, chances are you are ingesting enough of them in your diet to cause harm. Antibiotic use on farms grew from about 18 million pounds in 1999 to nearly 30 million pounds in 2011. Almost 80 percent of all antibiotics sold in the United States are used to increase growth in farm animals and are present in nonorganic meats, eggs, milk, and cheese. Subtherapeutic antibiotic growth promoters (AGPs) work in part by reducing the activity of an intestinal enzyme that inhibits fat digestion, so animals digest more fat and gain more weight. Just as antibiotics cause animals to gain weight, they do the same in humans. Though the FDA requires that farmers have a "washout time" between the last dose of antibiotics and the time an animal is slaughtered, this is rarely monitored. Foods in the grocery store are allowed maximum antibiotic residue limits but have been found to exceed these amounts almost 10 percent of the time. Two cups of milk, for example, can contain more than 50 micrograms of tetracycline, a drug that damages DNA and is not recommended for children under the age of eight years due to side effects, including dental complications. We can't emphasize enough the importance of choosing organic, always. So what are the alternatives to antibiotics? The following herbs have been used by humans for thousands of years. Talk to your primary care provider about using these before jumping on the antibiotic bus to microbe desolation land.

Herbs with Natural Antibiotic Properties

While there is certainly a time and place for antibiotics, their overuse is causing the current emergent crisis of superbugs, DNA damage, autoimmune conditions, and cancer. For all of human existence, plants have been used as the front-line medicinal treatment for everything from pain to digestive complaints. And because we all have an ancient genome, certain properties from the plants with which we have coevolved are still able to exert medicinal qualities against modern pathologies.

From a food perspective, there is a trio of herbs that have incredible natural antibiotic features that spare—and even support—microbes and mitochondria from damage: garlic, horseradish, and oregano. Even better, all three have benefits that extend beyond the microbiome, offering powerful immune and other anticancer benefits.

Garlic has certain antimicrobial properties that, paradoxically, are good for our microbiomes. One study shows that garlic hurts some of the bad bacteria in our guts while leaving the good guys intact. In fact three cloves of garlic contain the same antibacterial potency as an adult dose of penicillin. (Before penicillin, raw garlic was used to treat infected wounds.) Common pathological bacteria are a thousand times more likely to develop resistance to antibiotics than to garlic.[18] It doesn't stop there: Garlic has been found to inhibit tumor cell growth, induce tumor stress, and also stimulate the mitochondrial pathway for apoptosis in certain cancer cells, including brain cancer. Garlic should be consumed on a daily basis![19]

Horseradish is a pungent perennial plant related to mustard, cabbage, and other cruciferous vegetables. We mentioned it briefly in the last chapter as supportive for detoxification. It has very potent antibiotic properties, and is approved in Germany to treat urinary and upper respiratory tract infections. Preparations that include horseradish have been found as effective as antibiotics in the treatment of ear infection, certain flu strains, gastrointestinal illnesses caused by bacterial exposure, and pneumonia.[20] Horseradish also contains large amounts of cancer-fighting compounds called *glucosinolates*, which can increase the liver's ability to detoxify carcinogens, modulate inflammation, increase resistance to cancer, and suppress the growth of tumors. We suggest adding a spoonful of horseradish to sardine salads or in vegetable-based drinks.

Oregano, the famous Italian spice, offers incredible intestinal infection protection by destroying *Candida albicans* (commonly called candida), which is a yeast component of the gut microflora. Several constituents of oregano oil, including carvacrol, have been found to inactivate dangerous microbes that have become drug-resistant. Researchers at Georgetown University Medical Center found oregano oil effective against antibiotic-resistant *Staphylococcus* bacteria.[21] Furthermore, oregano oil has been found to be a very powerful killing agent against colon, breast, and prostate cancers. We always look to plant- and food-based medicine as a front-line treatment. When these and all other attempts fail, that is when, and only when, antibiotics should be considered. Now let's examine the other threats to our microbiome.

Sterile Environments

According to the widely accepted "hygiene hypothesis," modern life in hyperhygienic environments is responsible for the spikes in prevalence of childhood allergies, asthma, and cancer. Inculcation of beneficial microbes is hindered by the plethora of antibacterial home products and cleaning chemicals. We've all seen the TV commercials about keeping the kids "safe" with antibacterial wipes, when the reality is the exact opposite. Historically, people washed bacteria from their bodies and homes first using only water, then vitamin D–containing lard-based soap. The first definite evidence of soap-making was in ancient Rome, where it was made from goat's tallow and wood ashes. Modern antibacterial soaps are chemical agents used to disinfect surfaces and eliminate bacteria. They also destroy the skin microbes that are needed to absorb vitamin D!

Triclosan is an antibacterial and antifungal agent widely used in many different products, such as hand soap and sanitizer, plastic kitchen tools, cutting boards, high chairs, pencils, deodorant, clothes, toys, bedding, and other fabrics. When bacteria are exposed to triclosan for long periods of time, genetic mutations can arise. A 2014 study published in the American Chemical Society's journal *Chemical Research in Toxicology* found that triclosan, as well as another commercial substance called octylphenol, promoted the growth of human breast cancer cells. We can get just as clean with good old soap and water as we can with these highly toxic antibacterial products. Fortunately, in the fall of 2016, the USDA banned nineteen of the chemicals being used in antibacterial soaps, including triclosan. Unfortunately, most companies are substituting immunotoxic benzalkonium chloride, also an antimicrobial.

Thieves Oil: The Original Hand Sanitizer

The story goes that during the plague outbreak in the fifteenth century, a group of thieves were caught robbing from the dead bodies. Their secret to evading contagion—despite obvious exposure—was using a blend of clove, lemon, cinnamon, eucalyptus, and rosemary oils. In 1996, a lab test found a commercial thieves oil formula had a 90 percent effective rate against airborne bacteria.[22] We rub it on our hands and neck during airplane travel and use it to clean countertops. We have our patients diffuse it in the air at work during cold and flu season. It smells wonderful!

There are commercial blends available, or you can make your own. Here is the classic recipe:

40 drops organic clove bud essential oil
35 drops organic lemon essential oil
20 drops organic cinnamon bark essential oil
15 drops organic eucalyptus essential oil
10 drops organic rosemary essential oil

Mix all essential oils together in a dark glass bottle. Customize this by adjusting the quantities or adding other antibacterial essential oils such as oregano, thyme, or tea tree.

Medications and Chemotherapy

Anti-inflammatories, acid-blocking drugs, and chemotherapies can all damage gut microflora. There is a profound disruption of the intestinal microbiome, known as gastrointestinal mucositis, that is caused by chemotherapeutic agents. This is why probiotic, not antibiotic, therapy during chemotherapy treatment is especially important to maintain immune function. Chemotherapy and radiation treatments alter the population of gut bacteria in a way

Taking It Further: Testing

If you are looking for advanced ways to assess the state of your microbiome, you might check UBIOME, or ask your health care provider about a comprehensive stool analysis, a parasitology assessment, or a SIBO test. The American Gut Project, lead by Jeff Leach, author of *Bloom: Reconnecting with Your Primal Gut in A Modern World*, offered testing as of 2016, and results are going toward a large-scale research project.

that reduces the key bacterial strains involved in food metabolism. This can be a main contributor to weight loss and subsequent cachexia. Proton-pump inhibitor (PPI) use is associated with a significant decrease in microbial diversity, and users have a significant increase in pathogenic bacteria, including *Streptococcus*. Use of PPIs like esomeprazole (Nexium) has been linked to increased risk of bacterial infections, including *C. difficile*, yet they are the second-most prescribed drug in the United States. In many cases acid reflux can be easily treated with, you guessed it, probiotics!

The Metabolic Microbiome Reboot Plan

By now, we hope we have clearly established the critical role your microbiome plays in your overall health as well as both cancer prevention and progression. Because our mitochondria are actually microbial in nature, taking dietary measures to balance and repopulate our microbiome is one of the most powerful metabolic cancer deterrents around. So how do we use deep nutrition to optimize the health of the microbiome? By targeting the three main channels: specific foods, pre- and probiotic therapy, and changes to lifestyle, including hygiene practices. (That's right, we don't *need* daily showers, hand sanitizers, and antibacterial wipes. Let yourself get a little dirty!)

Of course, what you eat has the greatest influence on the composition of microbial communities within your gut. Numerous studies have compared the effects of a low-fat, high-fiber diet to an all-American Westernized diet. The composition of the microbiome shifts, in some cases within a matter of days; some species go up in number while others go down. The microbiome's dynamic ability to respond to diet is why our bodies can adapt to so many different ways of eating, regardless of how long it might take for our genes to catch up. And our microbes and genome have a lot to do with what diet best matches our current and long-term metabolic needs. The foods listed below are absolutely critical for feeding our beneficial bacteria and repairing damage done from the many threats to our microbiome.

Fiber

Dietary fibers are the structural parts of plants and are found in all plant-derived foods—namely vegetables and fruits—but are also present in (nonrecommended) foods such as grains and beans. Dietary fibers are non-starch polysaccharides, and cannot be broken down by digestive enzymes. Fiber therefore passes all the way through our stomach and small intestine like a scrub brush and proceeds to our large intestine, still largely intact. Then, in the large intestine, fiber is consumed by microbiota.

There are two types of fiber, soluble and insoluble. Soluble fiber dissolves in water, forms a gel, and is easily digested (fermented) by microbes in the colon. The best sources of soluble fiber are brussels sprouts, flaxseeds, and asparagus. Insoluble fiber meanwhile does not dissolve in water, does not form a gel, and is less readily fermented by bacteria. Insoluble fiber helps control the consistency of food in our digestive tract as well as the pace at which it passes through. Cabbage and celery are recommended sources. Both fiber types are important.

In addition to slowing the rate at which carbohydrates are converted to glucose, fiber also acts as the primary fuel for the growth of "friendly" bacteria. Some of the bacterial species in our gut are so specialized that they even digest specific subtypes of fiber. When food fibers are fermented in the large intestine by bacteria, their metabolism creates certain by-products, including short-chain fatty acids (SCFAs). Several SCFAs, butyric acid in particular, have been found to be critical for colonic health and reducing the risk of colon cancer. As it happens, butyric acid also prevents development of insulin resistance and promotes mitochondrial function.[23] Butyric acid plays major roles in metabolism and mitochondrial activity. A high-fiber diet, as you've heard even in mainstream recommendations, is therefore a key element to preventing and managing cancer. Try to consume as wide a variety of vegetables as possible. If supporting your microbiome is your top priority, then strive to eat at least thirty to forty *different* plants a week, and 40 grams of fiber a day. (Be aware that one common side effect of the ketogenic diet is constipation as the diet shifts from fibrous grains to high-fat foods. Adding the vegetables recommended below in addition to ground flaxseed and soluble fiber from psyllium seed husks, along with plentiful hydration, can help prevent this.)

Incidentally, there are resistant starches that also escape digestion and absorption in the small intestine. Recently there has been a buzz in the Paleo Diet and weight-loss circles about the benefits of resistant starch. Many followers of this trend have glommed onto something called industrial resistant starch. This is a chemically prepared, GMO "hi-maize"–resistant starch—in other words—a commercially produced potato starch. From what we have learned and observed, consuming isolated forms of resistant starch completely backfires when it comes to the health of our microbes, and we do not recommend it. Eat the whole plant!

Prebiotics vs. Probiotics

According to the WHO, *probiotics* are defined as live microorganisms that, when taken in adequate amounts, offer a health benefit to the host. *Prebiotics* are a category of nutritional compounds with the ability to promote the growth of commensal gut bacteria, especially lactobacilli and bifidobacteria. Simply put, probiotics are living microbes, and prebiotics are their food.

Prebiotics, inulin and fructooligosaccharides for example, are able to discourage growth of clostridia, prevent constipation and diarrhea, help keep blood sugar levels stable, and have even been found helpful in lowering ammonia levels for people with liver disease. Prebiotics are antagonistic to at least eight pathogenic bacteria, including *Salmonella listeria* and *Campylobacter*.

If supplementing with pre- and probiotics, which is usually warranted either during chemotherapy or after a course of antibiotics, we recommend a dose of 80–100 billion colony-forming units (CFUs) a day. (Note that use of either or both can cause gas or cramping for the first three or four days due to the demise of bad bacteria. These symptoms often dissipate after three or four days of continued or lowered use.)

Try to look for as many different strains of bacteria in supplements as possible. Research has found that our microbiota is most active at night, so the ideal time to take pro- and prebiotics is before bed. Rotate your brand of probiotics every ninety days to get the most benefit from the various strains. Probiotic supplements are excellent especially if you are unable to consume at least two or three of the foods listed below every day. And while any type of vegetable is going to be great for you, keep in mind that cooking foods reduces existing prebiotic content by 25–75 percent, so consuming foods in their raw state is optimal.

Top (Low-Glycemic) Foods for the Microbiome

It is essential to integrate microbiome-supportive foods on a daily basis, ideally with every meal. Here are the top microbiome-benefiting foods that contain probiotics, prebiotics, or both.

Leeks

The fiber content, vitamin K, and other anticancer properties make this vegetable a microbiome superfood. A member of the allium vegetable family, leeks are a great addition to soups or scrambled eggs. Note that ½ cup of leeks contains 6 grams of carbohydrates, so if you are on a low-carb diet, eat in moderation. Microbiome researcher Jeff Leach of the Human Food Project suggests consuming a leek a week.

Jerusalem Artichokes

Animal studies have found that consumption of Jerusalem artichokes adds significant microbial diversity to the gastrointestinal tract, in particular, bifidobacteria and lactobacilli. These potatoish-looking vegetables are very high in the soluble fiber inulin, a naturally occurring oligosaccharide belonging to a group of carbohydrates known as fructans. Start with very small amounts (¼ has 6.5 grams of carbohydrates, and they can cause gas), slice them thin, and sauté them with garlic and olive oil.

Fermented and Cultured Foods

In ancient diets around the globe, dairy products, fruits, vegetables, meats, and seafood were all fermented as a preservation technique. It is believed that hunter-gatherers would have eaten rotten and fermented fruits during times of scarcity, and repeated consumption could have created a taste for fermented fruits. Evidence of fermentation has been found to have occurred mainly within the last seven thousand years or so. Originally, fermenting kept food available for longer, an evolutionarily advantageous technique, and one that also came with health benefits. Fermented vegetables such as sauerkraut and kimchi—standard foods at every meal in some countries—teem with probiotics. Cultured condiments such as lacto-fermented mayonnaise, mustard, horseradish, hot sauce, relish, salsa, guacamole, and salad dressing can all provide billions of naturally occurring probiotics.

Garos and garum, the first known fish sauces, were prepared by fermenting fish blood and intestines in a salt brine. *Ketchup* comes from a Chinese word that means, literally, "brine of pickled fish." For a modern (and more palatable) approach to cultured foods, try fermented cabbage (sauerkraut), garlic, and radishes. If you buy commercial brands of fermented foods, make sure they are not pasteurized; this would mean that the food had been heated to a high temperature, destroying all live bacteria.

Wild and Garden Asparagus

Asparagus has a long history of use in India and other parts of Asia as a botanical medicine and is prized for its content of a phytonutrients called saponins. Saponins have been shown to induce apoptosis in human gastric adenoma cells among other anticancer activities. It has also been found that saponins are a major part of the asparagus plant's active immune system, acting as a "natural antibiotic," and in research they have been shown to exert antibacterial properties. Also very high in microbe-loving fiber, a whole cup of asparagus contains only 5 grams of carbohydrates, making it a great addition to a ketogenic diet.

Fermented Fish

Cultures that continue to incorporate fermented fish into their diet have some of the lowest rates of cancer worldwide. Popular fermented Japanese fish dishes include *funazushi* (carp), *gyosho* (fish sauce), and *shiokara* (salted fish guts). *Surströmming*, Swedish for "sour herring," are fermented Baltic Sea herring, a staple of traditional northern Swedish cuisine since at least the sixteenth century. *Rakfisk* is Norwegian fermented trout. It is interesting to learn that fermentation of protein-rich foods (like fish) not only enhances the overall protein content and bioavailability but also reduces toxic components such as heavy metals.[24]

Umeboshi Vinegar (Also Called Ume Plum Vinegar)

This fermented vinegar has an alkalinizing effect on the body; it can neutralize fatigue, act as a digestive aid, and prevent nausea. Beverages made with umeboshi vinegar should be a daily staple for those undergoing conventional cancer treatments as it reduces systemic toxicity. The citric acid component is believed to act as an antibacterial, helping to increase saliva production and aid in food digestion and nutrient absorption. Umeboshi vinegar has a very tangy taste that makes it an excellent dressing for crisp vegetables, like radishes.

Radishes

These easy-to-grow vegetables are a great source of the unique dietary fiber called arabinogalactans. In addition to boosting the activity of NK cells, which can attack tumor cells, arabinogalactans provides many other potent anticancer actions, including the inhibition of metastasis and protection against radiation-induced damage.[25] The fibers in radishes also help produce butyrate, the mitrochrondria-supporting short-chain fatty acid we mentioned earlier. Radishes are very low in carbohydrate and are a very powerful vegetable to include on a ketogenic diet.

Black Raspberries

One cup of this low-glycemic fruit contains 8 grams of soluble fiber and is a rich supply of ellagic acid. Ellagic acid is a compound known to be a potent antibacterial, antiviral, and anticarcinogen. No wonder our microbiome loves these! Phytonutrients like the ellagitannins found in black raspberries may decrease cancer cell numbers by sending signals that encourage apoptosis.[26] Black raspberry phytochemicals also protect the oral microbiome of smokers and may lower their risk of developing oral cancer. Studies at Ohio State University showed a 60–80 percent reduction in colon tumors in rats fed a diet with added black raspberries. The antioxidant content of black raspberries is about three times higher than blueberries, and they are extremely tasty!

Final Words on Fiber

We have no doubt that we will continue to learn more and more about the mighty microbiome and its role in health and cancer. It seems new research is published every day! But we cannot delay in taking action to help support the overall health of our microbes. Avoiding GM foods and animals treated with antibiotics while increasing fiber and fermented foods is the core of this terrain element's dietary approach.

With our fledgling understanding of how microbes help to train the immune system, we next take a closer look at particular cells of the immune system and the nutrients they require to function. Step by step, system by system, by addressing each one of these ten terrain elements, the body becomes more resilient. And cancer becomes weaker, one dirt-covered, fiber-rich vegetable at a time.

CHAPTER 7

Immune Function
Get on Guard with Deep Nutrition

Nature is a numbers game. We need all the support we can get as our immune systems and health are under assault from pollution, stress, contaminated food and age-related diseases as lifespans increase.

—PAUL STAMETS, *mycologist, author, and advocate of medicinal mushrooms*

Provided one has the correct level of vitamin, mineral, and nutritional input, the body can overcome disease.

—LINUS PAULING, *two-time Nobel Prize winner (1954, Chemistry; 1962, Peace)*

Right now, even as you are reading this sentence, your immune system is hard at work. Millions of cells are circulating through your bloodstream and functioning like your very own Homeland Security team. They are looking for and destroying foreign external and internal invaders like bacteria or viruses and also damaged and rapidly dividing cancer cells. In order to identify these harmful interlopers, immune cells need to distinguish between cells that are supposed to be in the body and those that should not. To do this, they need to know the difference between what is "self" and what is "nonself," and as we just learned, the microbiome provides this instruction. It is similar to the way competing sports teams wear two differently colored jerseys. Foreign elements (infectious organisms, foreign proteins) that are not supposed to be in the body wear a differently colored jersey than cells and proteins that belong in the body. The jerseys (in this case they're called *tags*) alert immune cells to the presence of a foreign invader to tackle. Sounds simple, right? Shouldn't the body's immune system be able to beat *all* disease then, as a rule? As simple as it may sound, this process can get tricky, since cancer cells have an incredible capacity to disguise themselves, suppress immune functioning, and even recruit immune cells to play on their side. Normally, though, it is the immune system's job to monitor all cells in the body to make sure they haven't become cancerous. This process is called *immune surveillance*, and confers important protection against the development of cancer. But because cancer is such a formidable opponent, our immune system needs to be at the very top of its game in order to trounce the competition.

Today our immune systems are in trouble. They've become unarmed, depleted, and confused by a variety of modern lifestyle and nutrition hab-its, including grain and sugar overload, stress, nutrient depletion, microbial depletion, and medications. Their ability to fight cancer has significantly decreased, and our immune surveillance systems have become weakened. Modern foods actually create a Code Red attack on our immune systems. Swarms of terrorist-like antigens invade our bodies on a daily basis with every bite of the standard American diet. Sounds overly dramatic, but it's true. Modern foods that are nonnative to our genes and gastrointestinal tracts— grains, beans, food colorings, and emulsifiers—cause intestinal permeability, also known as leaky gut syndrome (LGS). LGS is the root cause of modern immune distress and is a major focus of this chapter. LGS, in combination with a severely nutrient-deficient American diet, causes widespread malnour-ishment among our immune team. For example, an estimated 75–97 percent of Americans are deficient in vitamin D.[1] Scientists have found that vitamin D is crucial to activating our immune defenses and that without sufficient intake certain immune cells are unable to react to and fight off serious infec-tions—or cancer—in the body. These cells, called T lymphocytes or T cells, a type of white blood cell, are some of the most powerful cancer-fighting cells we have, and without vitamin D they are not activated—like hockey players without sticks.[2] (We discuss the role of specific nutrients in more depth later in this chapter. But already, now that you have learned about the significance of vitamin D, if you are pretty sure your doctor thinks nutrition has nothing to do with cancer, you may want to consider finding a new one.)

Because of the many factors we discuss, including a diet high in sugar, most Americans have chronically depressed immune systems. The evidence is everywhere. Immune conditions (both related and unrelated to cancer) are on the rise, and the statistics tell all: Between 2000 and 2009 autoimmune diseases increased by almost 25 percent. (An autoimmune condition occurs when the body mistakes self for nonself and begins to actively destroy its own tissues.) Autoimmune conditions, which include such disorders as type 1 diabetes, celiac disease, rheumatoid arthritis, Hashimoto's thyroiditis, and multiple sclerosis, now affect one in five people.

Immunodeficiency disorders also prevent the body from adequately fighting infections and diseases. The most common of these include varieties of leukemia and lymphoma, which have increased 20 percent since 1973. According to projections made by the Leukemia and Lymphoma Society, a combined total of 171,550 people in the United States alone will be diagnosed with leukemia, lymphoma, or myeloma in 2016. Approximately every nine minutes, someone in the United States dies from a blood cancer. In blood cancers like leukemia, a rapid production of abnormal immune cells occurs, and these cells are not able to fight infection the way healthy immune cells do. A healthy immune system is constantly providing surveillance and destruction of the many cancer cells naturally produced by the body before they have a chance to congregate and form a tumor. Therefore, keeping our immune system healthy is the cornerstone to cancer prevention and management.

Along with the extreme diet changes that have occurred over the last fifteen thousand years—with dizzying acceleration in the past two hundred—the human population has been exposed to escalated stress, widespread use of prescription medications, chemotherapy, vaccinations, sugar, fever suppression, microbiome eradication, and widespread nutrient depletion. It is no wonder our immune cells are overrun, tired, and confused; the hits just keep coming. Over time a weak immune system becomes more prone to infection, and chronic infection leads to further immune depletion, creating an environment that is very hospitable to cancer.

An estimated 5–15 percent of all human cancers worldwide are attributed to viruses. A virus is a small infectious agent that replicates only inside the living cells of other organisms. Because they have existed on Earth since its inception, it is highly likely that viruses may have been a primary cause of the earliest cases of cancer, those that arose before the Agricultural Revolution. In this chapter, we will give a general overview of how the immune system works and how cancer can block its kicks. We will detail the major threats to immune function, including ingredients found in almost all processed foods, even organic ones. And we will discuss Western medicine's approach to activating the immune system using targeted immunotherapies versus a natural approach to immune stimulation: mistletoe.

Here's the good news: With deep nutrition focused on repairing the intestinal tract through an autoimmune elimination diet, infusion with the top nutrients depleted in all cancer patients, including vitamin D and selenium, medicinal mushrooms, and lifestyle approaches like forest bathing, your immune system can get back in the game. If you scored high in the immune assessment section, and seem to have either frequent or no colds and flus (either can signal an immune problem), have an autoimmune condition, or chronic viral infection, then this chapter is of special importance to you. Your body has an incredible ability to heal. It just needs the right tools!

How the Immune System Works

The human immune system involves several organs including the thymus, spleen, tonsils, and lymph nodes. Lymphatic vessels, many types of white blood cells, and specialized cells that live in tissues all work together to form our immune system. The thymus gland, located in the center of the chest just above the heart, is the primary gland of the immune system. Thymus hormones stimulate the development of the major immune cells that regulate immune function. These cells (T cells) mature and receive their training in the thymus and then are released into the rest of the body. Go ahead and tap on your chest like Tarzan for a minute or so. You just activated your immune system a little bit through a process called "thymus-thumping." Thymus activity is highest after a child is born and its function decreases with age, so a little thumping never hurts. Another key immune organ is the

TABLE 7.1. KEY IMMUNE CELLS AND THEIR FUNCTIONS

Types of Immune Cell	Function
Natural killer (NK) cell	NK cells are a type of white blood cell and a component of the innate (nonspecific) immune system. NK cells are very proficient at destroying cancer cells and clearing them from the bloodstream.
B cell	B cells are a type of lymphocyte that can produce antibodies in response to the presence of an antigen. Memory B cells are a specific subtype of B cell that can remember a pathogen and produce antibodies more quickly in case of a repeat infection.
T cell	T cells are developed by the thymus gland. There are three main subtypes:
	Helper T (T_H) cells: These recognize antigens and help stimulate antibody production by B cells. They produce cytokines that activate other T cells and are required for almost all adaptive immune responses. There are two groups of T_H cells, T_H1 and T_H2. T_H1 is more involved with cell-mediated immunity and can be considered the anticancer mode, and T_H2 is more involved with humoral-mediated immunity processes and can be considered the autoimmune or antibody mode.
	Regulatory T cells (T_{Reg}s): Formerly known as suppressor T cells, T_{Reg} cells can suppress, modulate, or turn off the immune response.
	Killer T cells: Also known as cytotoxic T cells, these cells can kill cells that are infected, damaged, or cancerous.
Macrophage	An immune cell responsible for detecting, engulfing, and destroying pathogens and cancer cells.

spleen, located in the upper left abdomen. This is where many lymphocytes and other immunity-enhancing compounds are stored. With all these cells, organs, and glands, we can see why it's called an immune *system*.

As you may know, a variety of white blood cells are involved in the immune process. White blood cells, also called *leukocytes*, are the cells of the immune system that protect the body against infectious disease and other foreign invaders. All white blood cells—including B cells, T cells, and NK cells—are derived from stem cells located in the bone marrow.

Innate vs. Adaptive Immunity

The immune system is generally divided into two categories: *innate* and *adaptive*. As we learned in the last chapter our microbes also make up a third, critical arm of our immune system. In fact, our microbes essentially serve as the coaches for all immune cells. Without our microbes, our immune cells would look like a bunch of four-year-olds playing soccer: unorganized, untrained, and kicking the ball into their own goal. The innate immune system is one we are born with and consists of many elements including the skin and the mucous membranes found in the lungs, the nasal cavity, and the lining of the gut. The innate immune system is the first responder and offensive line when it comes to antigen detection. When this happens, cells like the macrophages and NK cells help by stimulating an inflammatory response (including fever and tissue swelling), during which the majority of pathogens and antigens are destroyed.

The *adaptive* (or *acquired*) arm of the immune system is an antigen-specific immune response that develops over time with exposures to different invaders, including the environmental microbes found in food and dirt. Once an antigen has been recognized, the adaptive immune system creates an army of immune cells specifically designed to attack that specific antigen or pathogen. Adaptive immune cells can retain a "memory" of a specific antigen, which allows future responses against the same invader to be faster and more effective. This is the concept behind how vaccinations work. It is estimated that the human body can create enough antibodies to recognize a total of one billion different targets. Pretty impressive. By means of both the placenta and breast milk, a mother transfers sufficient antibodies to her infant to protect the child against an antigen the mother was exposed to many years before. On the flip side, a mother who avoided dangerous childhood infections through herd immunity could put her child at risk by being unable to transfer specific protective antibodies.[3] In some cases, precluding development of immunity by avoiding exposure to certain viruses may not promote long-term immune health. Remember, humans lived without vaccinations for a couple million years. When we consider that autoimmune diseases did not appear until around 1900, which happens also to be when humans began actively vaccinating, we begin to wonder if we might not be enhancing our immune function in the best possible way.

T$_H$1 and T$_H$2 Balance in Cancer

In a healthy immune system both types of T helper cells—T helper 1 (T$_H$1) cells and T helper 2 cells (T$_H$2)—work together like a brother and sister on a seesaw to help keep immune responses balanced. T$_H$1 cells drive the innate immunity response and typically fight viral and bacterial infections inside cells. They also eliminate cancerous cells. A T$_H$1 response activates immune cells, including NK cells, killer T cells, other T helper cells, T$_{Reg}$ cells, macrophages, and IL-2 cytokines. T$_H$2 cells drive the adaptive immunity pathways, up-regulating antibody production to fight external threats like toxins and allergens. The primary immune cells involved in a T$_H$2 immune response are B cells, which produce antibodies.

A healthy immune system can "choose" which types of cells to produce and can easily switch back and forth between T$_H$1- and T$_H$2-type responses. Conversely, an unhealthy immune system can get "stuck" in one type of response, leading to excessive production of only one type of immune cell. Like one sibling's weight holding the other sibling in the air for too long, one response can prevail. When one of these systems is more active, it can suppress the activity of the other, causing what is known as either T$_H$1 or T$_H$2 dominance. When the T$_H$1 and T$_H$2 systems become imbalanced, inflammation increases and effective immune function decreases.

Autoimmune conditions, where the body mistakes self for nonself, are typical of T$_H$1 immune dominance. This response has been linked to gluten and other food allergies. T$_H$2-dominant conditions have been linked to the overuse of antibiotics and pesticides. When we are exposed to an allergen, the T$_H$2 system goes into overdrive and causes a massive inflammatory response. Subsequently the ability of the immune system to kill cancer cells is repressed. Most people in the developed world are stuck in T$_H$2 dominance. This is because our bodies are not exposed to as many parasites and bacteria as in the past (thanks to excessive use of hand sanitizers, soaps, and antibiotics) and our immune systems haven't had as much training or development. A mounting body of research is finding that deliberately exposing infants to germs offers them greater protection from illnesses such as allergies, asthma, and autoimmune diseases later on in life.

As the T$_H$1 mode is considered the anticancer mode, when people are stuck in T$_H$2, their ability to rid the body of cancer cells is diminished and the risk of developing cancer increases. Luckily, certain compounds have been found capable of stimulating both cell populations, T_H1 and T_H2. Even more fortunate is that there are compounds that regulate what's considered the fulcrum of the seesaw—and these include vitamin D, probiotics, and mistletoe. But first let's learn a little more about how cancer cells can successfully evade immune destruction and recruit immune cells to work for them, as well as the role nutrition plays in the process.

Cancer and the Immune System

Most cancer cells are actually very similar in appearance to normal cells. Like a person dressed in black and hiding in the shadows, cancer cells are able to create disguises that shield them from immune system detection and destruction. When a cancer grows, its ability to evade the immune system increases even more, despite increased size. This happens in a number of different ways. First, cancer cells can produce the inflammatory cytokines we just learned about as well as other substances that paralyze the activity of NK cells. This is not good because NK cells are like the Navy SEALs of the immune system—they are able to wipe out metastatic cancer and have a key role in preventing cancer recurrence and dissemination. Yet NK activity can be inhibited by a low-protein diet, stress, and exposure to toxins.[4]

Cancer cells are also clever at being able to get certain immune cells to switch teams, join them, and help promote their growth. Specific types of macrophages can embed inside tumors with the intention of activating a destructive immune response but end up helping tumors grow. These culprits are called tumor-associated macrophages (TAMs) and they secrete growth factors, stimulate angiogenesis, secrete enzymes that aid in metastasis, and suppress the adaptive immune system, neutralizing any cancer-killing activity. TAMs are found in most malignant tumors, and in some instances can compose up to 50 percent of the tumor mass. When they are working correctly, macrophages can literally eat cancer cells, which is what we want them to do. But the level and functioning of macrophages are compromised when vitamin B_{12} or B_6 consumption is low or when the individual has food allergies.[5]

Certain areas of the body, such as the lung and the gut, are more problematic from an immune surveillance perspective because they are relatively open to the environment and exposed to a larger amount of antigens than closed areas of the body, like bones. Because of its role in absorbing food, the gastrointestinal tract has an enormous surface area. The small intestine alone has a surface area two hundred times larger than the skin. Sections of the small intestine are lined with areas of lymphatic tissue called Peyer's patches that filter out dead cells, including cancer cells, and harbor a large number of lymphocytes. When the digestive system encounters a harmful or pathogenic antigen, cells in the Peyer's patches alert other T cells and instruct B cells to start producing antibodies in order to eliminate it. But the gut is continually being exposed to an unending number of antigens, thanks to a diet that is so rich in grains, beans, sugar, food additives, and colorings. This creates a chronic immune and inflammatory response—and allows cancer to escape amid the confusion. Perhaps you are wondering exactly how something as innocent as a piece of whole grain bread could devastate the immune system? We'll try to explain.

Causes of Immune System Impairment

We know that lifestyle choices such as smoking, drinking alcohol, having a sedentary lifestyle, and practicing excessive hygiene all contribute to immune dysregulation. And it should go without saying that all things on that list should be avoided. We further know that conventional treatments such as chemotherapy and radiation also significantly depress immune function, and we take specific precautions with our patients who are undergoing those treatments. As we noted earlier, sugar consumption severely hampers our immune function. When sugar enters the body, it basically pepper-sprays immune cells, paralyzing them for several hours following consumption. This is why cold and flu season generally kicks off right around Halloween: Not only are vitamin D levels dropping due to the lessened amounts of sunlight, but we celebrate a "holiday" centered on eating gobs of candy. The hard cold truth is that the high-sugar diet of so many Americans causes a chronically depressed immune system function. But also, not enough emphasis has yet been placed on grains, lectins, emulsifiers, and food colorings—additional elements of our non-natural diet—as well as nutrient deficiencies and medication overuse, all of which conspire to suppress immunity. We need to understand how each of these factors contributes to lowering our immune function in order to avoid them and begin to rebalance.

Immune System Offender #1: Food Allergens and Leaky Gut

Food delivers the greatest foreign antigenic load and presents the biggest challenge for the immune system. Every bite of food and sip of drink that goes into our mouths passes through the digestive tract, where an immune barrier works diligently to keep pathogenic invaders separate from the body. Basically, from mouth to anus, the long tube that is our digestive tract is lined with a single layer of specialized epithelial cells that constitute a protective barrier separating us from the external environment. This cells that form this protective layer are held together by structures called *tight junctions*. These tight junctions allow macro- and micronutrients like vitamins and amino acids to pass from the inside of the tube through the lining into the bloodstream, while keeping toxic particles like pesticides out. If this layer of cells and tight junctions develops a rupture, then the vast number of foreign antigens found in modern food suddenly gain access to the bloodstream. And these holes happen all the time. This phenomenon is called *intestinal permeability*, or leaky gut syndrome (LGS), and it is estimated that as much as 80 percent of the US population suffers from it.

Think of the plumbing system in your house. The pipes are designed to carry water to and from your sink, bath, or toilet. But when one of the pipes springs a leak, water can spill onto and damage the surrounding surfaces. That is what happens in LGS (though the holes in our guts are much smaller). Large food particles, pesticides, toxins, hormones, GMOs, antibiotics, and so on are not supposed to escape from the digestive tract. But when they do, it sounds an alarm to the entire immune system and, over time, results in a chronic T_H2 response. But what causes these holes, these breached tight junctions? Many things can, but gluten, legumes, emulsifiers, and solvents— staples of the standard American diet—are the biggest offenders. In essence, these foods contain proteins or other active substances that can create holes in our guts, and we need to avoid them at all cost!

Gluten

Gluten (from the Latin word for "glue") is a protein found in many grains, including wheat, barley, and rye. Researchers have demonstrated that eating these gluten-containing grains results in an increase in the level of the protein zonulin. This happens in everyone, whether or not they have celiac disease. As zonulin levels rise, the seal between intestinal cells is dissolved, creating spaces between cells that allow antigens to pass right through. The immune system then mounts an attack on these antigens, leading to food sensitivities, inflammation, autoimmunity, and cancer.[6] In fact, zonulin dysregulation has been observed in glioma patients and is correlated with a higher degree of malignancy of brain cancers.[7] Zonulin activity has also been linked to oral squamous cell carcinoma, lung, and pancreatic cancers.[8] Wheat proteins have also been associated with over seventeen different types of autoimmune conditions, including type 1 diabetes.[9] If you are not already convinced that a wheat- and grain-free diet is absolutely critical for cancer prevention, then read on.

Lectins and Emulsifiers

Lectins are sticky little proteins found in large numbers in many foods that have also been found to cause intestinal barrier permeability and immune system dysregulation. They have an affinity for binding to different body tissues. When lectins enter the bloodstream because of a leaky gut, they stick themselves onto multiple organs and tissues, such as the thyroid, liver, kidney, prostate, breast, pituitary gland, and pancreas. When this happens, the immune response against the lectins inadvertently causes inflammation to the tissue to which the lectin is bound. The result is organ-specific autoimmune conditions, like Hashimoto's thyroiditis, and the development of organ-specific cancers. In addition, the lectins that are found in cereal grains and legumes have been found to inhibit lymphocyte production and stimulate TNF, furthering both immune dysregulation and autoimmune processes.[10] For this reason, we advise our patients to avoid all legumes; this includes cashews, peanuts, chickpeas, lentils, black beans, pinto beans, soybeans, and kidney beans. Not only are beans a relatively new food to humans, but they are also high in carbohydrate, not protein. One cup of lentils, one of the highest-protein beans, contains 40 grams of carbohydrate and only 18 grams of protein. As a comparison, a cup of sardines contains 0 grams of carbohydrate and 37 grams of protein.

Another gut insult comes from the synthetic food additives that have found their way into almost all processed foods: *emulsifiers*. The most common emulsifiers in food use are mono- and di-glycerides, polysorbate-80 (P80), soy lecithin, and carboxymethylcellulose (CMC). Emulsifiers, too, have been found to cause increased gut permeability, alter gut bacteria, and directly contribute to colitis. Emulsifiers are a type of surfactant that allows oil and water to mix together and stay that way. (Think of trying to shake oil and vinegar together; they separate within a few minutes unless an emulsifier is added, right?) Emulsifiers inhibit separation, a task that for years humans used eggs to accomplish. Today the synthetic emulsifier market is considered to be the fastest-growing segment of the food additives market. These chemical versions are widely used in breads, chocolate, dairy products, sodas, salad dressings, and ice cream. Soy lecithins are found in many health foods, so while you think you may be safe shopping at your local co-op, it's more complicated than you think. It's hard to find an organic, fair-trade chocolate bar without it. So look for these ingredients on your food labels. There are many foods that do not contain synthetic emulsifiers; they are called whole foods.

Artificial Food Dyes

Last but not least in our list of LGS promoters are artificial food dyes. Colors like FD&C yellow no. 5, used widely in such products as yogurts, cereals, Play-Doh, and candy, are made from petroleum. Yes, the same substance that makes gasoline is in Froot Loops! In the last fifty years, the use of synthetic dye in food has increased 500 percent. Studies have found that exposure to food colorings can cause structural damage not only to the intestine, but to the spleen and thymus gland. Research has also found that food coloring binds directly with certain immunity-enhancing amino acids, lysine and arginine, and also causes a lowered serum albumin level (albumin is a form of protein). Insufficient albumin is very undesirable for anyone with cachexia. Meanwhile, food colorings are also linked to major immune problems such as dermatitis, rhinitis, and asthma attacks. The association of food dyes with behavior problems in children is undeniable. There are many natural ways to color food, and organic food companies use things like beet juice in products targeted for kids.

Now that we have identified the main culprits involved in causing LGS, it's important to understand another factor in lowered immunity: nutrient depletion. Americans are already poorly nourished from their processed-food-laden diets; LGS further exacerbates this by preventing the absorption of key vitamins and minerals that are required for the immune system to function efficiently. Next up we identify the nutrients that our immune system depends on so we can start eating more of the foods in which they are found.

Immune System Offender #2: Nutrient Deficiencies

A sufficiency of both macro- and micronutrients is required for a healthy immune system. Deficiency of just one nutrient results in altered immune responses, an effect that can occur even when the deficiency state is relatively mild.[11] The connection between nutrients and immunity is definitive, and nutrient deficiencies are the most frequent cause of depressed immunity.[12] Undernourishment and vitamin deficiencies arise from underconsumption of nutrient-dense whole plant and animal foods. Specific micronutrients (vitamins and minerals) and macronutrients (including the amino acids found in protein) are known requirements for immune system function. The five main immune micronutrients are vitamins A, C, and D, and the minerals selenium and zinc. These nutrients, along with complete proteins, support the immune system by a number of different mechanisms, among them modulating immune cell function, supporting an anticancer T_H1 immune response, producing antibodies and cytokines, and activating T cells, B cells, NK cells, and macrophages.[13]

Several clinical studies have also pinpointed the specific role each amino acid plays in various immune responses. Arginine, for example, has been demonstrated to enhance cellular immune mechanisms, in particular T cell function. In a study on postoperative surgical patients, arginine supplementation enhanced T cell response and increased the number of T helper cells, eliciting a more rapid return to normal T cell function when compared with the control group. The researchers found that arginine supplementation enhanced immune function in high-risk surgical patients and improved their capacity to resist infection.[14] Insufficiency of the sulfur-containing amino acids—methionine, cysteine, homocysteine, and taurine—adversely affects the functioning of T cells. Activated T cells can kill cancerous tumor cells both directly and indirectly. T cell activation is exactly what the new targeted immunotherapy drugs like pembrolizumab (more on immunotherapies in a minute) are designed to do. So why not give your immune system a boost with a little bite of arginine- and sulfur-rich Alaskan king crab or shrimp?

One of the scary aspects of a vegetarian or vegan diet is its effect on the immune system. A deficiency of dietary proteins has long been known to impair immune function and increase the susceptibility of humans to infectious disease.[15] Protein energy malnutrition causes immunodeficiency, which leads to increased frequency and severity of infection, thymus atrophy, and wasting of lymphoid tissue.[16] It causes the depletion of immune cells and an inability to make antibodies. Studies have shown that the immune system can be significantly compromised with even a 25 percent reduction in adequate protein intake. It is not only a deficiency of amino acids that can compromise the immune system, but an imbalance in the ratios among amino acids. Do you really want to take a chance with combining high-glycemic, lectin-laden grains in hopes of making a complete protein? No. Your immune system, just like your DNA, needs all amino acids present and accounted for in order to function. One of the very best foods you can eat for your immune system is broth made from the bones of a pastured chicken. There's a good reason why Grandma made chicken soup when her kids were sick: Several components of bone broth have been found to activate T cells and B cells!

When it comes to immune system nutrients, our bodies need a whole lot more than a daily multivitamin (which may or may not even contain bioavailable forms of the vitamins). The base camp of immune system nutrients should come from the diet—the way they did for the last couple of million years. The reason—as will become clear below—is that just as a full complement of amino acids must be present to work, there are incredible synergies between vitamins and minerals. In many cases they each require the other in order to function.

Vitamin A

Vitamin A is more than one vitamin; rather, it is a group of related fat-soluble nutrients. (Reminder: *Fat-soluble* means dietary fat must be present in order for absorption to occur, therefore these food sources and supplements should always be taken in tandem with dietary fats.) There are two main categories of vitamin A: *retinoids* and *carotenoids*. Retinoids are preformed sources of vitamin A and are found in animal products such as liver, kidneys, and butter.

Carotenoids, including beta-carotene and lutein, are found in plants. The plants with the highest content of ketogenic-friendly carotenoids include dandelion root, collard greens, kale, and spinach. Carotenoids can be converted by the body into retinoid forms. However, this conversion is inhibited by genetic mutations, insufficient bile acids, imbalanced microbes, excessive alcohol consumption, exposure to toxic chemicals, low protein status, low zinc status, imbalanced thyroid hormones, and the use of certain over-the-counter and prescription medications.[17] Long story short, in modern life, much of the time the conversion of plant beta-carotene to an active form of vitamin A doesn't occur. So we cannot depend on plant sources for retinoids.

Both retinoids and carotenoids provide the body with different types of anticancer benefits, but specific immune, inflammatory, and genetic benefits can only be obtained from the retinoid forms of the vitamin, specifically retinoic acid.[18] When it comes to the immune system, the retinol forms of vitamin A perform many functions. For starters, a deficiency impairs mucosal epithelial regeneration. This means that without enough vitamin A, those leaky tight junctions cannot be repaired. In addition, preformed sources of vitamin A enhance antibody responses, tumor cytotoxicity, and NK cell activity, and control leukocyte and T_{Reg} cell function. Unfortunately, a 2012 NHANES survey showed that more than 50 percent of Americans were deficient in *all* forms of vitamin A. We need to eat more of these foods. A retinoid- and carotenoid-rich meal would look something like a liver and dandelion root saffron sauté with a few dark cherry tomatoes.

Vitamin C

Even if they are resistant to natural medicine, most Americans are familiar with vitamin C and will take it—or (mistakenly) drink orange juice to try to get it—when they have a cold or flu. Known as the immune vitamin for good reason, vitamin C has a highly integral relationship with the immune system. It has also been shown to have potent anticancer actions, so it is unfortunate that over 40 percent of Americans have a deficiency of this vitamin, and over 75 percent of cancer patients have low levels—an indicator of poor prognosis. Not only do Americans not eat enough vitamin C–rich foods, which include the Barbados cherry, broccoli, red bell pepper, rose hips, and brussels sprouts, but vitamin C—a water-soluble vitamin—is also rapidly depleted during times of stress. When the body experiences any type of stress, our adrenal glands eat up vitamin C stores like it's going out of style, which explains why most people get sick after a stressful event.

Before we go on to explain how incredible vitamin C is, let's quickly talk about orange juice, since many people assume they are getting an immune benefit from drinking it when in reality, it's the opposite. Orange juice loses almost a third of its vitamin C (in the form of ascorbic acid) content after three days of being in a box; by the time most people buy it, it's been in the box for over five days.[19] (A sliced cantaloupe, by the way, loses more than 30 percent of its vitamin C content in fewer than twenty-four hours.) Furthermore, 8 ounces of orange juice contains 24 grams of sugar and is the equivalent of four oranges—without the fiber. We're pretty sure our ancestors were not juicing! Compare that 8 ounces of juice with a whole orange, which contains 7 grams of sugar and 2 grams of fiber, not to mention the anticancerous terpenes and the flavone-rich spongy white tissue found in the rind, and we see the whole orange is a far better choice for the immune system. Blood oranges are the most nutrient-dense varieties and have less sugar than the common navel variety.

This conversation brings us to a great example of how sugar depletes the immune system: Sugar and vitamin C have similar chemical structures and compete for absorption in white blood cells. They are both trying to enter through the same door, but there is only room for one. Even modest blood glucose elevations competitively impair the transport of vitamin C into immune cells. Sugar essentially negates the immune benefit of vitamin C. If you drink a liter of soda or eat 100 grams of sugar, the reactivity of white blood cells is reduced by 40 percent.[20] This is obviously problematic, since a high intake of vitamin C has been proven to reduce the risk of pretty much every type of cancer there is, including breast, colon, and pancreatic.

Vitamin C was first introduced in the world of cancer treatment in the mid-1970s by two-time Nobel Prize–winning biochemist Dr. Linus Pauling and a physician colleague, Dr. Ewan Cameron. In a comparison study, Pauling and Cameron gave one group of terminally ill patients 10 grams (10,000 milligrams) of vitamin C a day and another group no vitamin C. Survival rates among the patients who received vitamin C were almost five times higher than in those who received none.[21]

During the last forty years, we have learned that vitamin C has many immune-boosting and anticancer actions. Vitamin C

- has antiviral and antibacterial properties
- increases levels of interferon (a signaling protein produced in response to development of tumors)
- selectively increases the poisoning of cancer cells
- reduces the carcinogenic effect of toxins on DNA
- increases NK cell activity
- increases antibody responses and is required for the creation of immunoglobulins
- is anti-angiogenic, anti-inflammatory, and at lower oral doses works as a powerful antioxidant

Because it has been shown to exert all these impressive effects, vitamin C is now administered intravenously in progressive cancer clinics and is being actively studied in clinical trials around the world. At higher doses than can be tolerated orally, intravenous vitamin C (IVC) becomes a pro-oxidant, working similar to chemotherapy but offering greater protection to healthy cells. IVC has been found to stabilize many cancer cases, stopping the growth and spread of tumors, and enhancing response to chemotherapy. Before patients are considered eligible for IVC they must first be screened for a glucose-6-phosphatase deficiency (G6PD); those with this inherited metabolic disorder cannot tolerate such high doses of vitamin C and may experience hemolysis (red blood cell rupture) or severe kidney problems. A final word: If you take a vitamin C supplement, be sure it comes from a clean source; most vitamin C supplements are derived from genetically modified corn.

Vitamin D

Right up with vitamin C, vitamin D is also gaining a well-deserved limelight in the immune world. A deficiency in the "sunshine vitamin" (which is also considered a hormone) has been correlated with a higher susceptibility to many types of cancer, including colon, breast, prostate, and ovarian.[22] A vitamin D deficiency is also associated with increased autoimmunity problems and susceptibility to infection.[23] Low vitamin D levels can be the result of many factors:

SNPs; eating food products fortified with vitamin D_2 instead of D_3; not eating enough of the few vitamin D–rich foods; sunscreen use (human skin cells make vitamin D from sunlight) or insufficient time in the sun; and using harsh soaps that strip the key microbiota that help synthesize vitamin D from our skin. (To avoid this, Dr. Nasha likes to tell people, "Only soap up your pits and parts!")

Ultraviolet B light reaching the skin is needed to synthesize vitamin D_3—the active precursor form of vitamin D—and this cannot happen in places like the Northeast between November and March. This may be why more cancers are diagnosed in the winter than in the summer.[24] Everyday use of sunscreens that provide a high level of protection against the sun—and are used by more than half the US population—completely block photosynthesis of vitamin D and reduce circulating vitamin D metabolites. This results in a deficiency of the usable form unless there is adequate oral intake. Remember, sunscreen wasn't invented until 1936. Until then, humans not only spent far more time outdoors, but they also didn't wear sunscreen. The first proven case of melanoma was in 1987. We're certainly not saying that it's a good idea to get sunburned, but avoiding all sun exposure can also be very harmful. When you consider that most Americans spend less than fifteen minutes a day outside, you can see why we are having problems.

So for starters, many people don't expose themselves to the sun and also do not eat vitamin D–containing foods. There are two "food" forms of vitamin D: the synthetic vitamin D_2 (ergocalciferol) and the naturally occurring and more potent form, vitamin D_3 (cholecalciferol). Vitamin D_2 was first produced in the early 1920s, and is derived from irradiated ergosterol, a substance extracted from a mold called ergot that grows on rye and wheat.[25] This process was patented and licensed to pharmaceutical companies, which led to the development of a medicinal preparation of vitamin D_2 called Viosterol. Vitamin D_2 is now found in most fortified milks, cereals, and vitamins. It has far less bioactivity than the naturally occurring vitamin D_3, which is found in highest concentrations in cod liver oil; cold-water fish like salmon, sardines, mackerel, and herring; butter; and egg yolks. In the 1930s clinical trials found that cod liver oil could reduce the incidence of colds by a third. This was because of the vitamin D_3 content, yes, but also because cod liver oil is high in vitamin A. Studies suggest that vitamin D may be able to activate its receptor only with the direct cooperation of vitamin A. The role of food synergies should not go unrecognized, nor should we continue to isolate and extract vitamins and other compounds from food. Rather, we need to focus on the foods themselves.[26]

Regarding vitamin D's role in cancer and the immune system, a receptor for vitamin D is expressed on both B cells and T cells, and the activity of these immunologic cells can be turned up or down based on the presence or absence of this potent vitamin. This is how vitamin D modulates *both* the innate and adaptive immune responses, making it very useful as a T_H1–T_H2 balancer.

Up to 95 percent of the US population is deficient in vitamin D, therefore testing vitamin D levels is a cancer prevention strategy easily as important as mammograms, if not more so in our opinion. It is also important to test for SNPs that can impact vitamin D receptor sites. We see vitamin D receptor SNPs in almost all of our patients, and these folks often need significantly higher amounts of supplemental vitamin D than those who do not have the SNPs. Vitamin D receptor polymorphisms are also associated with more severe forms of malignancies in many cancers including prostate.[27]

Selenium

For a trace mineral, selenium has massive immune impacts. Low selenium intake is associated with an increased risk of all types of cancer. This is not surprising when we recognize that selenium is needed for the activity of glutathione peroxidase, our main antioxidant enzyme that protects us from inflammation-derived cancer. A selenium deficiency results in immune suppression, including impairment of NK cell activity. One study found that 200 micrograms of selenium daily increased the activity of NK cells by 80 percent and increased the tumor-killing ability of lymphocytes by 118 percent! This mineral can also protect the body from the damaging effects of the heavy metals mercury and lead. Selenium also exerts genetic protection. Those with mutations in their *BRCA1* gene have significantly greater frequencies of double-stranded DNA breaks per cell than healthy noncarrier relatives, but the frequency of these breaks is greatly reduced by selenium supplementation.[28]

The best food source of selenium is Brazil nuts. One of our most common nutrition prescriptions for cancer patients is to eat six Brazil nuts every other day. This serving provides 700 percent of the RDA for selenium, 19 grams of fat, and only 3 grams of carbohydrate, making Brazil nuts a ketogenic diet staple. Eating Brazil nuts is also important during chemotherapy, when selenium requirements go up. Other excellent sources of selenium include shrimp, lamb kidney, and skipjack tuna. Plant sources of selenium include asparagus and shiitake mushrooms. (If you are advised to take a selenium supplement, be sure it is in a methylated form.)

Zinc

Our final immune nutrient superstar is zinc. Zinc is involved in practically every aspect of immune function. It is crucial for normal development and function of neutrophils (another type of white blood cell) and NK cells. A zinc deficiency affects acquired immunity by preventing certain functions of T cells and T_H1 cytokine production.[29] Zinc improves thymus function and can restore immune function, making it particularly useful during cold and flu season. What's also helpful with zinc is that it competes with copper for absorption. High copper levels are a driver for many cancers, therefore balancing with zinc can be advantageous. Zinc also merits attention when evaluating the nutritional adequacy (rather, the inadequacy) of vegetarian and vegan diets. Animal products provide the most zinc, and the best sources are oysters, beef, fish, and shellfish. Diets high in legumes and whole grains are high in phytic acid, an inhibitor of zinc bioavailability.[30] Other ketogenic-diet-friendly sources of zinc include pumpkin seeds and pecans, which can be soaked overnight to reduce their phytic acid content.

———————

In summary, one of the best places to start boosting your immune system is by adding foods rich in the these vitamins and minerals into your diet. *Every* day, not just when you feel a cold or flu coming on. Now we'll take a closer look at the most common prescription medications used in America today and the effect they have on our immune systems.

Immune System Offender #3: Nutrient-Depleting Medications

There is certainly a time and place for prescription medications, and we are definitely not suggesting anyone discontinue their medications without consulting with their doctor. Many medications help save lives, and we are very thankful that they are available. However, it is important to understand how these medications affect our immune system and may cause immune suppression, especially when you consider the prevalence of use. Nearly three in five American adults take a prescription drug. A 2015 study published in the *Journal of the American Medical Association* reported the prevalence of prescription drug use among people ages twenty and older had risen to 59 percent of the population in 2012. The amount of Americans taking five or more prescription drugs is 15 percent. Prescription spending is also through the roof. In 2014 we spent over $374 billion on prescription drugs according to a report by the IMS Institute for Healthcare Informatics. Again, we have a drug problem.

And while these drugs do have the potential to do good, the majority of them are designed to suppress or inhibit actions or symptoms that are important messages from our body. Antacids, antihistamines, antibiotics, hormones, NSAIDS, steroids, antidepressants, and thyroid- and cholesterol-lowering medications are among the most commonly used drugs. In chapter 6 we referred to prescription medications as the leading cause of mitochondrial damage. We have also explored the destructive effects of antibiotics. The point is, many medications are overprescribed and overused, and in many, many cases they result in drug-induced nutrient depletion.

For example, antacids, histamine H2-receptor antagonists (H2 blockers), and proton-pump inhibitors are medications commonly prescribed for treating heartburn, GERD, and peptic ulcers. According to the labels, they are supposed to be used for a maximum of two weeks. However, most people use them for much longer. Numerous studies have found that these drugs can cause several nutrient deficiencies: They significantly increase the risk of vitamin B_{12} deficiency and decrease the absorption of folate, iron, and zinc. So not only are methyl donors getting depleted, but key immune nutrients are also falling short.

Women on either hormone replacement therapy (HRT) or birth control pills become depleted in vitamins B_6 and B_{12}, folate, and magnesium. As you would imagine, when the main methyl donors and immune nutrients get used up quickly, in the absence of a therapeutic diet or supplementation we see immune deficiencies. The common cocktail of diuretics and beta-blockers for high blood pressure frequently causes side effects like fatigue, anxiety, and insomnia—often leading to the prescribing of even more drugs. However, these drugs deplete the body of magnesium and zinc, both of which are needed for immunity and mental-emotional balance.

Nutrients are essential to every metabolic activity of every cell in the body. They are used up in metabolic processes and need to be replaced by new nutrients found in food or, in some cases, supplements. Some drugs deplete nutrients by speeding up their rate of metabolism, but the nutrients are rarely prescribed in tandem. (There are entire reference books on the topic of drug/vitamin interactions if you are curious to learn if your medication may be causing a nutrient depletion, including the *A–Z Guide to Drug-Herb-Vitamin Interactions Revised and Expanded 2nd Edition: Improve Your Health and Avoid Side Effects When Using Common Medications and Natural Supplements Together*, by Alan R. Gaby.)

In addition to prescription medications, the overuse of over-the-counter medications is also having a major impact on our immune systems—especially when these medications are given to children.

The Dangers of Acetaminophen for Fever Reduction

A large study of over twenty thousand children suggested that the use of acetaminophen (Tylenol, in the United States), even as infrequently as once a year, could have permanent, life-threatening health effects. The researchers at the University of A Coruña in Spain surveyed parents of 10,371 children ages six and seven years and 10,372 adolescents ages thirteen and fourteen years to see if their children had asthma and also to determine how often they had taken acetaminophen during infancy or within the prior year. Children in the younger age group who took acetaminophen only once a year were found to have a 70 percent greater risk for asthma. The children who received acetaminophen once a month or more were five times more likely to have asthma. Not only does acetaminophen cause immune problems, but it also causes direct DNA damage.[31]

Curiously, acetaminophen is most often taken to lower a fever. The irony is, we should be delighted to have a fever. Fever is actually a signal that the immune system is working *well*. We only started suppressing fevers in the 1970s and '80s; it is a completely modern idea. In the majority of cases, fever is a positive sign, and strong evidence that the child or adult has an active immune system. As Hippocrates reportedly said, "Give me a fever and I can cure any disease." Fever acts like a natural water purifier; it kills bacteria, viruses, and damaged cells, and induces apoptosis in cells running about that shouldn't be there. When we suppress a fever, we are suppressing the body's ability to fight off illness. Often the concern about a high fever is the possibility of a seizure, yet these types of seizures do not cause long-term damage. They are scary as can be to witness, but think of them as the body's way of shaking down a thermometer, cooling things down.

Suppression of a fever can also lead to viral shedding, which can facilitate increased dissemination of the illness. Dr. Nasha never considers suppressing a fever less than 102.5°F (depending on the comfort of patient and practitioner) and is comfortable working with temperatures much higher. It is scarier for her if a cancer patient does *not* mount a good fever; in this case she has to worry about immune system malfunction. Fevers actually upgrade and up-regulate the immune system. In fact, the use of applied heat to *induce* a fever has been used for a long time as a cancer therapy, and with great success.

Heat-Inducing Treatments: Coley's Toxin and Hyperthermia

In 1891 Dr. William B. Coley, who has been called the father of immunotherapy, injected streptococcal organisms into a patient who had an inoperable cancer. He hypothesized that the fever produced by the infection might, as a side effect, shrink the malignant tumor. And he was right. This is one of the first examples of immunotherapy. Immunotherapy is based on the idea that a patient's immune system can be stimulated or enhanced to attack tumors. Some clinics in Germany and Mexico still use "Coley's toxin," along with newer generations of fever-inducing therapies.

Meanwhile, there are hospitals in Germany that use high heat (106–109°F) to induce whole-body hyperthermia along with the administration of chemotherapy. In fact, many cancer clinics in Europe offer hyperthermia along with treatments like radiation, chemotherapy, mistletoe, vitamin C, and more. Hyperthermia therapy is rarely used on its own. It acts more like a Trojan horse, allowing the treatment of choice to enter the cancer cell to induce cell death. Heat changes the microcirculation of the body and helps to overcome drug resistance. Dr. Nasha has known several patients with stage IV diagnoses who had exhausted all other options and then achieved a complete remission with the help of hyperthermia. Heat is helpful as an immune therapy, so discuss options with your doctor, and think twice before suppressing a low fever!

The New Western Panacea for Cancer Treatments: Immunomodulation Therapies

As we have learned, our immune systems have massive potential to destroy tumors without harming healthy tissues. But we also realize there is much more to cancer than the immune system working alone; the other terrain areas are always at play. This is one of the limitations of immunotherapy, the new "cure-all"; it is an example of a targeted therapy that looks at only one aspect of the cancer as opposed to the whole terrain. Certainly the science of immunotherapy is changing the conversation in a great way for the first time since Nixon's War on Cancer back in 1971. We believe that hearts and pocketbooks are in the right place with the desire to learn more about immunotherapy, but while some assert that immunotherapy will overtake chemotherapy in the next decade, this shoot-for-the-moon initiative is largely missing the mark. There are several different types of immunotherapies. Monoclonal antibodies are one. These are synthetic versions of immune system proteins that are designed to attack a very specific part of a cancer cell. Yet despite this approach being spot-on in theory, a critical aspect of immunotherapy is that if an individual's immune system is not intact, or they have an ongoing autoimmune process, even powerful immunotherapies will not work and may in fact be extremely toxic, including causing severe autoimmune-stimulated organ failure of the kidney, lung, or liver.

A significant proportion of lung cancer patients also have autoimmune diseases, which makes them unsuitable candidates for these increasingly popular immunotherapy treatments. Dr. Saad Khan, an oncologist and researcher at UT Southwestern Medical Center's Harold C. Simmons Comprehensive Cancer Center, reported in the summer of 2016: "Immunotherapy treatments convey the risk of unpredictable, possibly severe, and potentially irreversible autoimmune toxicities affecting a variety of organs. With combination immunotherapy regimens, rates of these adverse events may exceed 50 percent."

The answer is to solve the problem of cancer from within, not to put yet another bandage on the bruise. Where we need to focus is on intrinsic immunomodulation therapies like deep nutrition—and also on mistletoe, the original immunotherapy.

Mistletoe: The Original—and Nontoxic—Immunotherapy

The white-berried European mistletoe (in Latin, *Viscum album*) has been used successfully with cancer patients since 1917, though as a treatment for diseases of the spleen it can be traced as far back as the time of Hippocrates (c. 460–370 BC). It is the most studied integrative cancer therapy in the world, with over seven thousand studies published to date. It is also the most utilized: 80–85 percent of German and Swiss and 60–70 percent of the rest of Europe's medical doctors integrate the use of mistletoe during chemotherapy and radiation. It is known to reduce adverse side effects—such as anemia, neutropenia, thrombocytopenia, hepatic toxicity, nausea, and vomiting—and also offer palliative support, improve quality of life, treat pain, reduce ascites, and increase survival. Mistletoe has the following mechanisms of actions and indications:

- Mistletoe lectins are directly cytotoxic to the cancer cell membranes
- Anti-angiogenic by lowering VEGF
- Stabilizes/repairs DNA
- Inhibits cancer spread
- Anti-inflammatory
- Immunomodulates (stimulates macrophages, T cells, NK cells, dendritic cells, cytokines, etc.)
- Acts as a fever-inducing therapy similar to that of Coley's toxin
- Enhances overall quality of life
- Can be administered subcutaneously, intravenously, directly into the tumor, and into abdominal ascites and pleural effusion

Dr. Nasha helped consult on a phase 1 clinical trial at Johns Hopkins University using mistletoe for all solid tumors. She has also been using it in private practice since 2006 with great success and continues to train doctors at clinics around the United States on its proper use. Mistletoe is an incredibly powerful immunotherapy that can help in the treatment of a variety of cancers. There are many other options out there, too, that can provide a boost to the immune system in a nontoxic way. Now let's turn to another method: a deep nutrition focus to optimize immune function.

A Metabolic Immune System Reboot

If you had a high score in the immune section of the questionnaire, have an autoimmune condition, hope to prevent cancer or halt it, or are looking to replenish your immune system following chemotherapy, then the following approaches are a great place to start. It is amazing how many foods possess the ability to support a healthy immune system. Of course, avoiding food altogether through fasting is perhaps the most effective way to rebuild your immune system. Several studies have found that fasting for at least two days can regenerate an immune system damaged by chemotherapy and cancer. What researchers have found is that fasting essentially "flips a regenerative switch" that prompts stem cells to create new white blood cells, completely repopulating the entire immune system. We detailed the benefits of fasting in chapter 5 in our discussion of detoxification, but there is also a major immune benefit from fasting as well. Here we discuss nutritional and lifestyle approaches that support the immune system, including following an elimination diet, the use of medicinal mushrooms, forest bathing, and hydrotherapy. These are all things you can implement through your food choices and choices for daily living. They are proven immune-boosting approaches that also happen to be side effect free!

The Elimination Diet and Gut Repair

One of the best ways to give your immune system both the nutrients it needs to heal as well as some rest—especially if you have an autoimmune disorder—is to follow a thirty- to ninety-day, Paleo-type, autoimmune elimination diet. There are many different ways to approach an elimination diet—which is why we recommend working with a nutrition-savvy practitioner—but the general concept remains the same. For thirty days or longer (the longer the better) follow a grain-, bean-, sugar-, and dairy-free diet. Also avoid all lectins, which includes nuts and seeds, eggs, all processed foods, and all members of the nightshade family. This includes tomatoes, white potatoes, eggplants, tomatillos, bell and hot peppers (not black pepper), and chili-based spices (including paprika). Nightshades can be problematic for many people due to their lectin and solanine content, both of which have been shown to contribute to intestinal permeability and increased inflammation. These compounds act as a defense mechanism for the plant against insects, disease, and predators. They are basically inherent poisons that protect the plant from predators, but are not so helpful for people with inflammatory autoimmune conditions like rheumatoid arthritis.

For some, an elimination diet provokes the same side effects as discontinuing drugs or alcohol. Some of our patients have reported headaches, fatigue, changes in bowel function, irritability, intense cravings, and other detox symptoms. Stick with it, though, and let your naturopathic doctor know about your symptoms. Some symptoms occur because people crave what they are most allergic to. When your immune system is used to fighting certain antigens on a daily basis, and then suddenly the antigens are removed, it will trigger cravings. Folks with blood sugar imbalances and high-gluten diets may experience carbohydrate withdrawal when gluten is removed. At first, patients will tell us things like, "My body just doesn't function without grains, I am too tired and hungry." But this is incorrect, and usually is an indication of an advanced degree of insulin resistance—even more reason to avoid lectin-rich grains! Additionally, because gluten works as an opiate in the brain, when it is removed people can feel extremely depressed. The food sources of opiates are gone! (Foods definitely can have druglike effects on the body. For more, read the excellent book *Grain Brain*, by neurologist David Perlmutter.) As you follow your elimination diet, adding foods like bone broth, foods high in zinc like oysters, and pre- and probiotic-rich foods like leeks and sauerkraut can all help with gut repair. (There are many wonderful books and cookbooks that can help you through an elimination diet. Two we like are *The Autoimmune Paleo Cookbook*, by Mickey Trescott, and *The Wahls Protocol*, by Dr. Terry Wahls.)

The provocation stage of this diet is when you begin to add foods back into your diet one at a time, in three-day increments, to see if they elicit a response. In general, we recommend keeping certain foods out permanently, but if you are curious to see if a particular food triggers a response, this is the way to approach it. When adding foods back in you may experience a headache, cough, digestive upset, abdominal pain, joint pain, or other complaints. Symptoms can appear within thirty minutes of ingestion or as delayed as three days later (these are immediate- versus delayed-onset allergies), which is why it is best to wait three days before adding each new food. We generally recommend at least thirty days of the elimination and repair diet before beginning a food-allergy test. If you have LGS and take a food-allergy test too quickly, most of the foods you regularly eat may show up as allergenic for you, and that can be quite depressing! Instead, take them all out for a significant period of time, repair your gut, then reintroduce them. The good news is that most people report feeling so much better once these foods are removed, they have no interest adding them back in! You are your own best doctor, and your body will let you know if it doesn't like a specific food.

Medicinal Mushrooms

Another approach to boosting your immune function is through the use of medicinal mushrooms. Since time immemorial, mushrooms have been valued as medicinal in Eastern medicine practices. They are one of the most powerful immune-enhancing foods there are. Mushrooms contain multiple bioactive metabolites that both invigorate and modulate our immune systems. Numerous clinical trials, both past and present, have or are currently assessing the benefits of using medicinal mushroom extracts in the treatment of cancer. And many benefits, both on their own and as adjuncts to cancer therapy, have emerged. Mushrooms have been found to complement chemotherapy and radiation therapy by countering several of the side effects of these modalities, including nausea, bone marrow suppression, anemia, and lowered resistance.[32] A couple of types to highlight first are the turkey tail mushroom and the maitake, both of which have shown powerful immune-boosting and anticancer activity—including blocking the formation of tumors. These mushrooms contain polysaccharides, substances that increase immune defense by enhancing the function of macrophages and NK cells.

We recommend incorporating medicinal mushrooms into your diet daily, but there is also some evidence that a monthly "mushroom feast"—eating a variety of mushrooms over a three-day period, almost like a mushroom fast—can be quite supportive of the immune system. Just as you rotate probiotics, it's a good idea to rotate the variety of mushrooms you consume to derive the most benefit. Fresh, dried, and powdered varieties of these mushrooms are wonderful in stir-fries and soups. We recommend the whole mushroom, best with stems and even part of the mycelium when possible, as opposed to extracts.

Many supermarkets carry mushrooms (just make sure they are organic!), and local farmers markets are also a great place to source uncommon mushrooms. (Before starting on any type of mushroom supplement, be sure to consult with your naturopathic doctor, as some can interfere with certain medications. Also, never pick a mushroom in the wild unless advised by an expert, and never eat raw button mushrooms; they can be carcinogenic, and it is best to roast them.)

Now we'll give a summary of just a few of the most studied and potent mushrooms used in oncology.

Turkey Tail

A seven-year clinical study funded by the National Institutes of Health and jointly conducted by the University of Minnesota and Bastyr University in Seattle found that turkey tail mushroom, in freeze-dried form, dramatically boosted immune function for women with stages I, II, and III breast cancer and also contributed to tumor shrinkage.[33]

Maitake

This mushroom, also known as hen of the woods, grows in clusters at the base of trees. This mushroom has been found to inhibit tumor growth in human clinical trials. It has also been found to increase the production of interleukins, neutrophils, T cells, and macrophages while ameliorating side effects of chemotherapy.[34]

Shiitake

A 2015 University of Florida study showed increased immunity in people who ate a cooked shiitake mushroom every day for four weeks.[35] By comparing blood tests obtained both before and after the experiment, researchers saw better-functioning immune cells and reductions in inflammatory proteins.

Reishi ("Mushroom of Immortality")

Reishi mushrooms contain beta glucans, a type of polysaccharide that has demonstrated antitumor and immunostimulating activity. Recent findings indicate that reishi mushrooms may increase NK cell cytotoxicity against various cancer cell lines. They may also protect against radiation damage.[36]

Lion's Mane

Lion's mane mushrooms have been demonstrated to stimulate NK and macrophage activity and also to inhibit angiogenesis, contributing to reduction of tumor size. It was also discovered that when the mushroom was combined with the chemotherapy drug doxorubicin, an otherwise drug-resistant human liver cancer became treatable.[37]

Cordyceps

Evidence shows that cordyceps is an immune modulator with potentiating and suppressive effects on both innate and adaptive immunity. It enhances the activity of NK cells and has been found to initiate T cell responses against microbial pathogens and tumors.[38]

Lifestyle Nature Cures: Forest Bathing and Hydrotherapy

There are many ways to boost your immune system through simple daily practices. In fact, many seem so simple it's hard to believe they actually work. *Shinrin yoku*, the Japanese art of "forest bathing," is one example. These contemplative walks, or moving meditations through the woods, are designed to reconnect people with nature and have been found to boost the immune system. In 2005 a small group of adult Japanese, both male and female, participated in a series of studies aimed at investigating the effect of forest bathing trips on human immune function. During this study subjects experienced a three-day/two-night trip to forest areas, and samples of blood and urine were obtained on Days 2 and 3 as well as twice during the month after the trips. It was discovered that forest bathing unintentionally promotes the inhalation of antimicrobial volatile substances called phytoncides (wood essential oils) derived from trees. Two such substances are α-pinene and limonene. Increased NK activity was found to last at least thirty days after the trip, suggesting that a forest bathing trip once a month would enable individuals to maintain a higher level of NK activity.[39] This is a wonderful and exciting example of the importance of spending time in nature for the health of your terrain!

The Wet-Sock Treatment

The wet-sock treatment, also known as the warming sock treatment, is indicated for sore throat (or any inflammation or infection of the throat), neck pain, ear infection, headache, migraine, nasal congestion, upper respiratory infection, cough, bronchitis, and sinus infections and works best if repeated until you are feeling completely better.

SUPPLIES

1 pair white cotton socks
1 pair thick wool socks
Towel
Bowl large enough to hold soaking socks
Several ice cubes
Enough cold water to fill the bowl

DIRECTIONS

Soak the cotton socks completely in the cold water. Wring the socks out thoroughly until they do not drip. Warm your feet. *(This is very important! The treatment will not be as effective and could be harmful if your feet are not warmed first.)* Warming can be accomplished by soaking your feet in warm water or taking a warm bath for five to ten minutes. Dry your feet and body with a dry towel. Put the cold wet socks on your feet first and pull the wool socks on on top of them. Go directly to bed. Avoid getting chilled. Keep the socks on all night. You will find that the wet cotton socks will be dry in the morning and you may sleep better.

Another natural element, water, and its therapeutic use, *hydrotherapy*, has been in use throughout human history. Today it is one of the most basic methods of treatment widely used in the practice of natural medicine. Hydrotherapy is the external or internal use of water in any of its forms (water, ice, steam) at various temperatures and pressures and sites for varying lengths of time. One popular regimen is a three-minute hot-water shower followed by a thirty-second cold-water shower, repeated several times.

Constitutional hydrotherapy, another method, stimulates the immune system by the application of hot and cold towels to the torso in a particular fashion. A wet-sock or warming sock therapy is home-based self-applied application of hydrotherapy. This practice involves going to bed wearing ice-cold wet cotton socks with dry wool socks over them. In the morning the feet are warm and the immune system is revitalized! Dr. Nasha has used this therapy with many patients, even children, for years with great success in aiding in the recovery from viral and bacterial illnesses or for anyone with a weakened immune system. Daily brief cold-water stress over a period of many months has been found to enhance antitumor immunity and improve nonlymphoid cancer survival rate.[40] There is good science behind the "bio-hacking" trend of cold-water plunges after all!

Winding Up Immunity

Our immune systems are critical when it comes to immune surveillance, our body's recognition of and response to cancer growth. But they are becoming weakened by modern diets high in sugar, grains, lectins, and artificial food dyes. These foods can cause LGS, which can both severely incapacitate and overstimulate immune responses and reactions. Modern diets are typically low in nutrient-rich vegetables and high in medications, resulting in danger-ously low levels of the vitamins and minerals that are required for a healthy immune system.

Following an elimination diet, with the subsequent addition of mush-rooms and key foods to provide immune nutrients on a daily basis, as well as spending time out in nature, can give your immune system what it needs to get back in the game. It's really possible! The immune system and our next terrain topic are very connected. We have learned how the immune system relies on inflammation to exert its effects. We now turn to the process that is considered the biggest driver of cancer—inflammation—also, as it happens, a process that is, you guessed it, profoundly affected by diet. Low immunity gives cancer cells a hall pass to run wild, while inflammation gives them the sneakers to help them run.

CHAPTER 8

The Inflammation-Oxidation Association

Extinguishing the Fires of Cancer with Food

Don't dig your grave with your own fork and knife.

—*English proverb*

The more severe the pain or illness, the more severe will be the necessary changes. These may involve breaking bad habits, or acquiring some new and better ones.

—PETER McWILLIAMS, *author and marijuana legalization advocate*

You can't start a fire without a spark.

—BRUCE SPRINGSTEEN

This chapter is a tale of two intertwined cancer-promoting events—both of which are a result of modern, imbalanced diets. Here inflammation and oxidation are bad influences on each other, together forming a vicious cycle that is at the root of the development of cancer. Inflammation is considered cancer's primary precursor; genetic damage is the match that lights the fire, and inflammation the gas that sustains it. When inflammation gets under way it stimulates the production of highly destructive free radicals (molecules with unpaired electrons) called reactive oxygen species (ROS). When there is an imbalance between the amount of ROS present in the body and the amount of antioxidants, their dietary counteragents, the result is *oxidative stress*. Oxidative stress causes both genetic and mitochondrial damage, which in turns signals NF-κB, the master protein that directs all inflammatory processes, to unleash the inflammatory cascade. One hits the other and the other hits back.

The most common disorders and diseases of today are all inflammation-oxidation based: arthritis, infections, allergies, autoimmune conditions, sinusitis, cardiovascular disease, colitis, and cancer.[1] Humans have gone from living in fear of infectious disease to aching in an age of inflammation. Americans are on fire, and our poor diet is fostering this rampant inflammation-oxidation cycle. Dietary factors are the primary contributors to inflammation and oxidative stress—the two main culprits are the overconsumption of inflammatory fats and the underconsumption of plant-based antioxidants. American meals are laden with synthetic inflammatory and trans fats found in such processed foods as salad dressing, barbecue sauce, corn oil, soybean oil, safflower oil, cottonseed oil, microwave meals, breads, chips, pizzas, french fries, cookies, ice cream, pastries, margarine, butter replacers, and fast food. Meanwhile, our meals remain largely devoid of the healthy omega-3 fats found in foods such as cold-water fish, olive oil, walnuts, and dark greens. Which have you consumed more of today?

Unfortunately, this dangerous imbalance of fatty acids stimulates the production of cyclooxygenase-2 (COX-2), the enzyme associated with inflammation and pain. (Small wonder that aspirin, ibuprofen, and naproxen sodium—all COX-2 inhibitors—are the most commonly sold over-the-counter drugs in the country.) Our Paleolithic ancestors ate a ratio of about 1:1, omega-6 to omega-3, while modern diets are closer to 20:1, sometimes higher. Our consumption of anti-inflammatory fats has dropped by almost a fifth since the 1850s, while our consumption of omega-6 pro-inflammatory fats has doubled in that time.[2]

This modern dietary trend, the root cause of inflammation, can be reversed only by the adoption ancestral dietary approaches. Yet the Western medical model uses drug-based treatments that merely mask the chronic pain so many Americans live with. We simply cannot go on with the all-too-familiar "take two aspirin and call me in the morning" approach. Especially when we are aware that chronic inflammation causes DNA damage; immune suppression; resistance to chemotherapy; inhibition of apoptosis; tumor promotion, proliferation, and invasion; angiogenesis; and metastasis.[3] As the burning embers of an omega-6-laden diet smolder on, high amounts of the inflammatory by-product ROS are generated. But many Americans are not eating enough dietary antioxidants—phytonutrients like vitamin C and the carotenoids found in berries, raw cocoa, and pecans—to counteract the inflammation. These foods, once staples in our diet, are now practically extinct on many modern plates. Reports from the CDC estimate that more than 90 percent of Americans fail to eat adequate amounts of dietary antioxidants, while only 9 percent consume 2–3 cups of vegetables every day.[4] And every time a chip is selected over a collard green, those DNA-damaging ROSs start to outnumber antioxidants, and genetic damage ensues. However, as we demonstrate in this chapter, given the right foods at the right doses, both inflammation and oxidative stress are preventable processes.

In fact, therapeutic doses of anti-inflammatory and antioxidant-rich foods ought to be mandatory cancer treatments. Why? Because our bodies are under constant attack from inflammatory agents. Eating to prevent inflammation and oxidation absolutely needs to be deliberate. We've covered a variety of inflammation-related topics already in reference to other terrain elements, so by now you understand that overeating foods such as gluten and grains causes LGS, a huge factor in the promotion of inflammation. Exposure to toxic chemicals not only causes inflammation but also generates a massive amount of free radicals. Excess weight—found on nearly two-thirds of the American population—causes the production of an inflammatory molecule called IL-6 as well as C-reactive protein (CRP), which a key indicator of inflammation.

But we have yet to deeply venture into the somewhat confusing world of *fats*. Since eating a high-fat diet is the centerpiece of our recommended ketogenic diet, it is essential to know the difference between—in the words of Udo Erasmus, one of the first "fat pioneers"—"the fats that heal and the fats that kill."

The whole good fat / bad fat controversy remains murky for many Americans. We have been bottle-fed misinformation regarding fat ever since Ancel Keys's fat-causes-heart-disease hypothesis, back in the 1970s. Over the years false fat fables trickled down through erroneous mainstream media reporting and eventually to doctors too untrained in nutrition to question the concept.

Unfortunately, the majority of the US population may still be confused about the positive effect certain fats such as those in eggs and LDL cholesterol can have on human health. Fortunately, it has recently been confirmed that the Sugar Association, a sugar trade group, paid three Harvard scientists to publish a review minimizing the link between sugar and heart health while vilifying saturated fat (this leak was published in *JAMA Internal Medicine* in the fall of 2016). The uncovering of these blatant conspiracies and cover-ups (and there are more!) is finally shedding light on just how unfounded the low-fat scam has been. Put simply, when we stopped eating the fats that had always been naturally present in the human diet (such as good fatty fish) and began eating synthetic fats, chronic inflammation, heart disease, and cancer ensued. Nothing has fueled inflammation more than the breakfast switch from eggs to oatmeal. High-carbohydrate grains promote weight gain and blood sugar disorders, while the loss of healthy fats has set us ablaze.

There is one simple biochemical aspect of fat that many seem to have overlooked for the past fifty years: Cholesterol is required to make all of our stress and sex hormones. It is so important to our terrain that our livers make it naturally. What is bad for heart health is sugar. Period. There are now hundreds of studies to prove it. (To learn more, read the bestselling *Big Fat Surprise*, by Nina Teicholz, or *Good Calories, Bad Calories*, by Gary Taubes.) Lard and butter are, and always will be, better than margarine.

In this chapter we discuss how the inflammation and oxidation processes work in a little more detail and how Western medicine's approaches to placate them are failing. We clarify the great antioxidant debate by offering evidence that supports the consumption of dietary antioxidants during chemotherapy and radiation, foods commonly discouraged by medical doctors not versed in nutrition science. We discuss the essential fatty acids, and debunk the myth that flax is a great source of omega-3 fatty acids (it is not, although it *is* great for hormones). Our metabolic approach to extinguishing the inflammation-oxidation terrain mutineers focuses on omega-3 foods, key antioxidants, edible herbs, and the remerging concept of earthing (skin-to-ground contact).

Now let's take a look at how inflammation works, its role in the cancer process, how exactly modern foods cause inflammation, and how Western medicine's drug-centered approach is not only failing to heal us, but making us worse.

Inflammation: The Wound That Does Not Heal

Inflammation is actually a normal and protective process designed to help safeguard tissues and promote healing during injury or infection. When you stub your toe, our old acquaintance NF-κB switches on the four cardinal signs of acute inflammation: redness (*rubor* in Latin), caused by blood vessel dilation; heat (*calor*); swelling (*tumor*); and pain (*dolor*). Typically a stubbed toe immediately turns red and warm to the touch, swells, and is painful and throbbing. These are a protective responses that help injured tissues repair and regenerate while protecting them from microbial infection. When NF-κB jumps in, it stimulates a variety of compounds—including ROS, neutrophils, COX-2 enzymes, interleukins, prostaglandins, and cytokines, including TNF—while activating angiogenesis, the production of new blood vessels, to the injured site.

Acute inflammation, in the case of the stubbed toe, is a good thing and persists only for a short amount of time, days to weeks. Where inflammation becomes problematic is when it shifts from acute to chronic. A chronic stimulation of blood vessel growth provides growing cancer cells nonstop food and oxygen, which is why cancer is often called a "wound that does not heal." So what causes chronic inflammation? Eating modern processed fats, grains, and sugar. Daily consumption of these foods is like stubbing your toe every day, month after month, year after year. Sadly, the standard American diet is the primary cause of chronic inflammation, heart disease, and cancer. Studies have found that those with diets higher in inflammation-promoting omega-6 fatty acids had forty times as much DNA damage as those with balanced ratios.[5]

In fact, chronic inflammation is considered a main precursor for cancer development, contributing to at least 25 percent of cases. Chronic inflammation can also lead to -*itis* diseases such as arthritis and colitis. (-*Itis* is a suffix meaning "inflammation.") Many cancerous tumors are preceded by chronic inflammation in a given organ. For example, people with chronic bronchitis are 15–20 percent more likely to develop lung cancer. And those with gastritis are more prone to the development of gastric cancer. In chronic inflammation, the agents engaged to reduce the acute inflammatory response stick around because the inflammatory trigger is never turned off. The daily stubbed toe, the daily bagel.

Constant activation of NF-κB in cancer cells is linked to elevated production of inflammatory mediators such as TNF, interleukin 6, prostaglandin E2 (PGE2), and ROS. Here the function of front-line inflammatory responders switches from protective to pestiferous, as they become promoters of tumor growth by activating genes involved in cell proliferation and carcinogenesis. When TNF lingers as a chronic, low-level presence in the body, it promotes cancer by encouraging the conversion of precancerous tissue into fully malignant cancers. In fact, tumor-promoting inflammation is one of the ten hallmarks shared by all cancer cells. The activation of NF-κB attracts those turncoat immune cells discussed in the last chapter called tumor-associated macrophages (TAMs) into a tumor. TAMs are dangerous because they produce the inflammatory cytokine IL-6, which in turn stimulates production of CRP, the well-known marker of inflammation. Not only are levels of CRP associated with resistance to chemotherapy, but both IL-6 and CRP can stimulate the production of ROS and impair antioxidant defenses.[6] This is a perfect example of how interconnected the Terrain Ten are. Here the inflammatory process and the immune system can together provoke oxidative stress. This is also another reason why we cannot tackle cancer with a one molecule–one target mind-set; it clearly must be a metabolic approach that addresses the whole terrain, not just the tumor.

Cachexia Is an Inflammatory Process

Inflammation also drives cachexia, the most deadly aspect of cancer. Cachexia is when cancer patients experience "wasting from within," a syndrome that is responsible for eventually killing an estimated 50–80 percent of patients. Cachexia is a multifactorial process that causes involuntary and continuous weight loss accompanied by systemic inflammation. It starts when cancerous tumor cells send out inflammatory cytokines, including IL-6, that release proteins from muscles and other places.[7] These proteins are sent to the liver, where they are transformed into glucose to feed the growing tumor. Cachexia is the reason behind the urgent exhortations not to lose weight during cancer treatment. "Eat whatever you want, just don't lose weight!" is the most common, and sometimes only, nutrition advice a cancer patient will get.

It is essential to understand that cachexia is in fact metabolism-based, *not* calorie-based, and research has proven that cachectic patients rarely respond to increased caloric intake alone.[8] This is important because practitioners of Western oncological medicine want to force-feed cachectic patients with high-sugar foods and inflammatory drinks like Boost—which only make it worse. Cachexia, like cancer itself, significantly alters a patient's metabolism, and it simply cannot be resolved using the calories in = calories out equation. During cachexia there is both a depression in protein synthesis and an increase in protein degradation, so making sure amino acid (that is, quality protein) consumption is high and complete becomes of utmost importance, while also keeping glucose low. Studies have also found that the ketogenic diet not only diminishes tumor growth and proliferation but also inhibits cancer-induced cachexia.[9] The "milk shakes to gain weight" model is actually lethal.

When it comes to weight loss, it is important to distinguish between the two types: pathological weight loss (cachexia) and therapeutic weight loss, which is beneficial. Practically every patient we have placed on a ketogenic diet has lost weight, at least ten pounds, very quickly. This is therapeutic weight loss, and a good thing. Typically, it's ten pounds of inflammation! Healthily thin and cachectic are not in same category whatsoever—and that's the conversation we have with patients and their family members who get nervous when weight loss occurs. The fact is this: It is more effective to stabilize and reverse cachexia by fasting than by repeatedly eating the wrong thing. By consuming the wrong foods (sugar and carbohydrates) the only ones benefiting from the glucose fuel are the cancerous hijackers, not the healthy cell hostages. While Western oncology has been beating the "eat as much as you can to prevent weight loss" drum, recent studies have shown that weight loss is actually beneficial in many cancer cases.

There are tests that can tell us if a patient is cachectic or just losing unhealthy, inflammation-promoting weight. The lab markers that show if the body has been "hijacked" by cachexia include albumin, protein, and CRP. If these labs confirm the patient is cachectic, we immediately become very aggressive with nutrition, and by that we don't mean calorie- or carbohydrate-dense, but ketogenic. There simply cannot be an insulin response during cachexia, that's the killer. Continuing to eat a pro-inflammatory and high-sugar diet only speeds the rate of cachexia's tissue destruction. This is a real paradigm-changing concept, and one that is deeply entrenched in Western medicine. But clearly eating ice cream when you have cancer is not working. Where we turn next is to how dietary fats cause inflammation and cancerous sparks to fly throughout our bodies.

Prostaglandins and Essential Fatty Acids

Good fats are critical to health, and their main function is to create the shape and structural stability of every cell in the body. The body makes all of its own fatty acids except for two that must be supplied by the diet, and are therefore named "essential" fatty acids: omega-3 and omega-6. Using these fats our bodies use multistep processes to create powerful, hormone-like end products called *prostaglandins* (PGs). There are three main groups of PGs, series 1, 2, and 3. Omega-6 fats are needed to make series 1 PGs, which are *anti*-inflammatory, via the action of COX-1 enzyme. But omega-6 fatty acids are also used in the manufacture of *pro*-inflammatory series 2 PGs via the action of COX-2 enzymes, which are derived from arachidonic acid. Series 2 PGs can counteract the effects of series 1 PGs, especially when series 1 PGs are outnumbered, an imbalance that promotes inflammation. The omega-3 fats make *anti*-inflammatory series 3 PGs, also via the action of COX-1 enzymes.

Here we want to briefly mention a talking point that the vegetarian community often hangs their hat on: Arachidonic acid mainly comes from beef, chicken, eggs, and pork. In commercially raised and even some organic animals fed a non-natural diet of organic corn and soy, the content of omega-6 fats is far higher and thus promotes inflammation. But in March 2010 *The Nutrition Journal* published a review of fatty acid profiles and antioxidant content in grass-fed and grain-fed beef and determined that grass-fed beef contains two to five times more omega-3s than grain-fed beef. Several studies also have found that exclusively grass-fed animals have higher levels of vitamin A, as well as increased amounts of the cancer-fighting antioxidants glutathione and superoxide dismutase, when compared with their grain-fed counterparts.

Foods in their natural state always provide more anti-inflammatory and antioxidant benefit. Even farmed "organic" fish (also fed grain) can have 20 percent less protein, twice as many inflammation-promoting omega-6 fatty acids, fewer usable omega-3s, and fewer nutrients overall than their wild cousins. If meat were the root cause of inflammation, then our ancestors—and the indigenous peoples of the Arctic who eat meat-centered diets—would have soaring rates of cardiovascular disease. But they don't. Cardiovascular disease did not appear until *after* the Agricultural Revolution. In short, eat your meat—but make sure it's organic and either grass-fed or wild.

To summarize the PG story, pro-inflammatory series 2 PGs are made by COX-2 enzymes (the primary target of NSAIDs, also known as COX-2 inhibitors) using omega-6 fatty acids. Anti-inflammatory series 1 and 3 PGs are made by COX-1 enzymes, using primarily omega-3 fatty acids. The main function of series 1 and 3 PGs is to block the series 2 PGs from being created. When there are not enough omega-3s in our diet, series 2 PGs predominate, thus igniting the wildfires of inflammation.

Another hurdle the body has to get over to create the very beneficial anti-inflammatory series 3 PGs is that a number of vitamin and mineral cofactors are also required. When the body does not contain sufficient amounts of vitamins C, B_6, B_3, magnesium, melatonin, and zinc, production of series 3 PGs is halted. It is halted because two enzymes that are critical to the creation pathway cannot be synthesized: the delta-5 and delta-6 desaturases (D5D and D6D). And as we learned in chapter 7, most Americans are highly depleted in vitamin C and zinc. This is where the inflammation problem becomes compounded. Consumption of trans fats (the type found in fried foods, chips, and more), radiation exposure, aging, and alcohol further inhibit the production of anti-inflammatory PGs by causing a significant loss of delta-6 desaturase activity and are associated with both inflammation and tumorigenesis.[10]

Debunking the Budwig Diet

Here is where a critique of the Budwig Diet, a frequently touted anticancer treatment, will be enlightening. In the 1950s German biochemist Dr. Johanna Budwig laid the groundwork for what we know today about the role flax plays in health. According to her research, people with cancer consistently lacked the essential fatty acids that are required to maintain the integrity of cell membranes. She noted that they were also deficient in albumin, a protein made by the liver. The lack of albumin explained the frequent anemia and cachexia she saw in cancer patients. Blood oxygen levels also become low in cancer because fats are required for the production of hemoglobin, the transporter of oxygen in the bloodstream. Budwig concluded that cancer must then provoke a dietary deficiency of essential fatty acids and hypothesized that replenishing the body with fats would help treat the cancer. Drawing from her hypothesis she prescribed her terminal cancer patients a mixture of a cream-cheese-like skimmed-milk protein called quark (*kwark* in Dutch) and flax oil. She also recommended carrot juice, buckwheat, rainbow trout, fresh greens, and flax oil enemas. She had the right idea, when it comes to fat, but unfortunately without the proper function of the D5D and D6D enzymes, flax oil remains in an omega-6 state, causing more inflammation, an effect that is further intensified if someone is going through radiation. The only preformed sources of omega-3 fats that do not require D5D and D6D enzymatic activity in order to produce anti-inflammatory prostaglandins come from deepwater oily fish. This may help explain why we generally don't recommend flax oil, but prefer high-quality fish oil to combat the production of pro-inflammatory series 2 PGs in cancer patients.

From Seed to Oil: Poisonous Processed Oil

Modern fats are also inflammatory because of how they are processed, and what they truly are: non-foods that are foreign to the human genome. Hydrogenated vegetable oil was invented in 1907, and in 1910 Procter & Gamble (a soap manufacturer at the time) filed a patent application to make it. They were motivated because they believed these oils would provide them with a less expensive product to use in place of lard in soap-making and cooking. Its original description was "a food product consisting of a vegetable oil, preferably cottonseed oil, partially hydrogenated, and hardened to a homogeneous white or yellowish semi-solid closely resembling lard. The special object of the invention is to provide a new food product for a shortening in cooking." Once the patent was approved, Procter & Gamble undertook a massive marketing effort to persuade homemakers to ditch butter and lard in favor of the new trans fat, Crisco. Yet another marketing scam that defamed animal fats in favor of industrial foods.

A trans fat is created when hydrogen is added to vegetable oil (a process called *hydrogenation*) to make it more solid. Partially hydrogenated oils are used by food manufacturers to improve the texture, shelf life, and flavor stability of foods. Partially hydrogenated oil is the reason modern bread

Snake Oil Salesmen:
The Original Omega-3 Fat Peddlers

Snake oil, derived from the water snake, has been a folk remedy in Chinese medicine for centuries, used primarily to treat joint pains, such as arthritis and bursitis. Its introduction to the United States occurred in the mid-1800s, with the arrival of Chinese laborers who came to build the Transcontinental Railroad. Astonishingly, the snake oil marketed by the original Chinese purveyors did exactly what they claimed it would: It relieved workers of the pains of their railway-building labors.

It has since been discovered that the soothing benefits of water snake oil are attributable to the plentiful omega-3 fatty acids that proliferate in cold-blooded creatures living in cooler environments. Omega-3 fatty acids don't harden in chilly water the way omega-6 fatty acids do. According to a 1989 analysis published in the *Western Journal of Medicine,* Chinese water snake oil contains 20 percent eicosapentaenoic acid (EPA), one of the two types of omega-3 fatty acids most readily used by our bodies.[11] For comparison, salmon, one of the most popular food sources of omega-3s, contains a maximum of 18 percent EPA.

Alas, most of the nineteenth-century snake oil salesmen found it more remunerative to harvest a less beneficial oil from a different type of snake, and this is probably why they got their bad reputation.

products can sit on the shelf for months without rotting like they should. Thankfully, in the summer of 2015 the FDA took a step in the right direction: It mandated that food manufacturers remove all partially hydrogenated oil from their products within three years. (As of this printing they still exist in many foods.) Yet what is still allows in food products are oils made from genetically modified, inflammatory sources. These include cottonseed (known as the "male birth control pill" for its negative effects on hormones), soybean, corn, canola, safflower, and others, and they exist in the majority of all processed foods. Just start reading labels; you'll be hard-pressed to find any packaged food that doesn't contain at least one of them. Even organic brands of processed foods rely heavily on these modern synthetic oils. (Hint: If it has a label, it's not a whole food.)

Traditionally oil was produced at home using mallets and manually operated wedge presses—and no heat. The stone mortars and presses used for olive oil extraction date back to 5000 BC and were used up until the Industrial Revolution. Now to become an oil, a bean or seed is exposed to toxic bleaching agents, deodorizers, solvents, high heat, and other "refining" processes. Processed oils are the liquid equivalent of white flour or white sugar: They are devoid of nutrients, noxious, and completely pro-inflammatory. What's more, when these oils are heated to high temperatures (as with frying or baking), they cause major oxidative stress in the body.

Selection of oils that have been properly extracted is paramount; cold-pressed with a "bottled on" date is key, and cooking them at the right temperature is also important. Low and slow is the theme for healthy cooking! We recommend avoiding all processed oils and making sure to buy food that doesn't have more than one ingredient—or if it does, that it doesn't contain any omega-6 oils. Olive, flax, and hemp oils should never be heated. Use coconut oil, grass-fed lard, tallow, or pastured butter instead.

The Western Medicine Approach to Inflammation

We have an inflammation epidemic in this country. More than thirty billion tablets of NSAIDS (aspirin and ibuprofen, for example) are sold every year, more than any other type of over-the-counter medication. In 2015 the arthritis drug adalimumab (Humira) was the bestselling prescription drug; its sales topped $8.6 billion. Adalimumab is an inhibitor of TNF (remember that TNF is the cytokine implicated in many inflammatory conditions, including rheumatoid arthritis and inflammatory bowel disease). The summary of a study reported in the December 2010 journal *Drug, Healthcare and Patient Safety* asserted that "TNF-α inhibitors are potent drugs and have theoretical and real risks in terms of decreasing tumor surveillance and allowing cancer cells to grow and proliferate. Clinical trials have shown that there is a higher than expected rate of lymphoid malignancies after TNF-α."[12] Yet another example of a drug being used to block or suppress a natural process of the body—in this case inflammation—that instead appears to cause cancer.

The reason NSAIDs are currently being studied in the prevention of cancer is because of their role in reducing inflammation. These drugs have been found to block carcinogenesis by reducing the production of certain pro-inflammatory cytokines such as IL-6 and TNF. However, they come with substantial side effects: alteration of the microbiome, inhibition of mitochondrial function, increased gastrointestinal bleeding. Aspirin was the first COX inhibitor, and now there are over fifty.

The main problem with many COX inhibitors is that they block both COX-1 and COX-2. COX-1 is critical for maintaining the integrity of the gastrointestinal lining, and use of an inhibiting medication therefore contributes to LGS.

Cortisone, a synthetic form of cortisol (the stress hormone), is a steroid used as an anti-inflammatory agent in the treatment of rheumatoid arthritis and is also often given as an adjuvant treatment in cancer. The problem with cortisone, hydrocortisone, and other corticosteroids is that that they cause short-term spikes in blood sugar levels, making it nearly impossible to achieve ketosis while on them. Further, their use also interferes with the metabolism of vitamin D, zinc, folic acid, B_6, and B_{12}, essentially halting methylation while causing immune and epigenetic problems. You might get an anticancer effect (read: reduced inflammation) in the short term, but long-term use of these drugs can cause more harm than good and is simply the wrong approach.[13]

In addition to the rampant overuse of COX inhibitors, steroids, and TNF blockers, Western medicine has also launched a new multimillion-dollar venture to treat inflammation with bioelectronic medicine. In 2015 the National Institutes of Health (NIH) announced a seven-year, $248 million program called SPARC (Stimulating Peripheral Activity to Relieve Conditions). In a nutshell, this approach uses implanted electrical nervous-system-stimulating devices, similar to pacemakers, to shunt the production of TNF. While this technology seems interesting and surely exciting for people living in chronic pain, it is missing the point, and—yet again—is treating the symptoms not the cause.

Meanwhile, from a nontoxic perspective, apigenin, a naturally occurring plant flavone abundantly present in parsley and chamomile tea, has been

TABLE 8.1. FOOD SOURCES OF OMEGA-3 AND OMEGA-6 FATTY ACIDS

Omega-3 Anti-Inflammatory Foods	Omega-6 Pro-Inflammatory Foods
Fish (salmon, sardines, mackerel, caviar)	Safflower and sunflower oils
Water snake oil	Canola oil
Flaxseed (in some cases) and hemp seed	Grapeseed oil
Chia and kukui (candlenut oil)	Vegetable oil
Walnuts	Wheat germ oil
Black currant seeds	Cottonseed oil
Fresh basil	Soybean oil
Sprouted radish seeds	Margarine
Pumpkin seed oil	Industrial shortening

found to exert potent anti-inflammatory activity by inhibiting NF-κB activation.[14] Luteolin, a flavonoid found in high concentrations in celery and green peppers, has been shown to reduce the production of IL-6.[15] The power of nutritional medicine is massive and far-reaching, but still largely ignored. It's time for that to end. We have to get out of the "treatment" mind-set and into prevention. Our metabolic approach gets at the root causes of inflammation, fatty acid imbalance and antioxidant scarcity.

Let's now turn to the role oxidative stress has in the cancer process and the dietary antioxidants that are the critical players in interrupting this damaging cycle.

Free Radicals, Mitochondria, and the Fasting Effect

As we have explained, oxidative stress occurs when there is an imbalance between the production of free radicals, namely ROS, and the body's ability to counteract their damaging effects through the neutralization action of antioxidants. A free radical is an atom or compound that is missing one or more electrons and goes about replacing it in an uncontrolled manner. Like a newly single person looking for an instant rebound partner, free radicals are highly unstable and are not selective about where they attain their missing electron. A free radical will steal an electron from the very first place it can. When free radicals take electrons from proteins, the loss causes tissue stiffening, the disabling of hormones and enzymes, and damage to cell structures.

DNA is also highly susceptible to free radical attacks, which cause genetic damage leading to cancer. The average rate of DNA damage inflicted by free radicals is actually quite high. It is estimated that more than ten thousand oxidative hits to the DNA of a human cell occur daily. With numbers like that, the importance of a high-antioxidant diet cannot be overstated. Free radicals and antioxidants are a 1:1 match: For every one free radical produced either through normal metabolism or external exposure to toxins such as processed oils, one antioxidant is used to squelch it. When not enough antioxidants are present, free radicals storm the body like angry protesters, damaging DNA, mitochondria, tissues, and cells.

The cell membrane is one of the most susceptible sites of free radical damage, and once free radicals break down the outer membrane of a cell, they are able to enter and cause damage to the mitochondria inside. Ironically, mitochondria are the main cellular organelles that incite free radical production yet they are also the most susceptible to oxidative damage. Damaged mitochondria are less able to utilize glucose and oxygen to generate energy, leading to fatigue, neuropathy, loss of memory, cognitive impairment, and of course the Warburg effect. Even beyond the Warburg effect, dysfunctional mitochondria are unable to modulate cell cycle, gene expression, metabolism, cell viability, and other established aspects of cell growth and stress responses, and free radicals are drawn to them.[16]

An observable example of oxidative stress is what happens to a slice of apple that turns brown from exposure to oxygen. When you squeeze lemon juice onto the apple (lemon juice is an antioxidant) the browning stops. Whenever you require your body to do work, as in exercising or eating, there is increased free radical production. ROS can be produced by both *endogenous* (internal) and exogenous (external) cellular substances. Potential endogenous sources include mitochondria, cytochrome P450 enzymes, and inflammatory cell activation. The most abundant source of free radical formation is in the mitochondria, which use more than 90 percent of the oxygen intake during metabolism to burn proteins, lipids, and carbohydrates and convert them to energy and water. This point alone completely solidifies the need for fasting and caloric restriction in the patient with an active cancer, as it reduces the need for mitochondria to convert food to energy, thereby reducing the production of free radicals.

The second source of free radicals is from environmental factors such as pesticides, alcohol, lack of sleep, chemical toxins, carcinogens, radiation exposure, cigarette smoke, and elevated iron levels. High blood sugar also accelerates the production of free radicals, and the extra weight that occurs as a result of high blood sugar causes increased and independent production of both CRP and IL-6.

As you can see, there are many ways these dangerous free radicals can be generated. Now let's meet their opponents, antioxidants.

Antioxidants: Their Anticancer Effects and Debate

How do we halt oxidative stress? Simple, by consuming antioxidants. Where do antioxidants come from? Easy: They come from plants that contain certain phytochemicals that act as antioxidants. Phytochemicals are compounds that occur naturally in plants (*phyto* means "plant" in Greek). There are thousands of different phytochemicals, and they are what give plants their color, odor, or flavor. The body makes some of its own antioxidants as well, including superoxide dismutase, glutathione peroxidase, melatonin, and COQ10. Glutathione is considered to be the most powerful, versatile, and important antioxidant made in the body. It plays many important roles in antioxidant defense, nutrient metabolism, and detoxification of carcinogens through phase 2 metabolism. It is also involved in the regulation of cellular events, including gene expression, DNA synthesis, and cytokine production. Glutathione is synthesized in the body from three amino acids: cysteine, glutamine, and glycine. Both animal and human studies demonstrate that adequate protein nutrition is crucial for the maintenance of adequate glutathione status (yet another strike against vegetarian and vegan diets).[17]

External sources of antioxidants include food in the forms of vitamin C and vitamin E, and also plant metabolites such as flavonoids, terpenoids, and coumarins. These antioxidants work by generously donating an electron, which neutralizes the damaging effect free radicals can have on proteins, DNA, lipids, and mitochondria. Their anticancer actions are no small potatoes! In fact, cancer chemoprevention using dietary phytochemical compounds is an emerging strategy to not only prevent but also to cure cancer.[18]Antioxidants have been found to exert the following anticancer benefits:

- Regulation of activities of the immune system
- Reduction in inflammation
- Modulation of hormones
- Tumor cytotoxicity
- Prevention of angiogenesis
- Prevention of side effects from chemotherapy
- Induction of apoptosis
- Inhibition of metastasis
- Support of DNA methylation and epigenetics

With all of the available evidence in support of the importance of consuming high-antioxidant foods (basically, lots of vegetables), their consumption remains a huge debate in the oncology world, and is even often discouraged. This is utterly erroneous. The controversial issue in the oncology world is whether using antioxidants in conjunction with radiation and chemotherapy is helpful or harmful. Because of this, consumption of antioxidant-rich foods and supplements is often discouraged to patients undergoing radiation or chemotherapy treatments. Jess has had several patients who were told by their conventional oncologists to avoid eating blueberries during their treatment regimen! However, ours and others' research tells a different story and has shown that antioxidants do not have a negative effect on the safety or efficacy of chemotherapy drugs. In fact, quite the opposite. The two in tandem can *increase* apoptosis of cancer cells while simultaneously protecting healthy cells and reducing side effects. Since antioxidants exist in all plant foods, to truly avoid them in your diet you would have to eat only distilled water and cardboard.

Keith Block, MD (medical director of the Block Center for Integrative Cancer Treatment in Evanston, Illinois, founder and editor in chief of the peer-reviewed medical journal *Integrative Cancer Therapies*, and author of the

Assessing Inflammation and Oxidation

Dr. Nasha has been using a set of three lab markers she calls "the trifecta" to assess a patient's inflammation level: c-reactive protein (CRP), erythrocyte sedimentation rate (ESR), and lactose dehydrogenase (LDH). Each marker provides insight into the level of inflammation, metabolic processes, and mitochondrial function and helps elucidate the amount of cancer activity or stability in the terrain at any given time. (She also recommends testing companies including Genova Diagnostics that offer oxidative stress panels.)

bestselling book *Life Over Cancer*), and his team at the Block Center took the most detailed look at this debate to date. They assessed more than 2,300 studies and nearly 5,000 patients, and *not a single study* they reviewed showed *any* clinical evidence of antioxidant use interfering with chemotherapy. "There is simply no evidence that antioxidants make chemotherapy less effective." Dr. Block wrote in his book. According to Dr. Neil McKinney, in his meticulously researched book *Naturopathic Oncology*, studies run around a hundred to one in favor of the use of antioxidants during chemotherapy for their ability to "enhance tolerability." Cytotoxic chemotherapy causes massive oxidative stress, leaving patients with severe deficits in antioxidants, which in turn—as we've just learned—promotes widespread inflammation. We typically advise eating foods high in antioxidants, like cocoa powder and capers, during both chemotherapy and radiation, and to consult with your individual practitioner depending on certain treatments with regard to supplementation.

The Metabolic Approach to Cooling the Inflammation-Oxidation Cycle

It has been said that if you can control inflammation, you can control cancer. Taking a metabolic approach to cancer means turning down the level of inflammation and oxidative stress with therapeutic nutrition. Without addressing the underlying cause of the inflammation, the fires of cancer will continue to get stoked. Medications may lessen the pain associated with inflammation, but they only mask a very destructive process that will continue, day in and day out. Because halting the inflammatory process prevents oxidation, and vice versa, focusing both on high-antioxidant *and* anti-inflammatory foods—often one and the same—is the key therapeutic approach of this terrain element. Specific antioxidant plant foods, fish, herbs, and lifestyle practices, including earthing, can significantly reduce inflammation and oxidative stress. Here are some of the specifics behind our approach to breaking the inflammation-oxidation cycle.

Step 1. Add Antioxidants and Anti-Inflammatory Plants to Your Diet

Antioxidants are present in foods and beverages of plant origin, including fruits, vegetables, herbs, spices, nuts, olives, chocolate, tea, and wine. These plant compounds have anti-inflammatory, antimicrobial, antiviral, anticancer, and immunomodulatory properties, all of which are beneficial to human health and further prove the benefits of a plant-focused diet. Additionally, because of their ability to affect the activity of multiple processes involved in cancer through direct modulation of gene expression, antioxidants have been found to also inhibit the growth of cancer cells.[19] There are thousands of different types of antioxidants—with more being discovered and studied all the time. To cover them all would easily fill a whole book. We will focus here two well-known antioxidants proven to be active inhibitors of both inflammation and oxidative stress: quercetin and resveratrol.[20]

QUERCETIN: CAPERS AND ONIONS FOR ALL

Quercetin is touted as the most powerful flavonoid known to man. It is certainly the most researched. Quercetin wears two hats—free radical scavenger and anti-inflammatory—and deserves its crowning as the inflammation-oxidation terrain superstar. It has been found to inhibit COX-2, NF-κB, and metastasis. When combined with the flavonoid epigallocatechin gallate (EGCG) found in green tea, it halts the growth of prostate cancer. Quercetin is found in highest concentrations in capers, organically grown apples (we recommend green and wild apples for their lower sugar content), and onions. (By the way, we can't say enough good things about onions. One of their phytonutrients, onionin A, was found to inhibit ovarian cancer progression by suppressing cancer cell proliferation. Onions should be on the menu, daily.) Other rich sources of quercetin are found in bilberries, black currants, black elderberry, and lingonberries. Bilberries have the highest COX-2 inhibitory effect.[21] Many of these berries might be unfamiliar to you; if so, start looking outside the supermarket and into farmers markets, ask naturalists in your area if any of these are native to your area, or grow your own!

RESVERATROL: THE TYPE OF WINE YOU DRINK MATTERS

Resveratrol is unique among antioxidants because it can cross the blood-brain barrier, the membrane that helps protect the brain and nervous system. When the anti-aging, antioxidant effects of resveratrol were fully realized in the 1990s, scientists believed they had discovered the key to the "French paradox." (You know what we mean: how the French are able to eat rich, fatty foods yet have an incidence of cardiovascular disease that is only a third of that in the United States.) *Their key is that they drink a resveratrol-rich red wine.* Resveratrol has been found to increase glutathione levels, minimize or prevent lipid oxidation, and act as a phytoestrogen. (Americans of course have since extracted resveratrol and turned it into a supplement, which doesn't show much—if any—benefit. Remember: The cornerstone of an effective metabolic approach is whole foods, not isolated components.) What's more, red wine also contains powerful tannins that have also been found to exert an anticancer effect.

While we do generally recommend a glass of organic, sustainably grown, and dry-farmed red wine two or three times a week, that recommendation does vary based on an individual's cancer type, liver function, and other factors. What's more, not all red wine is created equal. The Pesticide Action Network (PAN) found many pesticides used on wine grapes are listed as known or probable causes of cancer. Glyphosate is widely used on wine grapes in conventional farming. Also, the flame-retardant chemical 2,4,6-tribromophenol is sometimes used in the wooden barrels, racks, and crates used to transport wine or grapes. Again, it also comes back to quality.

Step 2. Add Key Anti-Inflammatory Herbs

Since the beginning of mankind, humans have used naturally occurring anti-inflammatory agents in the form of medicinal plants. These plants, specifically white willow and meadowsweet, created the foundation for what is the aspirin of today. Both herbs contain salicin, which has a very similar chemistry to aspirin (acetylsalicylic acid). Salicin also has the same antipyretic (fever-reducing), anti-inflammatory, and analgesic (pain-relieving) properties as aspirin; however, in contrast with synthetic aspirin, willow bark does not damage the gastrointestinal mucosa.[22]

There are several other culinary herbs that have been found to exert astonishing effects on both inflammation and oxidation. Black cumin seed oil is two hundred times more powerful than aspirin, and happens to be delicious in salad dressings. We are huge fans of herbs. Steve Ottersberg, Dr. Nasha's husband and a biochemist, refers to coriander, cumin, and turmeric as "the holy trinity" and adds the tasty combination of these three anti-inflammatory superstars to most all recipes. Jess named her daughter Pepper because compounds derived from black pepper can suppress TNF and NF-κB activation while also enhancing the potency of other herbs, including turmeric. No joke. The single largest step you can take in integrating the most powerful anticancer food into your diet is to add herbs, and lots of them. For the most complete guide to the medicinal properties of herbs, we highly recommend the book *Healing Spices* by Dr. Bharat B. Aggarwal and Debora Yost. Dr. Aggarwal has published numerous studies on the anti-inflammatory benefits of herbs. Thanks to his work and the work of other researchers that continue to explore the medicinal benefits of herbs and foods, we are at a new dawn of using nutritional medicine as a front-line approach for cancer. Let's take a closer look at some of these herbs.

TURMERIC: CANCER'S GREATEST EDIBLE ENEMY

Turmeric, the deep orange herb native to India and Southeast Asia, comes from the root (rhizome) portion of the plant *Curcuma longa* and has been used in Ayurvedic medicine for centuries. Turmeric, along with ginger and cardamom, is in the Zingiberaceae (ginger) family. Curcumin, the most studied extract from turmeric, has been found to possess an unprecedented amount of anticancer activities via its effect on biological pathways involved in mutagenesis, oncogene expression, cell cycle regulation, apoptosis, and metastasis.[23] Curcumin has shown antiproliferative effect in multiple cancers, and is an inhibitor of NF-κB. It is actually considered a "multifunctional" drug because of its ability to modulate the activity of multiple targets involved in carcinogenesis through direct interaction with gene expression. When combined with EGCG, curcumin suppressed breast cancer cell growth.

The best news is that the amount of turmeric needed in order to benefit from its anti-inflammatory benefits is minuscule. As little as 50 milligrams (approximately ⅓₀th of a teaspoon) of turmeric over a period of several months has been linked with health benefits. Of course we recommend more than that—at least 1 teaspoon a day of shavings from the whole root or dried powder. Whole turmeric of course provides a different set of benefits than curcumin extract alone because it contains three different curcuminoids (curcumin, bisdemethoxycurcumin, and demethoxycurcumin) and several volatile oils (including tumerone, atlantone, and zingiberone). Each of these different substances has been associated with anticancer properties. Turmeric is an excellent addition to egg dishes, stir-fries, medicinal smoothies, and golden milk. (A new trend in beverages, golden milk is a nut or seed milk warmed with turmeric added to it. It's wonderful.)

GINGER

This root is perhaps best known for its stomach-settling activity, and drinking ginger tea significantly helps reduce chemotherapy-related nausea. It also has very powerful anti-inflammatory actions, including the inhibition of both COX-2 and NF-κB. The root is rich in phytonutrients called gingerols, which have been found to raise levels of antioxidant enzymes including glutathione. Another ginger extract, zerumbone, was found to activate cancer-killing genes while also activating tumor-suppressor genes. Pickled ginger (look for brands that don't contain preservatives and colors, such as The Ginger People), kimchi, and fresh ginger minced in hot water are just a few ways you can enjoy this herb. It is also excellent with fish dishes.

BOSWELLIA

Boswellia is the name of the Indian plant or tree that produces the resin frankincense. Frankincense has been used as an ingredient in incense and perfumes for thousands of years, and at one time was so precious that the wise men of the New Testament reportedly gave it to the baby Jesus. Its anti-inflammatory activity has been attributed to its ability to inhibit TNF. It possesses antiproliferative and pro-apoptotic activities in rat astrocytoma and in human leukemia cell lines, reduces peritumoral edema in glioblastoma patients, reverses multiple brain metastases in breast cancer patients, and induces cell cycle arrest, cell growth suppression, and apoptosis in bladder cancer.[24] Place a couple of drops of a high-quality, therapeutic-grade oil under the tongue, or add a couple of drops to homemade salad dressing.

Step 3. Balance Your Fatty Acids: More Virgin, Less Shelf-Stable

It is abundantly clear that our modern diets are saturated (pun intended) with inflammatory fats. The road to reducing oxidative stress winds its way through the grocery aisles and back to your pantry. First, it is important to replace all vegetable oils found in condiments like mayonnaise, salad dressing, sauces, and dips as well as in processed, boxed foods (cookies, breads, et cetera). Anywhere you see canola, cottonseed, soybean, or corn, pack it up and either donate it to a food shelter or throw it away. Avoid fried foods, fast food, margarine, candy, chips, commercial meat products, and non-homemade baked goods. You may be surprised at how many places in the modern diet these fats are lurking. Read labels on *everything*, even at the health food store.

As you decrease these inflammatory fats, simultaneously increase your consumption of omega-3 fatty acids by eating fish like sardines, mackerel, herring, Arctic char, and wild salmon. Chia seeds, walnuts, cold-pressed extra-virgin olive oil (not used for high-heat cooking, though), and dark leafy greens are all also excellent sources of omega-3 fatty acids. Just 1 cup of the wild greens called shepherd's purse or purslane contains over 250 milligrams of omega-3 fatty acids.[25] Further, cooking fish over 300°F for thirty minutes can deplete its content of EPA and DHA by over 75 percent.[26]

The issue of mercury contamination in fish turns some people away from eating it, but that is unwise. First, smaller fish such as anchovies and sardines have less mercury contamination, and second, mercury toxicity is strongly influenced by selenium intake. Mercury and selenium have a chemical affinity for each other, and selenium binds to mercury and deactivates it. Fish, as it turns out, are very high in selenium. Fermented fish is also lower in heavy metals and is a great option.

Quality is very important with olive oil, which contains dozens of polyphenols, including the antioxidant vitamin E. Certain olive varieties contain

greater amounts of antioxidants than others, including Cornicabra, Cora-
tina, Moraiolo, and Koroneiki. The more bitter-tasting the oil, the higher
the polyphenol content. There is a good reason why olive oil is central to
the Mediterranean diet; another polyphenol found in olive oil (hydroxyty-
rosol) helps protect blood vessels from ROS damage. Other polyphenols,
including apigenin, oleuropein, and luteolin, have been shown to function
not only as antioxidants and anti-inflammatory nutrients but also as powerful inhibitors of angiogenesis and metastasis (which we cover in the next
chapter). When choosing high-quality olive oil, look for the "bottled on"
date, not the expiration date; be sure it is in a dark glass and is extra-virgin,
organic, and cold-pressed.

Step 4. Greens and Grass Help Inflammation Pass

Surprisingly, some wild plant foods can contain as much as 24 percent fat.
Greens such as kale, spinach, and wild grasses contain alpha-linolenic acid,
the building block of the omega-3 fatty acids—precisely why grass-fed animals contain almost six times more anti-inflammatory omega-3 fats than their
grain-fed counterparts. Animals labeled as organic often are also fed grains
like corn and soy, and even though these mixes are *technically* organic, we
still need to remember that grain is not the natural diet of ruminants (cows,
sheep, and goats). So don't be fooled by that label! Using their microbiome,
cows are able to derive nutrients from plant-based food by fermenting it in
a specialized stomach prior to digestion. A cow's natural diet is grass, with
some leaves, twigs, or bark. Not corn.

A 2001 peer-reviewed article in the journal *Science* concluded that grain-
based diets are "very stressful" for cattle. Not only that, but they also cause
ulcers and overgrowth of *E. coli* in the rumen. Cattle that are fed grain get
very sick, and therefore require more antibiotics to stay alive. So even organic
beef, even if the cow is fed 100 percent grain, is not the best choice. Organic
meat, eggs, and fish are just not good enough! Cows should be 100 percent
grass-fed and 100 percent grass-finished (even thirty days of corn finishing
will change the fatty acid profile to be higher in omega-6 fats than omega-3s).

Chickens are omnivores and should not be vegetarian; they enjoy
eating lizards and bugs just as much as the next bird. Chickens should be
pasture-raised and allowed to peck for bugs; if they are given any supplemental

TABLE 8.2. TYPES OF FATS AND FOOD SOURCES

Fatty Acid Family	Type of Fatty Acid	Food Sources
Omega-3	alpha-linolenic acid (LNA)	flaxseeds, walnut, hemp seeds, chia seeds, dark leafy greens
	stearidonic acid (SDA)	black currant seeds
	eicosapentaenoic acid (EPA), docosahexaenoic acid (DHA)	cold-water fish (e.g., sardines, salmon, trout, mackerel)
Omega-6	linoleic acid (LA)	soybean, safflower, sunflower, sesame
	gamma-linolenic acid (GLA)	borage oil, black currant seed oil, evening primrose oil
	arachidonic acid (AA)	commercially raised animal products
	caprylic acid (CA)	goat milk
Omega-7	palmitoleic acid (PA)	tropical oils (e.g., coconut and palm kernel)
Omega-9	oleic acid (OA)	olive, almond, avocado, filberts, macadamia nuts, lard, butter
Saturated fats	stearic acid (SA)	beef, pork, animal butters, cocoa butter, shea nut butter
	palmitic acid (PA)	tropical fats (e.g., coconut and palm kernel)
	butyric acid (BA)	butter
	medium-chain fatty acids	MCT oil
Trans fats	synthetically made partially hydrogenated oils	margarine, nondairy creamers, breakfast bars, shortening, baked goods

feed, it should be 100 percent organic—ideally without soy. Eggs should come from those same chickens.

Walnuts are also high in omega-3 fatty acids, while chia seeds, almonds, and pecans are high in antioxidants, including vitamin E. (In case you didn't know, pecans are the next walnut—they have the highest antioxidant value of all tree nuts!)

HAVE FUN WITH FENNEL

Arguably one of the most overlooked vegetables in the produce section is fennel. A light whitish green bulb with feathery, dill-like stems and a licorice taste, fennel is one of the most anti-inflammatory vegetables there is as well as a digestive aid. Chewing fennel seeds has been shown to be very effective against IBD pain and colic and is common practice in India. Fennel contains anethole, a powerful phytonutrient compound. In animal studies, anethole has repeatedly been shown to reduce inflammation and help prevent the occurrence of cancer through inhibiting TNF. (Fennel creates a wonderful dish when paired with sausage and cabbage, especially if you enjoy a crunch. Note: The longer you cook fennel, the less it tastes like licorice.)

EAT COCOA POWDER AND HIGH-QUALITY DARK CHOCOLATE

Since the seventeenth century, cocoa and chocolate have been considered medicinal, and chocolate lovers would agree. Cocoa contains more polyphenols and higher antioxidant capacity than green tea, black tea, or red wine. It also contains approximately 380 known phytochemicals, 10 of which are psychoactive compounds. Three groups of polyphenols can be identified in cocoa beans: catechins, which constitute about 37 percent of the polyphenol content in the beans, anthocyanidins (about 4 percent), and proanthocyanidins (about 58 percent). Cocoa polyphenols modulate intestinal inflammation and decrease the production of pro-inflammatory enzymes and cytokines. The phenolics in cocoa have antiproliferative, antimutagenic, and chemoprotective effects, in addition to their anticarcinogenic effects and ability to inhibit lipid peroxidation.[27] Cocoa polyphenols have even been found to inhibit the mutagenic activity of heterocyclic amines that are formed when meat is cooked to high temperatures. (Cocoa-dusted steaks are excellent.)

Cocoa powder also happens to be one of the best sources of magnesium. A 100-gram serving of raw cocoa powder provides almost 520 milligrams of magnesium. One study found that the inflammatory indicators CRP, TNF, and IL-6 were all reduced when magnesium intake was increased. In 2014 the *European Journal of Clinical Nutrition* published the results of a meta-analysis that revealed an association between increased dietary magnesium and lower levels of CRP.

There are several factors that can cause low magnesium, and these may be placed in one of two categories: diminished intake of magnesium or enhanced losses of magnesium (either through the gastrointestinal tract or through the kidneys). Examples of the first category are alcoholism (resulting in overall poor intake of nutrients) and a low intake of food sources of magnesium (cocoa, almonds, asparagus, coffee, and clams). Almost half (48 percent) of the US population consumed less than the RDA of magnesium from food in 2005–2006.[28] Examples of the second category include severe diarrheal states, stress, malabsorption, and antibiotic use.[29]

Unfortunately, by the time raw cocoa gets processed into a candy bar, most if not all of its antioxidant and anti-inflammatory compounds have been lost. The addition of the genetically modified emulsifier soy lecithin, conventional dairy products, and loads of sugar further negates any of the cocoa's benefits. Selecting high-quality chocolate of 85 percent cocoa or higher (with no soy lecithin), cocoa nibs, or pure cocoa powder are the best ways to garner the most benefit from cocoa. By the way, nibs are cocoa beans that have been separated from their husks and broken into smaller pieces. (Yes, you can still enjoy *real* chocolate on a ketogenic diet: 2 teaspoons of organic raw cocoa nibs—which may sound like a small amount but is all you need to deeply satisfy a chocolate craving—contains 2 grams of carbohydrates and 0 grams of sugar. Cocoa nibs actually make an excellent crouton replacement in salads, believe it or not.)

Earthing: An Anti-Inflammatory Lifestyle Focus

Humans started wearing shoes somewhere around forty thousand years ago, and sandals were the most common footwear in most early civilizations. Soft, moccasin-like shoes were first worn by Mesopotamian mountain folk. We have since developed thick-soled shoes and—for some bizarre reason—high heels. Our feet and bodies have slowly their lost direct connection to the earth. When is the last time you slept on the ground? Walked around barefoot? For most people, the answers are not in a long time, if ever. The concept of *earthing*, also known as *grounding*, means deliberately having direct skin contact with the surface of the Earth, such as with bare feet or hands, or using various grounding devices that have been created. Grounding has been found in studies to reduce or even prevent the four cardinal signs of inflammation following injury: redness, heat, swelling, and pain.[30]

In addition, some experts assert that the free radicals we build up throughout the day carry a positive charge, and since the Earth's surface is negatively charged connecting to it would exert a massive antioxidant effect. Jess has begun to experiment with thirty-minute barefoot walks in the woods in lieu of afternoon tea, and reports heightened energy, focus, and mood. Antioxidant activity has yet to be assessed, but for now, it certainly feels good and she performs her daily commute to work barefoot.

Cooling It All Down

Inflammation and oxidation are two processes that really poke a stick at cancer. Inflammatory conditions are rampant in the United States and, unfortunately, the modern medicine, drug-centered approach comes with side effects that include risk of developing cancer. Eating common fats like soybean oil that are highly processed causes inflammation, while oxidation—a side effect of inflammation—needs counterbalancing with plant-derived antioxidants. Managing both processes is possible through increasing omega-3 fatty acids and specific plants such as capers, onions, fennel, and herbs. The importance of achieving this balance cannot be overstated! Inflammation is one of the main drivers behind the two most deadly aspects of cancer: growth and spread. In the next chapter we take a close look at both angiogenesis and metastasis and the food factors that provoke and inhibit them.

CHAPTER 9

Cancer Growth and Spread
Halting Angiogenesis and Metastasis

Imagine that one medical advancement holds the promise to conquer cancer and more than 70 of life's most threatening conditions. This is the promise of angiogenesis.

—Dr. William Li, *President and Medical Director,*
The Angiogenesis Foundation

A biochemical vampire, the cancer cell's nectar of choice is blood.
—*From* The Definitive Guide to Cancer
by Lise Alschuler, Karolyn A. Gazella

Be still like a mountain and flow like a great river.

—Lao-tzu

In the last chapter we talked about inflammation, the spark that ignites the fire of cancer. Of the many negative effects inflammation has on the body and the cancer process, stimulating cancer cells to grow and spread is one of them. This chapter is about two processes that happen when cancer starts to get really out of control: angiogenesis, the formation of new blood vessels that help sustain a growing tumor, and metastasis, the development of the cancer in a new site. These two hallmarks of cancer, both involving blood and circulation, are the most deadly. But there are nontoxic and metabolic approaches that can halt both of these processes from occurring. Approaches that confer legitimate benefits to a component of our terrain where Western medicine falls short on treatment options, a component that cancer cells capitalize on and manipulate in order to grow and spread: the circulatory system.

Each of our bodies has enough blood vessels to circle the Earth twice—more than sixty thousand miles' worth. These blood vessels deliver oxygen and nutrients to tissues and organs throughout the body and carry away their metabolic waste products. Another way to think about it: Blood vessels act as both the milk deliverer and the trash collector. They keep the body both fed and clean. The human body, when in balance, runs like a perfect system, every cell doing its part to promote proper functioning, the milk delivery coming at the right time, and the trash picked up right on schedule. For the most part, everyone (meaning our organs and tissues) stays in their designated pickup or drop-off spot. (An exception is red and white blood cells.) The primary way the body is able to keep blood vessels, cells, and organs from taking a bad road trip through the body is by means of the *extracellular matrix* (ECM). This weblike matrix is made up of nonliving material that fills the spaces between cells, both protecting them and helping to hold them together. The ECM is the main reason that when you do a handstand, your stomach doesn't fall out of your mouth!

Outlaw cancer cells and tumors do not abide by these rules; they grow and spread outside of their designated areas. In fact, they have developed ways to acquire even more nutrients and oxygen by summoning new blood vessels to be built (angiogenesis) so that they can grow larger. They also use cunning tactics to break through the thick web of the ECM and spread throughout the body (metastasis). Once a cancer has metastasized, a patient's prognosis worsens. Over 90 percent of cancer deaths are due to metastasis formation, and despite the high mortality from metastatic cancer, therapeutic targets to prevent metastasis remain limited in the Western medical realm. In this chapter, we present the current evidence for a metabolic approach to preventing and halting growth and spread of cancer, a therapeutic option to accompany what Western medicine has to offer. When cancer is significantly progressed, the more options there are the better.

First we will discuss the mechanisms behind how cancer is able to accomplish such growth and spreading, and how circulation, clotting, and blood health contribute to the process. We will illuminate the shortcomings and dangers of some of the Western approaches to circulation. (For example, a 2013 study published in the *Journal of the American Medical Association* found that certain blood pressure medications increased the risk of breast cancer over two and a half times.[1]) We will also discuss the connections among high copper levels, "sticky" blood, fibrinogen, and angiogenesis, and pinpoint exercise as the ultimate antidote to these processes, not to mention for the general prevention of cancer. We highlight food compounds, including specific mushrooms and fatty acids, with the potential to inhibit key metastatic events. In fact, a multitude of food compounds have been identified that exert nontoxic angiogenesis- and metastatic-modulating effects on tumors. These include green tea, bone broth, aloe vera juice, and capsaicin from spicy peppers. More at the end of the chapter.

First let's review the processes and factors involved with cancer's growth and spread.

Blood: The Pathway for Circulation and Angiogenesis

In healthy adults, new blood vessels don't normally need to grow, with a few exceptions: the monthly growth of the uterine lining, which facilitates the menstrual cycle; pregnancy; and following an injury. And normally the body has a checkpoint system for regulating angiogenesis, a system comprising stimulators and inhibitors. When blood is needed, the body signals certain growth factors including vascular endothelial growth factor (VEGF), an angiogenesis stimulator, to make new vessels. TNF and IGF-1 are also able to stimulate the production of new blood vessels. Normally when vessels are no longer needed they are dissolved through the action of angiogenesis inhibitors. When these systems of checks and balances becomes dysregulated, however, cancer and other diseases can occur. Impaired blood vessel development results in arteriosclerosis and increased risk of stroke, while too many blood vessels are a cause of pulmonary hypertension and endometriosis. Dozens of diseases in addition to cancer are linked to angiogenesis.[2]

Cancer cells need a blood supply to grow and nourish their rapid metabolism. Like any organism, without food or oxygen they cannot survive. And any tumor that grows past a very small size (0.5–1 millimeter, approximately the size of the tip of a ballpoint pen) needs new blood. Like little vampires, tumor cells commandeer the normal process of angiogenesis for their own survival. Cancer cells are able to "switch on" angiogenesis and activate VEGF while at the same time deactivating angiogenesis inhibitors.

When microscopic cancers start out, they reach that ballpoint-pen size and then most cancers stop—a state called "cancer without disease." When the body is in balance, it doesn't provide blood supply to these tiny tumors, and they eventually die. But cancer cells get creative when they become *hypoxic*, meaning when they are deprived of oxygen. Hypoxia can occur when tumors grow and also with low blood pressure, chronic obstructive pulmonary disease (COPD), high altitude, and anemia. By activating a process called the *hypoxia stress response*, tumors emit signals to neighboring blood vessels, persuading them to throw them a "vessel extension lifeline" that will deliver needed oxygen and nutrients. Once cancer cells connect with new food and oxygen lifelines, not only do they grow, but they also like to travel. A growing tumor is rarely the main cause of death; it's when cancer metastasizes to a new location that it becomes a big problem.

That tumor "lifeline" formation is directed by VEGF, and therefore the majority of anti-angiogenesis drugs are VEGF inhibitors. The goal of angiogenesis inhibitors is to stop the growth and migration of new blood vessels. Bevacizumab, an angiogenesis inhibitor we discussed previously, has been shown to slightly improve survival rates in different types of cancer, yet also indiscriminately cuts off circulation in other areas of the body with serious side effects, including severe high blood pressure, bowel perforations, and hemorrhaging.

Metastasis:
How Cancer Cells Travel and Invade

Blood vessels serve as the body's highway system. Blood pumped from the heart is carried to distant tissues and organs by a vast network of blood vessels that includes nineteen billion capillaries. When a tumor metastasizes, a few cancer cells break away from the "primary tumor," the tumor they first formed, and enter either the blood vessel superhighway or the lymphatic system to travel to a new location. This is how they form new tumors, metastases, in other parts of the body. For example, breast cancer that has spread to the lung is called metastatic breast cancer, not lung cancer.

Like explorers hungry to discover new lands, a growing tumor will designate clusters of pioneer cells to travel to distant sites where they can form new settlements, or secondary tumors. It's how the West was won—not a new concept. But how do cancer cells go about it? Remember that a large proportion of human tissue consists of extracellular space filled with a mixture of carbohydrate and protein molecules called the ECM. The molecules that make up the ECM tether themselves to one another, forming thick weblike bonds. In order for cancer cells to metastasize, they must untether these bonds by creating protein-digesting enzymes. Like swordsmen through the jungle, cancer cells hack away at the thick matrix. Once they've escaped the matrix, metastatic cancer cells attempt to gain access to systemic circulation by one of two routes. For many cancer cells, their best opportunity to spread is by means of the lymphatic system (this is why lymph nodes are often biopsied or removed during surgery to assess if the cancer has spread; this information also determines the cancer's stage). Using the alternative route, cancer cells enter the bloodstream either indirectly through the lymph or directly through blood vessels.

Once these pioneer cancer cells arrive at a distant organ, they can grow into a metastatic tumor. But most of them do not. It has been estimated that between ten million and one billion cancer cells are released into the bloodstream by tumors on a daily basis, but only 0.001 percent go on to develop into metastatic colonies. A century ago Dr. Stephen Paget, a surgeon, asserted the "seed and soil" hypothesis. He theorized that the organ preference patterns of metastasizing tumors are due to symbiotic interactions between the metastatic tumor cell (the seed) and its potential new organ microenvironment (the soil). Some tumor types are able to form metastases in just about any organ in the body, but the most frequently targeted organs for metastasis are bone, brain, liver, and lung.[3] When a person's terrain is balanced and healthy, cancer *can't* form a metastatic tumor, as the new environment will not support it. Metastatic cancer cells are essentially seeds that grow into highly toxic, lethal plants only if they are planted in unhealthy soil.

A portion of the "soil" Dr. Paget referred is now known as the *tumor microenvironment*, or TME. The TME consists of all the noncancerous cells present within the tumor. These include immune cells, cytokines, growth factors, ROS, and other inflammatory compounds. One other compound found in the TME is the cancer-associated fibroblast (CAF). These are cells that promote the cancer process by encouraging tumor growth, angiogenesis, inflammation, and metastasis.[4] Since they are associated with cancer at all stages of progression—their production of growth factors facilitates angiogenesis—they have become an emerging target for cancer therapies.[5] In fact, normal fibroblasts (cells found in connective tissue that produce the collagen and fibers that make up the ECM) can be "educated" by cancer cells to express pro-inflammatory genes, further fueling the cancer process.[6]

There is a lot happening in the immediate surroundings, the soil, of a tumor that can help to either provoke or inhibit its growth. The seeds of metastatic cancer will thrive in an inflammatory, immune-compromised, and highly oxidative environment. Yet when the terrain is healthy, nourished, and optimized, those same bad seeds cannot sprout. Because blood and the circulatory system are the primary systems that can enable cancer's growth and spread, understanding how blood flow works—and how nutrition factors into it—is paramount.

Circulation: The Link Between Blood Viscosity ("Stickiness") and Cancer

According to Chinese medicine, stagnant blood, or what Western doctors call "sticky" blood, is one of the main causes of cancer. With blood stagnation, nutrients from the blood do not enter cells efficiently, cellular waste is not properly removed, and cells, basically, become sick. No milk delivery, no trash pickup. The term *viscosity* refers to the thickness and stickiness of a liquid. In the case of blood, its viscosity is directly correlated with its ability to flow through vessels. Blood should flow through our bodies like a river.

When the river gets dammed up or filled with debris and flow stops, then all sorts of things can grow. Think of the difference between a mud puddle and a clear stream. Over time, stagnant water becomes host for all sorts of pathogens and bacteria. In the case of cancer, after cachexia and infection, circulation issues are the third leading cause of death in cancer patients. Considering heart disease has been the number one killer in the United States for decades (though quickly being overtaken by cancer), we clearly have rampant circulation issues that are linked—unquestionably—to diet and lifestyle.

Blood that is sticky or stagnant means that it is more prone to clotting, or *coagulating*. Here is how that process works: Within a moment of getting a cut, for example, damaged skin tissue will activate platelets within the blood in the torn blood vessel—perhaps a vein or even an artery—to become sticky and to clump together like glue around the cut, forming a clot at the damaged part of the blood vessel. (Platelets, also called thrombocytes, are components of the blood that help it clot and are produced in the bone marrow.) Soon threadlike proteins called fibrins arrive to form a structural scaffolding throughout the clot to hold it in place (we will talk more about them in a minute).

A person's normal platelet count ranges from 150,000 to 450,000 platelets per microliter of blood. Having more than this is a condition called *thrombocytosis* and having less than this is known as *thrombocytopenia*. Thrombocytosis, a condition of having too many platelets, can increase risk of either spontaneous blood clotting or bleeding, depending on what is causing it.

Cancer and coagulation activation go hand in hand. Cancerous tumors can activate platelets, which help them to both grow and spread. These activated platelets form around tumors, shielding them from immune cells and also from chemotherapy drugs. Activated platelets also assist in metastasis and migration by creating pathways into the bloodstream and promoting angiogenesis. Again, a normal bodily process is hijacked and subverted by cancer cells.

Hypercoagulation also increases the production of fibrins, the structural proteins that help with clotting. Fibrin is formed from fibrinogen, a protein produced by the liver. When tissue damage results in bleeding, fibrinogen is converted into fibrin by the action of the enzyme thrombin. The drug heparin, an anticoagulant (or blood thinner), works, through a multistep pathway, by preventing the conversion of fibrinogen to fibrin. Heparin is used to treat and prevent blood clots in veins, arteries, and the lung and also decreases the spread of cancer; it works so well that Dr. Nasha actually considers it an underutilized antimetastatic pharmaceutical!

A high fibrinogen level indicates sticky blood and has been linked to reduced survival and poor response to treatments in certain cancers. Foods with a higher glycemic index, including sugars, are known to be associated with elevated fibrinogen.[7] Thus, one natural antigen to high fibrinogen is the elimination of sugar from the diet, and another is consuming coumarin-containing plants and herbs. Coumarin is a sweet-smelling compound found in aniseed, cassia cinnamon, dandelion, horseradish, and wild lettuce. Coumarin is used in topically in perfumes, but when ingested it has anticoagulant properties.

Top Causes of Dysregulated Blood Flow

We covered how harmful an unbalanced ratio of fatty acids was in the last chapter. Some of the same concepts apply to blood flow. Trans fats, especially the synthetic, partially hydrogenated oils found in baked goods, fried foods, margarines, and nondairy creamers, can increase factors involved in clotting and make blood more viscous. Synthetic fats coupled with high-sugar diets are the leading cause of both heart disease and cancer. Inflammatory omega-6 fats can induce production of a protein that stimulates the production of new platelets as well as increases platelet aggregation. This is one of the reasons why the American Heart Association recommends eating fatty fish (with its omega-3 fatty acid content) at least twice a week: to balance the pro-coagulation activity of omega-6 fats.

But there are two other much more basic but nevertheless hugely significant contributors not only to cardiovascular health but also to an anticancer lifestyle that many Americans do not practice, and these are: (1) drinking enough water, and (2) exercise. These two factors alone are the greatest contributors to sticky blood. Another factor, a high copper level, is also frequently found in metastatic cancer patients and can contribute to cancer growth and spread. Let's explore all three of these concepts in greater detail.

Dehydration and Angiogenesis

Dehydration, which is far more common than you might expect, can have far-reaching effects on the terrain and also supports cancer growth. Cancer treatments, and the side effects of vomiting and diarrhea, only increase dehydration among cancer patients. To maintain proper hydration, a person needs to drink at least half their body weight (measured in pounds) in ounces of clean, filtered water daily. (That is, a person who weighs 130 pounds needs to drink at least 65 ounces of water per day.) But not all water is the same quality! And quality matters. Tap water from city drinking systems can contain fluoride, for example, and several detrimental health effects of fluoride are beginning to surface, one of them being that it has been found to increase angiogenesis in the skin and bones.[8] With skin cancer the number one cancer today, further investigation into the role showering, bathing, and swimming in fluoridated water may have in promoting angiogenesis is warranted.

The primary issue with dehydration is that it causes increased histamine levels.[9] Histamine is a compound produced by mast cells as part of the local immune response. Mast cells are considered the "master regulators" of the immune system and are found in connective tissues, especially the skin, intestine, and lungs. When stimulated by a pathogen (including food allergens, such as wheat, cow milk, or soy), mast cells secrete both TNF and histamine.[10] This release of histamine causes capillaries to become more permeable and has been shown to induce an angiogenic response similar to that promoted by VEGF.[11] You can see how important it is not only to follow the allergen elimination diet outlined in chapter 7, but to remain very well hydrated in order to avoid increased angiogenesis.

The Importance of Exercise

There is an Eastern saying that goes, "A man will live a hundred years if he takes a hundred steps after every meal." We believe it. When it comes to cancer, optimizing diet and exercise are the two top ways to prevent the disease. As mentioned in the introductory chapters of this book, diet and lifestyle are estimated to cause more than 85 percent of all cancers. A sedentary lifestyle increases the risk of developing both cancer and cardio-vascular disease.[12] A CDC study estimated that nearly 80 percent of adult Americans in 2013 were not get the recommended amount of exercise each week.[13] In total, Americans are sitting an average of thirteen hours a day and sleeping an average of eight hours a night, resulting in being sedentary approximately twenty-one hours a day. Avoiding long periods of sitting down in the car or at a desk seems like a no-brainer, but in our modern (as Jess likes to say, "deskmesticated") times, most of us are seated all day.

In 2016 data gathered from 1.4 million people in the first-ever world-wide pooled analysis of physical activity and cancer incidence showed that exercise reduces the risk of thirteen types of cancer by 25–30 percent.[14] Physical activity decreases the risk of cancer recurrence and prolongs overall survival—especially in women with primary breast cancer—and evidence is now showing a benefit from exercise for people with metastatic cancer. In fact, exercising increases survival time by over 20 percent for those with any kind of metastatic cancer. But conventional exercise recommendations, similar to conventional dietary recommendations, fall short of optimal: Current recommendations are that adults get at least two and a half hours of moderate-intensity aerobic exercise *each week* or an hour and a quarter of vigorous-intensity activity. That's it.

This is a far cry from our activity levels of even thirty years ago, let alone our Paleo ancestors who would cover six miles a day, on average, for women, and ten for men. Really, movement should occur every two hours. Daily exercise should include at least thirty minutes of walking or running—which means getting winded and breaking a sweat. Standing desks, walking meetings, and daily exercise are a must. As we tell our patients: If you have time to watch TV, you have time to exercise.

Copper: The On Switch for Angiogenesis

Copper, an essential mineral, is a cofactor for the production of many promoters of angiogenesis, including VEGF.[15] Copper is widespread in the environment as a result of mining, emissions from factories that make or use copper metal or copper compounds, waste dumps, domestic wastewater, combustion of fossil fuels and wastes, wood production, and phosphate fertilizer production. Copper is used as a fungicide on tomatoes (approved, unfortunately, for organic gardening), older houses have copper piping, and of course there is copper cookware. According to the CDC, approximately 1.4 million pounds of copper were released into the environment by industries in 2000. We are unknowingly exposed to high levels of environmental copper all the time.

There are also many food sources that are high in copper. These include organ meats, shellfish, and liquid chlorophyll. However, these foods are also very high in zinc. Like other pairs of minerals that have balancing effects on each other (calcium and magnesium, sodium and potassium), zinc is the counterbalance to high copper levels. Nature has an amazing way of creating foods in perfect balance. You should talk to your doctor about testing copper levels and also about zinc supplementation should copper levels be in excess or if you have metastatic cancer. Currently Dwight McKee, MD, is researching a copper chelation method using pharmaceutical tetrathiomolybdenate (TM) as a treatment for copper excess angiogenesis, an option we are really excited to learn more about.

Sugar, Metastasis, and Hyperbaric Oxygen

As we learned in chapter 4, the single biggest cancer promoter is a high blood sugar level. Not only is sugar the preferred fuel source of cancer cells, but proteins that proliferate in the setting of extra glucose, like IGFs, suppress apoptosis, promote cell cycle progression, angiogenesis, and metastatic activities in various cancers.[16] You may remember that IGF-1 is a hormone similar in structure to insulin and works with growth hormone to reproduce and regenerate cells. It is often high in individuals with prediabetes or full-blown diabetes. IGF-1 has been shown to promote the growth and metastasis of liver, breast, pancreatic, and several other cancers.[17] Altered angiogenesis and insulin resistance are intimately related. The high sugar intake signature of the Western diet was found to increase the risk of breast cancer and metastasis to the lungs, according to a 2015 study done at the University of Texas MD Anderson Cancer Center.

To avoid the spread of cancer, eliminating all forms of sugar, grains, legumes, and other high-carbohydrate foods is unquestionably essential. Prolonged fasting, fasts of 48 to 120 hours, has been shown to effectively and rapidly reduce IGF-1 levels while also sensitizing cells to chemotherapy agents.[18] Combining a ketogenic diet with another nontoxic therapy called hyperbaric oxygen therapy also has significant emerging potential. Hyperbaric oxygen therapy saturates tumors with oxygen, which can reverse the cancer-promoting effects of tumor hypoxia we discussed earlier. In fact, a 2013 study published in the journal *PLOS ONE* by Angela Poff, Csilla Ari, Thomas Seyfried, and Dominic D'Agostino found that combining the ketogenic diet and hyperbaric oxygen therapy produced significant anticancer effects, including decreased blood glucose levels, reduced tumor growth rate, and a 77 percent increase in mean survival time in mice with systemic metastatic cancer when compared with controls.[19] This is big, and thankfully more research continues in these combined therapy areas. We highly recommend integrating the metabolic approaches of fasting and the ketogenic diet as a front-line treatment for angiogenesis and metastasis and also seeking out professionals trained in hyperbaric oxygen therapy.

Coagulation and the Vitamin K Controversy

On the opposite side of the blood viscosity coin is *hypo*coagulation, or when blood becomes too thin and cannot adequately form clots. Blood clotting (coagulation) prevents excessive bleeding when a blood vessel is injured. When platelet levels are lowered as a result of poor liver function, or due to chemotherapy, overuse of blood-thinning medications—either natural or pharmaceutical anticoagulants—the risk of hemorrhage, headaches, nosebleeds, easy bruising, and uncontrolled bleeding increases. A 2015 University of California study found that almost one-quarter of people with atrial fibrillation with a low risk of stroke were prescribed blood-thinning drugs they didn't need. An analysis of US government inspections performed between 2011 and 2014 revealed that approximately 165 nursing home residents were hospitalized or died due to errors involving the anticoagulant warfarin (Coumadin).[20] We are not saying blood thinners are bad, just that caution and regular monitoring need to be exercised when it comes to both hyper- and hypocoagulation, and there are many safer and just-as-effective natural substances to thin the blood.

Vitamin K Controversies

Inevitably when it come to the coagulation conversation, vitamin K always seems to come up—as it should, since it is required for the clotting process to work! Vitamin K, a fat-soluble vitamin, was given the designation of *K* (derived from the German word *koagulation*) because the liver uses it to make several blood-clotting proteins, including prothrombin. A low level of vitamin K results in a reduced ability to clot. Warfarin is a drug that works against vitamin K by reducing the liver's ability to use it. However, it is a common misconception that people taking warfarin should completely avoid naturally occurring vitamin K, which is found in kale, spinach, brussels sprouts, parsley, collard greens, mustard greens, chard, and green tea. What *should* be the goal is achieving equilibrium. First of all, if you have thin blood, or *hypo*coaguability, increasing your consumption of vitamin K–rich foods is a must (and happily these foods have anti-angiogenic properties as well). If you have *hyper*coagulation issues and are on medication for it, a sudden increase in vitamin K intake may decrease the effect of warfarin. On the other hand, greatly lowering your vitamin K intake could increase the effect of blood-thinning drugs. Because we want you to eat many of these vegetables—and most likely higher quantities that you already are—it is important to talk to your doctor about adjusting the dose of the anticoagulant. Over time, once you make the dietary changes outlined in this book, there is a chance your coagulation issues will resolve.

Vitamins K1 and K2 (MK-7), two natural forms of vitamin K, have also been noted to target cancer at multiple stages of development and to promote apoptosis. Vitamin K1 is found abundantly in the green vegetables mentioned above. Vitamin K2 is found in meat, egg yolk, organic chicken liver, and *natto*, a Japanese fermented soy product with enzymatic derivatives that have a powerful anticancer effect. In the wonderful world of synergies, vitamin K also plays an important role in the action of vitamin D, and the two should be taken together in both supplements and food. Believe it or not, sautéed Swiss chard and smoked salmon make an excellent breakfast.

Low Iron, High Ferritin,
Grains, and a Genetic Switch

Along with vitamin K, iron is another poorly understood and often incorrectly prescribed supplement. Just as the body requires vitamin K to clot, it requires iron to produce blood. Approximately 70 percent of the body's iron is located within the red blood cells, where it forms part of hemoglobin. Development of new red blood cells is dependent on sufficient stores of iron, and iron is also required in other cells' DNA replication and repair processes.[21] Important functions, but most people don't get enough of it. According to the World Health Organization, two billion people, over 30 percent of the world's population, are iron-deficient. It is the most common nutrient deficiency in the world.[22] When iron levels are low, oxygen delivery to cells and tissues is compromised, resulting in *anemic hypoxia*. Anemia—which contributes to tumor hypoxia—can impair the effectiveness of radiation and chemotherapy by depriving tumor cells of the oxygen essential for the cytotoxic activities of these treatments. The effects of hypoxia also cause increased invasiveness and metastatic potential, loss of apoptosis, and angiogenesis.[23] On a day-to-day level, low iron can cause fatigue, shortness of breath, and light-headedness.

Several factors lead to anemia: insufficient intake of iron (in the case of vegetarian or vegan diets), compromised absorption or utilization, blood loss, pregnancy, menstruation, and more. But the main reason iron deficiency is the most common worldwide nutrient deficiency is that when we transformed from hunter-gatherers to farmers fifteen thousand years ago, our diet shifted away from iron-rich meat to less iron-rich grains. Grain-based diets are also laden with phytic acid, the number one "antinutrient." Consumption of phytic acid can reduce iron absorption by 50 percent.[24] Phytic acid is also present in nuts and seeds, but the amount can be reduced by soaking or sprouting. Unfortunately most humans stopped soaking and sprouting grains around the time of the Industrial Revolution, while simultaneously increasing consumption of them.

There are two food sources of iron. One is called *heme* iron and comes from meat, while *non-heme* iron is found in plants, including grains. Heme iron is attached to proteins called heme proteins. It has been well established that heme forms of iron are significantly more bioavailable, whereas the plant forms readily oxidize (form free radicals) and are not directly available for absorption.[25] This is another example showing that when we actually get to the nutrition science we see that vitamins and minerals are complex, often have several forms, and are frequently more bioavailable coming from animal sources. The oxidation issue of plant-based non-heme iron has presented a problem in iron fortification of foods; the sources that are approved and on the FDA's "Generally Recognized as Safe" list (which, needless to say, doesn't make us feel all that safe) cause more problems from an inflammation-oxidation standpoint than they are worth. Synthetically fortified grains such as those found in breads and cereals should never be considered an optimal way to get adequate or bioavailable amounts of iron. Vegetarian diets do not provide adequate iron levels despite proponents who insist that plant sources offer sufficient iron. That is simply biochemically incorrect.

What plant sources of iron *can* boast, however, is that many come conveniently "packaged" with vitamin C. In addition to to the immune benefits, vitamin C has an enhancing effect on the absorption of dietary non-heme iron, while also reducing its oxidative effects. It should be noted that grains have little to no vitamin C content. One cup of durum wheat contains 0 milligrams of vitamin C, and the same is true for oats and rice. Therefore, the best plant sources of iron and vitamin C–rich foods are parsley, seaweeds like kelp, borage (a cucumber-flavored herb), and spinach.

While a low iron level is a problem, so is a high level—especially a high level of *ferritin*, which is the form of iron that gets stored in the body. Several lines of evidence have demonstrated that high ferritin plays a role in proliferation, oxidative stress, angiogenesis, and immunosuppression. Ferritin is detected at higher levels in many cancer patients, and higher levels correlate with a more aggressive disease and poorer clinical outcome.[26] This becomes a major problem when serum RBCs, hemoglobin, and/or hematocrit levels are low and doctors have failed to properly test ferritin levels before considering supplementation of iron. Often, in this situation, ferritin is high (about 35–75 is optimal). Adding more iron to an already high ferritin is like pouring gasoline on a fire, yet many cancer patients are prescribed iron supplements (especially if they complain of fatigue), despite the fact that research has shown that iron directly fuels the growth of certain cancers, including

Lab Assessments for Circulation

Because there are so many balancing acts to consider when it comes to circulation and metastasis, Dr. Nasha regularly obtains the following labs (in addition to a complete blood count (CBC):

Fibrinogen: A protein involved in coagulation. High levels can indicate thick/sticky blood, making a person more susceptible to clotting as well as fueling cancer growth.

Vascular Endothelial Growth Factor (VEGF): A marker of angiogenesis. Serum VEGF levels in gastric and other types of cancers are typically significantly higher than those in controls.

Serum copper and ceruloplasmin: An angiogenesis inducer.

Ferritin: An iron storage marker. High levels can feed and fuel growth of cancer cells and cause inflammation and oxidative stress. Excess iron has been shown to increase the risk of breast cancer.

As with all lab tests, be sure to consult with your primary care provider in order to decipher results and determine the appropriate interventions.

glioblastomas.[27] Symptoms of iron overload include joint pain and loss of sex drive (and also, paradoxically, fatigue).

So where do high ferritin levels come from? Those with an ancient DNA mutation to the *C282Y* gene absorb more iron than most, and the resulting condition (hereditary hemochromatosis) is among the most prevalent genetic diseases in the United States—affecting almost one in two hundred people. Theorists have conjectured that the C282Y mutation evolved when the pandemic of iron deficiency began in the Neolithic era, as diets bloated with grains replaced those rich in meat and fish. This mutation may have protected humans against the threat of a diet lower in heme iron. Today that same mutation can cause high iron levels that fuel cancer. Therefore, it is absolutely essential that doctors check ferritin levels of their patients with cancer. When we see patients with high ferritin, they need to avoid red meat and other high-iron foods, which helps to reduce their levels. This is where red meat consumption becomes highly bio-individualized. In the absence of genetic and lab value assessments, iron levels can exert a broad array of effects on the cancer process.

The Metabolic Approach to Halting Cancer Growth and Spread

While the prognosis of a rapidly growing or metastatic cancer sounds grim, it does not mean that remission cannot be achieved. Never, ever give up hope. Dr. Nasha starts every one of her cancer retreats with this Emily Dickinson quote: "'Hope' is the thing with feathers that perches in the soul— / and sings the tune without the words— / and never stops—at all—." Having overcome stage IV ovarian cancer herself, Dr. Nasha has also helped hundreds of other stage IV patients who were essentially "sent out to pasture" by their conventional oncologists. With the right foods, a therapeutically tailored diet, and nontoxic therapies—including mistletoe and hyperbaric oxygen—all working to optimize the terrain, cancer can be overcome. You just have to believe that it will.

Our food-focused metabolic approach to this terrain element is multi-tiered. When these advanced processes occur, we first recommend avoiding all dairy products. A colon cancer study published in 2003 found that pathogenic gut bacteria such as *E. coli*, *Salmonella*, *Listeria*, and others could convert beta-casein-derived proteins from milk into pro-invasive factors that stimulate cancer cell invasion and motility.[28] As we learned in chapter 6 when discussing the microbiome, many factors contribute to imbalanced gut bacteria, so we don't take chances.

Therapeutic use of protein-digesting enzymes—including nattokinase, a powerful enzyme derived from Japanese natto, and lumbrokinase, derived from earthworms—helps to break down the thick fibrin matrix, thus weakening that cancer-protecting microenvironment, while supporting healthy circulation. We recommend increasing intake of the top low-glycemic, anti-angiogenic foods, herbs, and phytonutrients. We also add cartilages and bone broths from pastured chickens and wild fish bones. Sipping aloe vera juice and different types of tea, including green, have all been found to exert highly therapeutic and nontoxic antimetastatic potential. Let's take closer look at how some of these nutrition therapy approaches can help prevent and reduce the rate of cancer's growth and spread.

Top Foods for Inhibiting Angiogenesis and Metastasis

A 2005 review article titled "Nutraceuticals as Anti-Angiogenic Agents: Hopes and Reality" in the *Journal of Physiology and Pharmacology* determined that specific plant agents can suppress cancer cell proliferation, inhibit growth factor signaling pathways, induce apoptosis, and inhibit angiogenesis. These include resveratrol (from organic red grapes and wine) and curcumin (from the spice turmeric), which we mentioned in the last chapter. Naringenin, one of the most abundant citrus bioflavonoids found in grapefruit peels, also significantly reduces metastases.[29] This is where modified citrus pectin, one of the most powerful natural antimetastatics available, comes from. Here we take a closer look at other foods whose compounds also convey anti-angiogenic properties—including apigenin (from parsley), lycopene (from cherry tomatoes), and capsaicin (from chili peppers)—as well as some of the properties of the chaga mushroom.

Dr. William Li, president and medical director of the Angiogenesis Foundation, gave an excellent TED Talk in 2010 titled "Can We Eat to Starve Cancer?" In it he presented a list of many foods and herbs that he and his team found inhibit angiogenesis better than many cancer drugs. Vitamin E, found in the highest amounts in sunflower seeds, topped the chart. The best part of these plant foods is that they exert chemoprotective effects beyond angiogenesis and metastasis, further enhancing the need to accept nutrition as a primary cancer therapy. Building from what research has already been done on food synergies, it is highly possible we will discover that consuming several of these foods together could provide an anti-angiogenic effect far greater than that of conventional therapies, and of course, without the toxic effects.

PARSLEY: A HIGHLY MEDICINAL GARNISH

Native to the Mediterranean, parsley was considered sacred to the ancient Greeks, who used it to adorn winners of athletic events and also as décor on tombs of the deceased. The practice of using parsley as a food garnish actually has a long history that can be traced back to the ancient Romans. It is often used today in tabbouleh, a Middle Eastern dish made of tomatoes, chopped parsley, mint, onion, and seasoned with olive oil, lemon juice, and salt. (Tabbouleh traditionally includes bulgur, a gluten-containing grain, but since every other ingredient is a superfood we have created a grain-free cauliflower version; see the full recipe in chapter 13.) Apigenin, a plant flavonoid found in parsley's stems and leaves (as well as in celery and chamomile tea), demonstrates cytotoxic activities against breast cancer, induces apoptosis in colon cancer cells, and inhibits metastasis in ovarian cancer; its cytotoxic activity has been found comparable to that of doxorubicin.[30] Parsley is also exceptionally high in vitamins K, C, A, and folate. Both flat leaf and curly parsley are excellent additions to many dishes.

CHERRY TOMATOES: LYCOPENE IN THE LIMELIGHT

Second to potatoes, tomatoes are the most consumed vegetable in the United States—albeit mainly in the form of ketchup and spaghetti sauce. Tomatoes are technically a berry and have been in the limelight recently for their prostate-cancer-preventing lycopene content. Lycopene is a bright red pigment and phytochemical found in tomatoes, red and purple carrots, and rose hips (which are also high in vitamin C). Lycopene has been found to inhibit cancer cell proliferation, and reduce the risk of prostate cancer by blocking angiogenesis.[31] The smaller and deeper red the tomato (even to purple hues), the higher the lycopene content—far higher than the large, flavorless, beefsteak variety most often seen in grocery stores. Currant and cherry tomato varieties pack the most nutrient density, and cherry tomatoes also have fewer carbohydrates than larger varieties; ½ cup contains only 3 grams of carbohydrates.

CHAGA MUSHROOM TEA: A CUP A DAY KEEPS CHEMO AWAY

Chaga is a fungus that grows on birch trees in cold regions such as Siberia, northern Canada, Alaska, and northern parts of the United States, including

Maine and Vermont. Siberian tribes would grind it up and add to stews, soups, and daily beverages. It purportedly helped prevent degenerative disease and promote long life, and in areas of daily chaga consumption, cancer rates are low to none. Studies have since uncovered many of the mechanisms of the mushroom, including having antioxidant effects, lowering blood sugar, and stimulating the immune system. Chaga is known for its very high content of superoxide dismutase, an enzyme that functions as a powerful antioxidant. It also contains high levels of beta glucans, the potent polysaccharide that can reduce tumor proliferation and prevent tumor metastasis.[32] According to Dr. Cass Ingram, chaga expert and author of the excellent book *The Cure Is in the Forest*, chaga tea should be consumed daily. He also recommends taking chaga together with wild oregano, a natural antifungal agent that helps stimulate the absorption of chaga's active ingredients. The power of traditional food pairings is just breathtaking sometimes!

CHILI PEPPERS: TOO HOT FOR CANCER TO THRIVE

Chili peppers belong to the family of foods with the Latin name *Capsicum*. Recent studies have shown that their capsaicin component not only has chemopreventive properties against certain carcinogens and mutagens but also exerts other anticancer activities. Specifically, this spice has been found to inhibit VEGF and was able to suppress tumor-induced angiogenesis.[33] It seems almost counterintuitive that something that makes you sweat and increases your circulation would *inhibit* angiogenesis but it does, just like exercise! A population-based prospective cohort study of 199,293 men and 288,082 women ages thirty to seventy-nine years published in the *British Medical Journal* in 2015 found that frequent consumption of spicy foods was associated with 14 percent less risk of dying from cancer, most likely due to its anti-inflammatory effects.[34]

The hottest varieties include red chili, habanero, and Scotch bonnet peppers. The hotter the chili pepper, the more capsaicin it contains. Harissa, a spicy chili paste made with garlic and olive oil, is a widely used staple in North African and Middle Eastern cooking. It not only is rich in capsaicin but also contains other powerful anticancer herbs, such as caraway. Time to add a little spice to your life! You get used to it the more you eat it, then start to crave it after a while. A spicy pepper addiction is one we wholeheartedly endorse.

CARTILAGE: STOPPING METASTASES BY EATING BONES

Earlier in this chapter we discussed how cancer cells are able to metastasize by breaking down the thick jungles of the surrounding ECM. This weblike matrix composed predominantly of collagens provides a structural and biochemical scaffolding that tries to prevent cancer cells from spreading by modulating cell proliferation and differentiation.[35] It also serves as a reservoir for growth factors. If you include collagen-rich foods in your diet, your body is able to regenerate degraded ECM, which helps to encapsulate tumors.

So, where does collagen come from? Bones. Until the last hundred years, humans ate bones in one form or another; no part of the animal went to waste. All edible parts of an animals were eaten, and the leftover bones were thrown into soup. Now, as we mentioned earlier, most Americans eat only animal muscle meat, while bones and organs are tossed in the trash. Yet glucosamine/chondroitin is one of the most consumed supplements in this country because it really helps ease the pain of arthritis. So why not just eat them in your food? The high glucosamine and chondroitin content in bone broth can stimulate the growth of new collagen, repair damaged joints, ease arthritis, and reduce pain and inflammation. Glucosamine is also known as a toxic agent for several malignant cell lines, with little toxicity to healthy tissues, and can halt metastatic progression in colon, breast, and prostate cancers.[36] While the body produces collagen naturally, the process slows with age. Adding mineral-rich bone broth can not only help support the integrity of the ECM, but also provide the DNA-protective measures discussed in chapter 3. We highly suggest fish-bone broth and broth made from pastured, organically raised chickens if ferritin levels are too high for beef-bone broth.

ALOE VERA JUICE: SOOTHER OF AGGRAVATED PLATELETS

Use of the prickly aloe vera, known as the plant of immortality, can be traced back six thousand years to early Egypt. It grows wild in tropical climates and is cultivated for both agricultural and medicinal uses. Today it's most popular as a sunburn remedy, but its extracts are also powerful antioxidants that can inhibit platelet aggregation and angiogenesis—a wise moisturizer choice, especially if showering in fluoride-treated water. Aloin, one of aloe's main components, has been found to inhibit the secretion of VEGF in cancer cells.[37] Taken internally, aloe helps with gastric inflammation and constipation. In aloe, there are over two hundred biologically active components—vitamins, enzymes, and amino acids—that convey detoxification and immune benefits. Despite its label as a "juice," it contains far less sugar and carbs than its fruit juice counterparts: 2 ounces of aloe vera juice contains 2 grams of carbohydrate and 6 grams of sugar—though it should still be consumed in moderation in order to stay in ketosis. If you have an aloe plant at home, you can make this powerful drink by scooping the gel out of the stems and mixing it with water or green tea, fresh lemon juice, and apple cider vinegar in the blender.

GREEN TEA: A POWERFUL GROWTH INHIBITOR

Green tea is probably the most well-known and widely accepted anticancer beverage, and for good reason. The catechins found in tea are the most extensively studied flavonoids that show anti-invasive and antimetastic activity. The journal *Cancer and Metastasis Reviews* published a paper in 2011 titled "Cancer and Metastasis: Prevention and Treatment by Green Tea." It summarizes the effects of green tea, as well as outlines the role of EGCG (the primary catechin) in inhibiting tumor invasion and angiogenesis.[38] The paper notes that EGCG has an antioxidant activity about twenty-five to a hundred times more effective than either vitamin C or E, and is a potent regulator of the signaling pathways that contribute to cancer metastasis. There have been so many research studies done on green tea it deserves a chapter of its own; but for now, just know that it is most likely the most potent antitumor and antimetastasis beverage you can consume.

All true teas come from the leaves of an evergreen tree called *Camellia sinensis*. It is the way the leaves are processed that determines whether it is a green, black, or oolong tea. Green tea is the least processed of all and provides the most antioxidant polyphenols. Green teas do absorb high pesticide loads, however, so buying organic is absolutely necessary. The highest-quality green teas are the Japanese varieties, such as *sencha*, *matcha*, and *gyokuro*. Of these, *gyokuro* is the best and is an intensely green and sweet tea that is slowly matured to enhance the leaves' flavonol and amino acid content. To properly brew green tea, let the water barely reach boiling, then allow to cool slightly before pouring over the tea. Let steep for three to ten minutes to release the catechins, then remove the tea leaves. The recommendation is five cups a day if possible!

GINSENG: AN HERBAL INVASION SUPPRESSOR

There are three different types of ginseng—panax, Siberian, and American—and each has different bioactive properties. Ginseng contains various active components, including ginsenosides, polysaccharides, flavonoids, volatile oils, amino acids, and vitamins. All three varieties can be helpful for restoring energy to fatigued cancer patients while also suppressing cancer invasion, metastasis, and angiogenesis. American ginseng contains a chemical group called ginsenosides that can affect insulin and help lower blood sugar levels. These compounds have also been found to inhibit tumor angiogenesis. Other active phytochemicals in ginseng include polysaccharides, which exert a positive effect on the immune system and are often used in combination with anticancer drugs to enhance chemotherapy and reduce toxicity. Combined therapy with ginseng and low-dose gemcitabine or cyclophosphamide has been found to produce significant anti-angiogenic effect without overt toxicity.[39] For those looking to wean off caffeine, ginseng tea is a wonderful replacement.

CHAMOMILE CALMS METASTASES

There are two chamomile plants: the more popular German chamomile, and the Roman, or English, chamomile. Like all foods we've mentioned before, chamomile has been used as a medicine for thousands of years, dating back to the ancient Egyptians, Romans, and Greeks. Like cherry tomatoes, chamomile also contains the phytochemical apigenin, which has been shown to inhibit cell growth, sensitize cancer cells to elimination by apoptosis, and hinder angiogenesis. It also has actions that alter the relationship of the cancer cells with their microenvironment, and is able to reduce cancer cell glucose uptake, slow progression, and inhibit metastasis.[40] Chamomile also helps with digestive upset and aids with relaxation. The incredible effects of these foods, herbs, broths, and teas are simply amazing, as long as they are high-quality organic. Tea time should be all the time!

Crystalizing Impacts of Cancer's Growth and Spread

Where angiogenesis and metastasis are two of the most lethal aspects of cancer, a metabolic approach can offer significant protection. Both processes are primarily activated by inflammation, dehydration, sedentary lifestyles, and high copper levels. Regular consumption of spicy peppers, chaga mushrooms, parsley, green tea, bone broth, and more have been found to reduce the spread of cancer and the growth of new blood vessels to feed it. A diet of green tea and a spicy fish-bone broth is a powerful protocol here.

The next terrain element, hormones, has much to do with cancer's growth and spread as well. Modern life is teeming with environmental estrogens that are fueling breast, prostate, and all other cancers to pandemic levels. Hormone balance is imperative, and while flaxseed is not the best source of anti-inflammatory omega-3 fatty acids, it is one of the best foods for hormone balance. Let's learn more about the role hormones play in cancer and, most important, how to balance them.

CHAPTER 10

Hungry for Hormone Balance

To control your hormones is to control your life.

—BARRY SEARS, PhD

The doctor of the future will no longer treat the human frame with drugs, but rather will cure and prevent disease with nutrition.

—THOMAS EDISON

Hormones are a whole lot more than what got us pleasantly hot and bothered as teenagers (and not so pleasantly during menopause). Hormones coordinate growth, fertility, immunity, and metabolism as they naturally fluctuate throughout a lifetime. These fluctuations are often more pronounced in women because of such phases including puberty, pregnancy, and menopause, but men are just as susceptible to hormonal imbalances as women. *Andropause*, "male menopause," is the gradual decline of testosterone that occurs as males age. Men who are overweight are also prone to estrogen dominance and its associated symptoms, including erectile dysfunction, low libido, and prostate cancer.[1] Neither sex is immune to the powerful effects of hormones, especially estrogen—we all experience its associated ups and downs, no matter how healthy we are.

Unfortunately, hormone-related and reproductive organ cancers are one of the most common cancers of our time. Breast and prostate cancers now affect one in seven of us. In addition to cancers of the reproductive organs, however, excess hormones can stimulate the growth of all types of cancers, including lung, the most common type of cancer worldwide. Where do all these hormones come from? The scary answer is they come from many common sources. Much of our food and many of the products we use in daily life contain synthetic chemicals called *xenoestrogens*. These compounds are as strong as the naturally occurring estrogen in our bodies—sometimes even stronger. The sharp rise in reproductive cancer rates has been glaringly concurrent with the approval and use of hormones and endocrine-disrupting chemicals in our food, household products, and hormone-based medications. Just look at the time line.

In 1947 sex hormones were approved and introduced to livestock production. In 1960, the birth control pill was approved for use. Since 1945 thousands of endocrine-disrupting chemicals have been released into the environment, and less than 5 percent of these have been safety-tested. From 1950 to 2000 rates of breast cancer increased 60 percent, and from 1973 to 1991 a 126 percent increase in prostate cancer occurred. Rates of testicular, ovarian, and endometrial cancers have also all been rapidly increasing over the past few decades. And we will explain why.

Imbalanced hormone-related signs and symptoms—including acne, autoimmune disease, depression, infertility, thyroid disorders, endometriosis, ovarian cysts, insomnia, low libido, early puberty, menopausal symptoms, and weight gain—are widespread in modern times. Infertility affects one in six couples. Thyroid disorders affect one in five women. More than 50 percent of women report menopausal symptoms including hot flashes, which is not normal. And speaking of not normal, breast development typical of eleven-year-olds a generation ago is now occurring in seven-year-olds, and those even as young as three years. It is time to start paying *very* close attention to what is causing this massive surge in hormone-related imbalances and cancers. As we will learn in this chapter, breast and prostate cancers are not simply "bad luck." They are a direct result of the hormones in our food, especially meat and dairy products, daily exposures to synthetic hormone-disrupting chemicals found in products from water bottles to shampoo, and the use of synthetic and bioidentical hormones in birth control and hormone replacement therapies. You have probably been exposed to over two hundred hormone-disrupting chemicals just today.

Hormones are so potent at driving cancer that it is a terrain area Western oncology commonly tests for and has developed drugs to combat. Yet these hormone blockade "life rings" are not helping those who are drowning in pools of estrogen. As much as cancer cells like sugar, they also love hormones, which stimulate them to become hot and bothered and reproduce. Approximately 70 percent of breast cancers are sensitive to estrogen, meaning estrogen makes the cancer grow. In nature, estrogen's job is to cause cells to proliferate, and *all* cancer cells will grow in response to this hormone, not just those diagnosed as hormone-sensitive. Estrogen drives angiogenesis, causes inflammation, and modulates metabolism.[2] So no more tiptoeing through the daisies like a starry-eyed teenager when it comes to hormones and cancer. Ridding our food and household products of hormones while taking nutritional steps to balance hormones is a critical terrain element.

Yet balancing hormones takes a lot of awareness and effort, as so many aspects of daily living result in overexposure to estrogen. Just the simple routine of taking a shower, washing your hair, putting on scent, popping a birth control pill, and having yogurt for breakfast is enough to whack your estrogen levels out of the park. As always, however, with the right nutrition and lifestyle modifications, balance is completely possible. A number of food-based compounds can help support hormone balance. These include proper use of phytoestrogens, fatty acids, certain seeds, phytonutrients, herbs, and specific cruciferous vegetable compounds, as well as the reduction of sugar and alcohol consumption (detailed at the end of the chapter). Hormonal health—like all other terrain elements—is completely dependent on good nutrition.

In this chapter we explain how hormones work in the body, their role in cancer, what throws them out of whack, ways to test them, and a proven plan for hormonal restoration. So take a cold shower and locate your flotation devices. We are going to pull you out of the estrogen pool and onto the warm beaches of hormone balance.

The Basics of Hormones and Cancer

The word *hormone* has Greek origins and means "to stir up" or "to urge on." Hormones are chemical messenger molecules that control and regulate the activities of cells, organs, and just about every process in the body, including digestion, metabolism, and reproduction. Hormones are produced by endocrine glands and travel through the bloodstream to their various cellular destinations. While all cells are exposed to circulating hormones, not all react, only those that have hormone-specific receptors. You can think of hormone receptors like a garage door that opens when a hormone pushes the matching opener button and allows the car to drive in. When a hormone binds to a receptor, like a car entering the garage, it causes a biological response that alters the behavior of the cell. For example, when estrogen binds to an estrogen receptor on a cell, it tells that cell to divide and grow. Too much estrogen equals too much growth, and that's a problem. Cells in the endometrium, breast, ovaries, kidney, brain, bone, heart, intestines, and prostate all have receptor sites for estrogen. Cells in each of those tissues will grow and divide when estrogen drives in.[3]

Since hormones are involved in most aspects of bodily function, it comes as no surprise that they are intricately involved with cancer progression. There are several ways in which estrogens and other hormones fuel the cancer process: They stimulate growth and division of cancerous cells, cause immune system suppression, promote inflammation, and increase blood flow to tumors. Incredibly, cancer cells are able to dictate the number of hormone receptor sites on their surfaces, just as they do with insulin receptors.

When a breast, ovarian, or prostate tumor is removed, the tissue is tested to determine if it has hormone receptors, which kind, and how many. If cancer cells have estrogen hormone receptors, that cancer is labeled ER-positive, or ER+. Concentrations of estrogens have been shown to be twentyfold higher in breast cancer tissues. If cancer cells have progesterone receptors, they are called PR-positive or PR+. This means that the hormone progesterone encourages their growth. A "triple negative" breast cancer diagnosis means that the tumor has neither estrogen nor progesterone receptors and is also negative for the *HER2* gene (a growth-promoting gene). This is viewed as a poor prognosis in Western medicine because the leading—and in some cases only—treatment options for breast cancer are hormone blockade therapies.

Anti-estrogen drugs, also known as *selective estrogen receptor modulators* (SERMs), work by blocking and deactivating the estrogen receptor on the surface of a cancer cell. Basically these drugs park a car in the garage and leave it there. One example of these drugs is tamoxifen; unfortunately, tamoxifen has also been found to cause cancer of the uterus, strokes, and blood clots in the lungs.[4] And despite the fact that tamoxifen is listed as a Group 1 carcinogen, it remains a front-line treatment for many breast cancers. There has to be a better way.

Male dominant hormones, androgens, are involved in promoting prostate cancer growth. Androgens are steroid hormones that confer masculinity, sexual development, and physique in men. They include testosterone, androstenedione, and dehydroepiandrosterone (DHEA). Androgens promote the growth of both normal and cancerous prostate cells by binding to and activating androgen receptors, just as estrogen and progesterone do with their receptors. Once activated, the androgen receptor stimulates the expression of specific genes that cause prostate cells to grow.[5] During early development, prostate cancers need relatively high levels of androgens to grow, and these prostate cancers are referred to as androgen-dependent or androgen-sensitive. Anti-androgen hormone therapy drugs bind to androgen receptors, blocking androgen uptake in androgen-sensitive prostate cancer cells. An example of this drug class is flutamide, used in advanced prostate cancers. It can also cause severe and sometimes fatal liver damage.

These drugs are merely a lid on a pressure cooker; they do not change the SNPs, the metabolic processes, or the terrain. Instead, in most cases they make the terrain worse off. We have to look at what we are eating and how we are living, because these two factors have everything to do with how hormones are created and used in the body. Let's take a closer look at estrogen, since this hormone—produced in both men and women and widespread in our environment—is hands down the most influential driver of cancer.

Estrogen

When we say estrogen, many people assume that it is a single hormone, but it actually comprises a class of over two dozen different types of estrogen hormone molecules. The most commonly known are estrone, estradiol, and estriol. Estradiol is the predominant form of estrogen in nonpregnant, reproductive females and primarily aids in the cyclic release of eggs from the ovaries (ovulation). It is the most potent of all the estrogens, meaning it has the ability to provoke the most growth in cells. Estrone is produced in the ovaries and by fat cells in both men and women, and is the dominant estrogen in postmenopausal women. Estriol is secreted in large quantities by the placenta during pregnancy. All types of estrogens are created from cholesterol via a hormonal domino effect. The first domino in line is pregnenolone, which converts into other hormones including DHEA, progesterone, testosterone, and the various forms of estrogen.

Aromatase is a very important enzyme that is responsible for converting androgen hormones into estrogens in both men and women. Aromatase-inhibiting drugs work by blocking the enzyme so that less estrogen is produced and available to stimulate the growth of estrogen-receptor-positive cancer cells. Drugs like this may have worthwhile function, but they are certainly not useful in preventing cancers from occurring in the first place, nor in stopping the mechanisms that are ultimately driving them. When you consider the amount of estrogens we are exposed to on a daily basis, it's like trying to stop Niagara Falls using a pin-sized plug.

After estrogens have completed their tasks in the body they are sent to the liver to be metabolized or deactivated and prepared for excretion through the feces or urine. This busy detoxification organ is also a hormone processor and director. It manufactures and regulates hormone levels and can also direct various hormones to perform their proper function in other parts of the body. When the body is exposed to excess toxins, the liver is not able to process hormones as quickly or efficiently, leading ultimately to hormonal imbalances. Defects in optimal detoxification can cause a hormone to be only partially metabolized, sort of like a dirty dish that gets put back in the cabinet. A partially metabolized hormone can cycle back into the bloodstream looking for receptor sites, but can't relay the intended message of a fully functioning hormone. It opens the garage door, but rather than saying, "Turn on the lights," it says, "Turn on the blanket." *Not* the intended result. The take-home message here is that optimizing liver function and integrating detoxification strategies is critical for the proper metabolism of hormones.

Estrogen Metabolites and Cruciferous Vegetables

The liver converts estrogens into estrogen metabolites through the actions of certain enzymes including COMT and CYP1B1.[6] Three of estrogen's metabolites, the breakdown products of this hormone, are 2-hydroxyestrone, 4-hydroxyestrone, and 16-alpha-hydroxyestrone. Since the 1980s, 2-hydroxyestrone has been considered a "good" or chemoprotective form of estrogen, while 16-alpha-hydroxyestrone has been associated with the development of cancer. It has tissue-stimulating effects similar to estradiol and can fuel the growth and division of hormone-dependent and other cancer cells more than the 2-hydroxyestrones can. The 2-hydroxyestrones, in contrast, have almost no estrogenic effect. Despite some mutterings to the contrary, prevailing evidence has shown that the ratio of 2-hydroxyestrone to 16-alpha-hydroxyestrone is relevant as a risk factor for estrogen-sensitive cancers, including breast and cervical cancers. Simply put, when it comes to estrogen metabolites, you want more 2s than 16s. And guess what can help the body do that? Cruciferous vegetables.

Two of the many active components in cruciferous vegetables are indole-3-carbinol (I3C) and diindolylmethane (DIM). Physiologically, DIM is the predominant active agent and I3C is the precursor. Studies have found that these compounds can inhibit the formation of the "bad" 16-alpha-hydroxyestrone estrogen metabolite.[7] One study found that DIM had the ability to decrease its production by 50 percent while increasing production of the "good" 2-hydroxyestrone metabolite by 75 percent. A placebo-controlled, double-blind study of women at increased risk for breast cancer found that four weeks of supplementation with I3C promoted favorable changes in the ratio of the two metabolites as measured in the urine. A pretty impressive feat, without side effects.

I3C is found in a number of cruciferous vegetables, including broccoli, brussels sprouts, cabbage, cauliflower, collard greens, kale, kohlrabi, mustard greens, radish, rutabaga, and turnip. The highest concentrations are found in garden cress (different from watercress) and mustard greens. I3C is released when these foods are chewed then converts to DIM by the action of stomach acid.[8] Use of antacids therefore prevents this conversion. Also, stomach acid levels naturally decline with age and also with stress. Optimizing digestive

Hormone Myth Buster #1:
Cruciferous Vegetables and Thyroid Function

In 1929 researchers from Johns Hopkins University fed rabbits a diet of cabbage, and the rabbits developed goiters (enlarged thyroid glands). Consequently, for decades many people with thyroid problems have been incorrectly advised to avoid cruciferous vegetables because of their *goitrogen* content. (Goitrogens are substances that can disrupt the production of thyroid hormones by interfering with iodine uptake by the thyroid gland and are present in drugs, chemicals, and food.) Cruciferous vegetables have been erroneously blamed for causing low iodine levels.

Fast-forward through eighty more years of thyroid research, and we can confirm that goiters are definitely not caused by eating cabbage. So please don't keep cruciferous vegetables off your plate! Goiters, and in some cases thyroid cancer, are caused by the autoimmune thyroid disease Hashimoto's thyroiditis and from goitrogenic xenobiotics.[9] Hashimoto's thyroiditis is responsible for close to 90 percent of all cases

pathways and secretions is clearly important when it comes to hormone balance. Talk to your primary care provider about what is right for you.

Estrogen, Apples, and the Microbiome

We've known since the 1970s that the composition of our microbiome impacts how estrogens are metabolized. These microbiota even have a name: the *estrobolome*. The estrobolome are beneficial bacteria in the gastrointestinal system that produce an essential enzyme that helps metabolize estrogen. The health of the estrobolome also affects one of the phase 2 liver detoxification pathways, glucuronidation, described in chapter 5. Glucuronidation is involved in the detoxification of xenoestrogens (synthetic or natural), human estrogens, drugs, chemical toxins, and more. Pathogenic bacteria of hypothyroidism. Perchlorate, a synthetic chemical released in 1952, has been found over and over to impair normal thyroid function by interfering with iodine uptake by the thyroid gland. Drugs such as benzodiazepines, calcium channel blockers, steroids, retinoids (synthetic vitamin A), and pesticides also are causes of thyroid dysregulation.

This low iodine thyroid myth has perpetuated a prevalent and dangerous recommendation in the natural medicine community, which is the recommendation of iodine supplementation for hormone balance. Iodine supplementation is often suggested to breast cancer patients and those with low-functioning thyroids, but it is critical to note that most of us actually have iodine *excess*. Proper iodine levels can be achieved by eating high-quality sea salt and occasional seaweed. Avoiding grains and fluoride-treated water (fluoride competes with iodine) also significantly enhances thyroid function. When patients who are hypothyroid are overtreated with iodine, we send them into autoimmune storms. We test thyroid antibodies in all patients before even considering adding iodine-rich foods to avoid damage to the thyroid gland.

in the intestines can produce an enzyme called β-glucuronidase that blocks this important estrogen detox process and allows partially metabolized hormones to be reabsorbed into the body. This causes all types of estrogens to accumulate and reach excessive levels.

High levels of β-glucuronidase are also associated with an increased risk for various cancers, particularly hormone-dependent cancers such as breast, prostate, and colon cancers. Thankfully, there is a nutrition antidote. Calcium-D-glucarate is the calcium salt of D-glucaric acid and is found in many fruits and vegetables, at the highest concentrations in apples. Calcium-D-glucarate increases glucuronidation and inhibits β-glucuronidase. It therefore enhances the body's ability to excrete estrogens and environmental toxins.[10] But keep in mind a few important points with apples: First, the best choice is the smaller, green, wild crab apples, which have less sugar than red apples and substantially more phytonutrients than modern varieties. Second, to avoid the sugar and get the most fiber benefit focus on the peel over the flesh; that is where most of the nutrients and fiber are found. Finally, commercially grown apples have some of the highest levels of pesticide residues, so choosing organic apples is paramount. A small, green, wild apple exerts extremely powerful chemopreventive effects!

Progesterone and Cholesterol

Every yin has a yang, and estrogen's yang is progesterone. Progesterone opposes estrogen, and it protects the body against its powerful growth effects. Estrogen dominance largely occurs when there is not enough progesterone present to counter excessive estrogen. In menstruating women, progesterone and estrogen are the two primary sex hormones produced during a monthly cycle by the ovaries. During the first fourteen days of the menstrual cycle, the ovaries secrete increasing amounts of estrogens. Halfway through a woman's cycle, around Day 14, one of her two ovaries will ovulate and release an egg. The portion of the menstrual cycle that follows ovulation is called the luteal phase and is orchestrated by progesterone. This is one of the many natural biorhythms the body follows in relation to the planet: a month is how long it takes for the moon to complete its orbit around the Earth.

When it comes to cancer, low progesterone is just as big a problem as high estrogen. One of the most significant studies of the relationship between low levels of natural progesterone and increased breast cancer risk was published in the *American Journal of Epidemiology* in 1981. The study followed 1,083 women with a history of difficulty becoming pregnant for periods ranging from thirteen to thirty-three years. The researchers found that infertile women who demonstrated a progesterone deficiency had a premenopausal breast cancer risk that was more than 500 percent greater than that of women whose infertility was due to nonhormonal causes. Furthermore, the women with a progesterone deficiency had a 1,000 percent greater chance of death from all types of cancer.[11] But what causes low progesterone? According to toxicology textbooks: chemical toxins, including pesticides.[12]

If you have spoken with your doctor, been tested, and determined that you do have a low progesterone level, then chasteberry tea might be worth considering. Used for twenty-five hundred years, chasteberry, also known as vitex, is the fruit of the chaste tree, a small shrublike tree native to Central Asia and the Mediterranean. Studies have demonstrated its ability to increase progesterone while decreasing estrogen. It has also demonstrated the ability to normalize abnormal cycles, improve premenstrual syndrome (PMS), and support fertility.

Hormone SNPs and Dietary Approaches

As we learned in chapter 5, the liver's many detox pathways and enzymes play a critical role in the body's detoxification of chemicals, in addition to the processing of hormones. We feel that it is malpractice not to assess SNPs, family history, hormone metabolites, steroid use, and history of hormone blockade therapies before putting anyone on hormone therapy. There are so many pieces of the puzzle that absolutely must be considered when it comes to hormones, and genetics is at the top.

For example, many SNPs have been identified as playing a role in estrogen metabolism and detoxification. For starters, the creation of the aromatase enzyme is made possible by the instructions contained in gene *CYP19*. When there are SNPs in this gene, estrogen production is altered. The CYP1 detox enzymes we discussed are also directly involved in the formation of estrogen metabolites and can cause the formation of more 16s than 2s. These CYP1 enzymes are also involved in the body's ability to detox (which is why we always look at detox SNPs before starting any detoxification plan). Food to the rescue! Various plants and phytonutrients have been found to alter CYP1 activity. Cruciferous vegetables and resveratrol-containing foods have been shown to act as activators of CYP1A1. Another compound, chrysoeriol, present in celery, can inhibit CYP1B1 and may be especially relevant to patients with CYP1B1 overactivity.[13] SNPs in the CYP2 family of enzymes can be supported with foods and phytonutrients such as quercetin, broccoli, and rosemary.[14]

By now, you can see that there is more to hormones and how the body processes them than we are often told. There is also a lot of power in good nutrition. The genome, microbiome, and detoxification systems are all intricately involved in hormone health. Assessing and monitoring hormone levels should be mandatory. Make sure you request this of your doctor before they place you on any type of hormone therapy, as most women have estrogen dominance, not depletion.

Hormone Testing

Testing hormone levels is critically important, especially for women considering hormone replacement therapy (HRT), and there are three main testing methods: serum (blood), urine, and saliva. There are benefits and drawbacks to each of these methods. Serum testing is the standard for measuring hormones in the conventional medical community and is ideal for testing certain hormones, like follicle-stimulating hormone (FSH), fasting insulin, and thyroid hormones. However, for sex hormones such as estrogen, progesterone, and testosterone, serum-testing validity is limited. Here's why: There are two types of hormones—bound and unbound. Approximately 95 percent of hormones are bound by proteins and are therefore not available for tissue use. The remaining 5 percent of hormones are unbound, remaining active and fully available for tissue use. Serum hormone testing doesn't make the distinction between bound and free hormone levels, and results often show normal or high-normal results because of the inclusion of bound hormones. Therefore, to get the real picture, blood is not best.

Saliva is better for evaluating estrogens and progesterone. Saliva tests measure free hormones, making this a more accurate measure than serum for evaluating hormone status. Measuring hormones in urine is less common in clinical practice, yet quite common in research. A twenty-four-hour urine collection (depositing pee in a cup for a full twenty-four-hour period) is the preferred method for testing hormones that are secreted during deep sleep, such as melatonin. An advantage of urine hormone collection is the ability to measure hormone metabolites like 2- and 16-hydroxyestrone. This is especially important when evaluating the adequacy and safety of exogenous estrogen drugs. (There are many different testing companies, but Dr. Nasha generally prefers to run the Meridian Valley 24-Hour Urine Test, Diagnos-Techs saliva hormone test, and/or the DUTCH dried urine test. We suggest that you consult with your naturopathic oncologist about the most appropriate testing option for you.)

Top Three Hormone Hijackers

Despite the shocking rates of prostate, breast, and other hormone-related cancers, most people are not aware of the everyday diet and lifestyle factors that are causing significant endocrine disruption in men, women, and children. There are many ways that we get exposed to estrogens in the environment, but the following three are the most common. In this section, we put our scuba tanks on and go deep into the waters of these hormonal growth factors. We want you to have the knowledge and tools to avoid these hormone-disrupting chemicals and also, hopefully, be able to share this information with others so we can start reversing the skyrocketing rates of cancers fueled by environmental estrogens. It can be stopped. It's time to put a kink in the hoses that are filling these pools of estrogens we are all bathing in.

Exposure to Environmental Estrogens in Everyday Products

Every day Americans use skin creams, shaving creams, bubble bath, lotions, perfumes, lipsticks, fingernail polishes, shower gel, makeup, shampoos, hair colors, deodorants, sunscreens, bug spray, household cleaning products, toys, clothes, bottled water, garden fertilizers, and more. These products can all contain endocrine-disrupting chemicals. On average, Americans are exposed to hundreds of these chemicals each day. From 1940 to 1982, the production of petroleum-derived chemicals increased 350 percent. These types of chemicals are also called xenoestrogens, xenobiotics, xenohormones, exogenous estrogens, or, the technical term, endocrine-disrupting chemicals (EDCs). They are synthetic chemicals that imitate and act like estrogen in the body and are widely used in just about every product of the modern age.

Many types of chemicals are considered EDCs, among them plastics, plasticizers, pesticides, and flame retardants. And just as with toxins, human exposure to EDCs occurs through ingestion, through inhalation, and through the skin. When we lather on lotions and sunscreens loaded with xenoestrogens, these chemicals are absorbed directly into bloodstream. Would we so readily slather sunscreen on our toast, or would we read the ingredients

TABLE 10.1. ENDOCRINE-DISRUPTING CHEMICALS, PRODUCTS OF ORIGIN, AND HOW TO AVOID THEM

Chemical	Product Sources	How to Avoid
Bisphenol-A	Plastic water bottles and cups Paper receipts Canned foods and drinks Dental sealants Plastic food wrap Wines fermented in vats lined with plastic	Use glass water containers. Have receipts emailed. Avoid all canned food and drinks. Speak with your dentist. Use glass food storage containers. Contact your favorite winemaker and inquire about their fermentation practices.
Dioxins	Bleached toilet paper White paper napkins and paper towels Tampons Bleached coffee filters Nonorganic beef and dairy consumption Herbicides widely used on cereal grains, including wheat, corn, oats, and rice Hand sanitizer	Use only nonbleached paper products, especially internally (i.e., tampons). Avoid all grains, especially those that are not organic. Use thieves oil (see chapter 6) or natural, non-triclosan-based hand sanitizers.
Phthalates	Synthetic fragrance (perfume, laundry detergent) Air fresheners Shower curtains Plastic baby toys Raincoats Carpet Intravenous drip bags and other medical devices	Avoid all products that use synthetic fragrance. Do not use plug-in or car air fresheners; opt for essential oils instead. Avoid all plastic baby and kid products. Use natural-fiber carpeting. Follow detox protocols under naturopathic medical supervision following medical procedures.

more carefully? It's almost the same thing (although people are slathering a lot more lotion on their body than they would ever eat).

In 2013 the World Health Organization and United Nations concluded: "Exposure to EDCs during fetal development and puberty plays a role in the increased incidences of reproductive diseases, endocrine-related cancers,

Chemical	Product Sources	How to Avoid
Perchlorate	Drinking water (especially high in Nevada, California, and Utah) Rocket fuel manufacturing and military operations Fireworks Blasting rocks Fertilizer used in tobacco and citrus fruit cultivation	Aggressive measures must be taken for filtering water (see chapter 13). Eat only organic fruits and vegetables. If you live near a military base, make sure to follow detox protocols every 2–3 months under a naturopathic provider's supervision.
Polybrominated diphenyl ethers (PBDEs), chemicals	Nonstick pans Children's pajamas Couches Mattresses New cars Airplane seats Computer monitors	Switch to stainless steel cookware. Buy organic cotton children's pajamas. Seek products that do not use flame-retardant chemicals. Use thieves oil during air travel.
Glycol ethers (including 2-butoxyethanol [EGBE] and methoxydiglycol [DEGME]).	Cleaning products Paint Liquid soaps Dry-cleaning chemicals Whiteboard cleaners Cosmetics	Opt for nontoxic cleaning products. Wear a respirator and gloves when using paint products. Do not have clothes dry-cleaned. Use nontoxic cosmetic products.
Parabens	Shampoos and conditioners Lotions and sunscreens Antiperspirants	Audit all personal care products and switch to brands that do not use parabens.

behavioral and learning problems, including ADHD, infections, asthma, and perhaps obesity and diabetes in humans." Some of these EDCs have been classified as *obesogens* and are dietary, pharmaceutical, and industrial compounds that alter metabolic processes and predispose some people to gain weight. *Phthalates* and *plasticizers*, for example, have been related to obesity in humans, as have scented items such as air fresheners, laundry products, and personal care products. Obesogens can affect the number and size of fat cells as well as the hormones that affect appetite, satiety, food preferences, and energy metabolism.[15]

In table 10.1 we outline a few of these chemicals, the places where we are exposed to them, and how to avoid them. Do note that there are excellent resources out there to learn more about EDCs, including the EWG, Safecosmetics.org, the Endocrine Disruption Exchange, and the Silent Spring Institute.

This list hopefully provides the needed "aha" moment about how many hormone-disrupting chemicals we are exposed to just in the course of a normal day. Of course it's overwhelming. But start by replacing one product at a time, or go through each room in the house and start switching out laundry, cleaning, and personal care products for brands that do not contain these ingredients. Next up, a look at the hormone component of modern food products.

Commercial Meat and Dairy Products

Since the 1950s the FDA has maintained approval of six growth-promoting steroid hormone drugs for use in beef cattle and sheep. Note that these are called growth promoters because that is what hormones such as estrogen—and antibiotics—do: They make tissues grow! The hormones used in commercial animal production can make animals grow up to 50 percent faster. The approved hormones are estradiol, progesterone, testosterone, and synthetic hormones, including the estrogen compound zeranol, the androgen trenbolone acetate, and progestin melengestrol acetate. The first synthetic estrogen used for this purpose, diethylstilbestrol (DES), was approved for use in beef cattle in 1940. An estimated two-thirds of the nation's beef cattle were treated with DES in 1956, and the NCI estimates that between five and ten million people were exposed to DES in the United States between 1938 and 1971.[16] During this time DES was also used in pregnant women to prevent miscarriage, their and their offsprings' cancer rates went completely through the roof, spurring the well-known epidemic of "DES babies."

DES was removed from use with cattle in 1972 after it was determined to cause cancer. Yet here in the United States we are still eating six hormones in commercially raised meat that other countries have flat-out banned and refused to import because their analyses have shown that they cause cancer. In 1981 the European Union (Germany, France, Italy, and seven other countries) banned the use of synthetic hormones and prohibited the import of animals and meat from animals that had been administered the hormones. The European Union's Committee for Veterinary Measures Relating to Public Health determined that these six commonly used growth hormones had the potential to cause "endocrine, developmental, immunological, neurobiological, immunotoxic, genotoxic and carcinogenic effects. Even exposure to small levels of residues in meat and meat products carries risks, and no threshold levels can be established for any of the six substances."[17]

In 1999 a European Union scientific committee reported evidence showing that the estradiol used in US cattle production is a "complete carcinogen." The report went on to say, "Estradiol exerts both tumor initiating and tumor promoting effects. In plain language, this means that even small additional doses of residues of this hormone in meat arising from its use as a growth promoter in cattle has an inherent risk of causing cancer."[18] Of course in the United States we don't even require labeling! The system is keeping our heads buried in the sands of deception despite conclusive research done in other countries that has definitively proven that hormone use in animal products causes cancer. And here's just one more: In a 2009 study published in the journal *Annals of Oncology* titled "Estrogen Concentrations in Beef and Human Hormone-Dependent Cancers," researchers found that beef raised in the United States contained 140 to 600 times more estrogen than Japanese beef. This study concluded that the "recent increase of hormone-dependent cancers roughly parallels the increasing consumption of US imported beef in Japan. During the past quarter century, hormone-dependent cancers have risen fivefold: 4 times in breast and ovarian cancer, 8 times in endometrial cancer, and 10 times in prostate cancer."[19]

One of the most common ways to force greater milk production is with injection of recombinant bovine growth hormone (rBGH), a genetically engineered artificial hormone. A Monsanto product, rBGH was approved by the FDA in 1993, but again, Canada and the European Union have banned its use in dairy cows due to its health risks both for humans and cows.

Meanwhile, with nonorganic cheese, yogurt, ice cream, butter, whey protein isolates, or any US product with milk derivatives that is not organic, there is a good chance it contains rBGH (and other growth-promoting hormones).

These products have been found to also contain higher levels of IGF-1, the hormone that regulates insulin function and carbohydrate metabolism and also causes the pituitary gland to induce cell growth and replication. Many studies have found higher levels of IGF-1 associated with increased risk of breast, prostate, and colorectal cancer. The primary action of the breast cancer drug tamoxifen is to reduce blood IGF-1 levels, so we know how powerful its effects are. In fact, IGF-1 is widely considered the number one driver of "triple negative" cancers and most ovarian cancers. If you currently have a high IGF-1 level, your first step should be to stop eating commercially raised animals and dairy products. If you have been eating very clean meat sources (100 percent pasture-raised, organic) and your IGF-1 levels are still high, then you want to drastically decrease meat consumption to approximately 5–10 percent or less of the diet and stick to eggs, fish, and chicken bone broth until levels drop. Meanwhile, for everyone else, there is never a time to eat or drink meat, milk, or milk by-products that are not labeled organic or have been treated with hormones. Ever.

Hormone Replacement Therapy and Birth Control Pills

Hormone replacement therapy (HRT) and oral contraceptives are exogenous hormones that have been studied extensively. Both have been conclusively found to increase the risk of various cancers, including breast, ovarian, cervical, endometrial, liver, and colorectal. In fact, both HRT and birth control pills are listed as Group 1 carcinogens by the IARC! A meta-analysis that included over 160,000 women showed that for current or recent use of HRT, the risk of breast cancer increased in relation to duration of use.[20] A 2008 NIH study concluded that health risks of long-term combination hormone therapy outweigh benefits for postmenopausal women. Women taking the combined HRT were 25 percent more likely to have an invasive breast cancer than women in the placebo group, 78 percent more likely to have cancer that had spread to the lymph nodes, and almost twice as likely as the placebo group to die of breast cancer (and 57 percent more likely to die of other causes).[21] Remember, use of hormone therapies is new to humans in the past hundred years.

Today approximately one in five postmenopausal American women takes HRT, largely to treat symptoms such as hot flashes, night sweats, and vaginal dryness. For some reason, we treat menopause like a disease, when in reality these symptoms prevalent in baby boomers are the direct result of the low-fat diet trend that started in the 1970s. (Remember that estrogen is made from cholesterol. When we follow a low-fat diet, we cannot make these hormones.) Additionally, menopausal symptoms are just as easily remedied with the approaches we outline at the end of this chapter as by taking synthetic hormone growth promoters. One of the most effective ways to reduce menopausal symptoms is by following the ketogenic diet!

Bioidentical hormones are no better, yet they are erroneously thought of by many as natural and healthy. These hormones are so similar to our own hormones that the body doesn't recognize them as "other." This is why autoimmune conditions are so much more common in women then men. The other problem with bioidentical hormones is that they bind more efficiently and irreversibly than our own hormones do. The bottom line is that bioidentical hormones are neither safer nor more natural than synthetic versions. Not to mention it misses the point—hormone metabolism and contributing Terrain Ten issues are where to direct our attention and treatment, not replacing function with hormone therapy.

At the other end of the hormone spectrum, we have teenage girls. The birth control pill and hormone-releasing IUDs have seemed to be the only answer to controlling reproduction. To reiterate, combined estrogen-progesterone contraceptives are listed as IARC Group 1, known human carcinogens. Despite this, the number of teenage girls on the birth control pill jumped 50 percent from 2002 to 2009 according to a study by Thomson Reuters. Today, one in five American girls between the ages of thirteen and eighteen, 2.5 million teens in all, are on the birth control pill, and the age at which teens start on the pill is getting younger and younger, at times as young as twelve. How on earth did we get so disconnected?

There are other, nonhormonal ways to prevent pregnancy. The fertility awareness method (FAM) is an option for young women to not only get in touch with their own cycles but also prevent pregnancy naturally. Also called

NuvaRing: A Deadly Choice?

This sidebar is dedicated to Karen and Erika Langhart

We'd like to honor a dear friend of Dr. Nasha's, Karen Langhart. Karen's daughter, Erika, was killed as a result of using the NuvaRing, which contains two kinds of female hormones: estrogen and etonogestrel (progestin). Erika had a double pulmonary embolism and died on Thanksgiving Day in 2011, which her doctors stated was a direct result of using this contraceptive. Sadly, Karen took her own life January 8, 2016, after a futile fight with the FDA trying to educate and empower the population on the dangers of these medications. The NuvaRing remains on the market. To learn more about Erika's story, contraception choices, and more, visit their website at www.informedchoiceforamerika.com.

natural family planning or the rhythm method, FAM is a way to predict fertile and infertile times during the female monthly cycle. FAM is based on such body signs as temperature and cervical position. According to a 2006 study published in *Oxford Journal*, 1.8 per 100 women of the cohort experienced an unintended pregnancy when using the FAM method for thirteen cycles. It's both effective and nontoxic. Another option is a copper IUD; we always test copper levels first and make sure that women are taking supplemental zinc, as copper will deplete stores of zinc.

As you can see from just these three endocrine hijackers (and there are many others; this book isn't big enough!), we are utterly bombarded with environmental estrogens. From the food we eat, to the pills we pop, to the products we put on our bodies, estrogen is everywhere, and it is responsible for driving the cancer process. Start reading labels and replacing your body care and cleaning products. Start buying organic and pasture-raised meat products. Start addressing your hormone cycles with natural medicine. Do this, and you will begin to reverse the rates. Let's now turn to what we can do to balance things out.

Balancing Hormones with Deep Nutrition

If you want to balance your hormone levels, optimize your diet and avoid endocrine-disrupting products. Diet and lifestyle approaches are *the most* effective ways to reduce exposure and effects from EDCs. In fact, diet is the *only* way to help your body properly metabolize estrogens and is a proven, side-effect-free way to tackle hormone imbalances. How empowering is that?

We have already covered a few strategies, including the microbiome benefits of apples and focusing on healthy fats, including pasture-raised, organic eggs to optimize cholesterol levels. Additionally, because the liver plays such a critical role in metabolizing and detoxing hormones, everything you learned about detoxification like saunas and fasting becomes that much more critical. We talked about how cruciferous vegetable compounds including I3C and its derivative DIM can have powerful hormone-modulating and chemopreventive properties. It's also important to know that boiling cruciferous vegetables from nine to fifteen minutes results in 18%–59% decreases in their total I3C content. We recommend cooking methods that use less water, such as steaming, to reduce losses. Consumption of raw cruciferous vegetables is ideal. Unfortunately, fermentation can reduce the concentration of health-promoting I3C in Brassica vegetables, so if they tend to give you gas, then a light steam or sauté is better than sauerkraut.[22]

In this section we look at a seed-based hormone balance protocol and flush out the confusing role of phytoestrogenic foods, including soy. We also cover a very powerful herb, rosemary, which may be more powerful—and certainly safer—than Group 1 carcinogen tamoxifen in blocking estrogen. Other powerful hormone-balancing foods and phytonutrients are also covered, including flax and flavonols. So let's get started!

Figuring Out Phytoestrogens

More than 160 plant compounds found in over 300 plant species have been identified as estrogenic. Phytoestrogens are weak forms of estrogens, equivalent in action to estriols, the least active form of human estrogen, and are not as stimulating as estradiol.[23] Phytoestrogens work the same way human estrogens do, by binding to receptor sites and signaling a message.

Phytoestrogens, however, are generally misunderstood by the Western medical community. Jess can't count the number of times patients have been told by doctors to avoid yams and sweet potatoes because they increase progesterone. This is just straight up wrong. Supermarket yams and wild yams are in completely different families of plants, and the supermarket yam has zero impact on hormones. The wild yam is a perennial vine that is not normally eaten, but rather used in a topical cream form. We've also had patients whose doctors have prescribed a wild yam cream as hormone therapy without first assessing their SNPs or terrain, landing them in an active cancer recurrence. Plants are powerful drugs, and therefore we must approach them on a highly bio-individualized and nuanced basis.

From an evolutionary medicine perspective, we know that humans have consumed plant phytoestrogens for millennia, therefore these natural compounds have been and should remain part of the human diet, not avoided altogether. It is the *chemicals* that are our estrogen problem, not the plants. If we eat a balanced diet with naturally occurring phytoestrogens, our hormones will be balanced. It's when we start megadosing with supplements and herbs that contain phytoestrogens that we run into difficulty. Scores of research studies have found that phytoestrogens can help prevent and treat cancer through a number of different mechanisms, including:

- Inducing apoptosis
- Reducing the generation of "bad" estrogen metabolites
- Exerting anti-angiogenic potential
- Acting like natural SERMs
- Enhancing the effectiveness of radiation treatment
- Inhibiting tumor growth, invasion, and metastases
- Inhibiting aromatase enzyme activity
- Reducing resistance to anticancer drugs
- Reducing cancer recurrence
- Reducing the production of estrogen

So what exactly are they? Phytoestrogens can be divided into five main categories: *isoflavones, lignans, coumestans, flavonols,* and *stilbenes*.[24] Within each of these categories are subcategories of hundreds compounds, with more surfacing all the time. There is a large body of evidence coming from epidemiologic studies showing that people who consume high amounts of phytoestrogens in their diets have lower rates of several cancers, including breast, prostate, and colon cancer.[25] We'll take a closer look at each of these, starting with the most controversial phytoestrogen on the block: soy.

Isoflavones and the Great Soy Debate

Close to six hundred different isoflavones have been identified, but *genistein*, *daidzein*, and *equol* are the most well known and well researched. Isoflavones are largely found in soy, especially in organic fermented miso and natto; fermentation has been shown to increase the bioavailability of isoflavones.[26] High concentrations of genistein and daidzein are also found in currants and psoralea (*bu gu zhi* in Chinese medicine).[27] Equol is the most powerful of all isoflavones, but it doesn't come from food. Rather, it is the end product of the intestinal bacterial metabolism of daidzein. Equol is superior to all other isoflavones because of its antioxidant activity, a greater affinity for estrogen receptors, and its anti-androgenic properties. Without the right intestinal microbiota, however, equol cannot be formed.

This is where "to soy or not to soy" starts to become very bio-individual. Only 30–40 percent of adults produce equol after eating soy, and it has been suggested, for obvious reasons, that those individuals are more likely to benefit from soy intake. Again, the ability to produce equol depends on the presence of equol-forming bacteria, and only a small percentage of humans harbor the gut bacteria (*Slackia*) that effect this biotransformation. This is most likely why research results have shown mixed benefit of soy consumption. The prevalence of equol producers is higher in Asian populations than in Caucasians.[28] Only 30–40 percent of the US Caucasian population is capable of converting daidzein to equol, compared with 40–60 percent of people of Asian descent. It has also been found that seaweed consumption can enhance intestinal production of equol, and therefore the presence of seaweed in the Asian diet may enhance intestinal conversion of phytoestrogens.[29]

Another important point to take into consideration on the topic of soy is the *type*. Soy intake studies that have shown increased cancer-protective benefits are reflected with one to two servings a day of traditional Asian soy products, which are fermented soybeans in the form of tofu, tempeh, and miso. Western soy products, including soy protein, soy milk, soy-based veggie burgers, tofu dogs, the ever-popular Tofurkey, and isoflavone supplements, can contain several-fold *higher* levels of genistein and therefore exert increased estrogenic effects. In America we are megadosing soy and being exposed to levels of isoflavones far higher than in the traditional Asian diet. What's more, soy was not a food consumed by ancient humans—its cultivation began only during the Agricultural Revolution and didn't make it to Europe until the mid-1700s. It's actually a modern food that contains high amounts of lectins (covered in chapter 7; see "Immune System Offender #1"). In summary, because of all these factors, we rarely recommend soy. What we do recommend for hormone balance—not inflammation—is ground flaxseed.

Sesame and Flax Balance Hormones Fast

Lignans represent one of the five major classes of phytoestrogens and are present in a wide variety of plant foods. The highest concentrations are found in flaxseeds, sesame seeds, and curly kale. When consumed, lignan precursors are converted by the intestinal microbiome to the biologically active phytoestrogens enterolignans, enterodiol, and enterolactone,. Flaxseeds have been found in some research to be just as effective as tamoxifen in reducing the recurrence of breast cancer and can slow the growth of breast cancer in women. In one study, thirty-two women awaiting surgery for breast cancer were randomized to receive a daily muffin either with or without 25 grams of flaxseeds. Analysis of the cancerous tissue after surgery revealed that markers of tumor growth were reduced by 30–71 percent in the flaxseed group, with no change noted in the control group. A comprehensive review of twenty-one studies found that postmenopausal women with higher lignan intake were significantly less likely to get breast cancer.[30]

Ground flaxseeds bind to estrogen in the bowel and help eliminate it, like helping to wash those dirty dishes of partially metabolized estrogens. Flaxseed lignans have also been shown to bind to male hormone receptors and promote the elimination of testosterone, deeming them also helpful for prostate cancer prevention and management. It's important to note that the highest concentrations of enterolignans were reached after supplementation with fresh ground flaxseeds. Flax oil and whole flaxseeds do not have as much

Seed Cycling for Hormone Balance

In the realms of naturopathic nutrition and herbal medicine, seed cycling for hormone balance has been shown to be a helpful and natural approach for hormone balance in both men and women. The seed cycling protocol uses specific seeds during specific times of the month in order to balance estrogen and progesterone. A pumpkin-and-flaxseed combo during the first two weeks after the new moon (for men) or following menstruation (for women) helps detoxify the extra estrogen that occurs this time of the month. A sunflower-and-sesame combo used in the second half of the twenty-eight day cycle is rich in selenium, which promotes progesterone production. Here's how seed cycling works:

> Days 1 through 14: Eat 1 tablespoon ground flaxseeds and 1 tablespoon ground pumpkin seeds every day.
>
> Days 15 through 28: Eat 1 tablespoon ground sunflower seeds and 1 tablespoon ground sesame seeds every day.

The seeds can be ground in a mortar and pestle, coffee grinder, or food processor and added to cold foods like smoothies or salads, or mixed with water. (See the recipe in chapter 13 under "Hormone Balance"). During the two-week follicular phase, avoid sunflower seeds and sesame seeds, and during the two-week luteal phase avoid flax and pumpkin. You can also add fish oil on Days 1 through 14 and evening primrose oil on Days 15 through 28 to further help balance fatty acids.

effect. Freshly ground flaxseeds are very easily oxidized (remember the apple flesh turning brown when exposed to oxygen) and should not be stored for longer than five hours or used in cooking. They are good for adding to cold beverages or smoothies, or sprinkling on top of salads.

The second-richest source of lignans is sesame seeds. Sesame lignans are called sesamin and sesamolin, and their metabolites include enterodiol and sesamol. Sesame has been evaluated for its estrogenic activities and found to have benefits equal to ground flaxseeds. Sesame seeds are thought to be one of humanity's oldest foods, and new research has found synergistic effects in sesame lignans' interaction with vitamin E, accounting for "the anti-aging effect of sesame." According to a Japanese review sesame lignans exert immunoregulatory and anticarcinogenic activity.[31] Like flaxseeds, sesame seeds are very susceptible to oxidation and should not be cooked at high temperatures.

Coumestans and Flavonols: Hormone-Balancing Superstars

Coumestans, including coumestrol, are found in a variety of plants. Food sources highest in coumestans include red clover sprouts, spinach, and brussels sprouts. Red clover and the phytoestrogens that it contains are well known for relieving menopausal symptoms and have strong inhibitory effects on the growth of three cancer cell lines, including ovarian. Red clover has a powerful effect, and you should work closely with your doctor to monitor your body's response.

Flavonols are phytochemical compounds found in high concentrations in a variety of food sources such as chocolate that is high in cacao content (over 85 percent), onions, chives, kale, cranberries, romaine lettuce, and turnip greens. Studies have found that dietary flavonols reduce breast and pancreatic cancer risk. Higher intake of flavonols is also associated with lower risk of ovarian cancer. Flavonols include the following compounds: quercitin, myricetin, and kaempferol. A 2004 study published in the journal *Cancer Research* found that kaempferol helped to reverse breast cancer resistance to several chemotherapy agents.[32] It's research like this that gives hope to those with chemoresistance: knowing that eating kale, which is highest in kaempferol, might help a body respond better to conventional medicine. Therapeutic nutrition simply must be included in everyone's cancer treatment plan.

Hormone Herbs: Rosemary and Thyme

Rosemary, long considered a sacred plant, has several different anticancer properties, including promoting hormone balance. Research at Rutgers University found that rosemary has the ability to inactivate estrogen hormones by stimulating liver enzymes that switch off aggressive estrogen types. It was shown that a 2 percent rosemary diet increased glucuronidation, the phase 2 detox process that helps remove estrogen. Rosemary's unique blend of anti-oxidants—carnosic acid, carnosol, and rosmarinic acid—protect against the cancer-causing heterocyclic amines (HCAs) that form on meat when cooked at high temperatures. In fact, one study found that adding rosemary extract to hamburgers significantly decreased or even eliminated levels of HCAs. This is a great herb to grow at home and enjoy all year long!

Thyme (from the Greek word *thymon*, meaning "to fumigate") has more than a hundred varieties. One of its active compounds is called thymol, a potent germ killer from the class of phytonutrients called *monoterpenes*. Monoterpenes have been found to protect DNA and have anticancer effects on liver, blood, skin, and uterine cancers. And the benefits of thyme don't stop there: A 2012 study published in *Nutrition and Cancer* found that thyme induced significant cytotoxicity in breast cancer cells.[33] The authors concluded that thyme "may be a promising candidate in the development of novel therapeutic drugs for breast cancer treatment." Freshly picked herbs can be added to eggs, stir-fries, and other dishes throughout the year. A meal is not complete without herbs, as we demonstrate throughout this book. Try adding sprigs of fresh thyme to warm lemon water in the morning with a splash of bitter herbs—a tonic like none other!

Balancing the Biorhythms of Hormones

If your hormones out of balance you need to ask yourself, what is the hidden message? A woman's (and man's) typical hormone cycle is twenty-eight days, the length of a full lunar cycle. Humans are designed to be at peak fertility and ovulation at the full moon when nights are brightest. Fertility is lowest during menstruation, and should naturally occur during the new moon when nights are darkest. Male fertility naturally follows the female's in this scenario so that we're all most fertile at the same time to enhance the chance of reproduction. Amazing, right? Because of this biorhythm that is innate to all humans, we love the concept of moon bathing as a natural way to balance hormones. Moon bathing is just that, lying outside naked during the full moon—a hormone-modulating practice that may also encourage conception!

With hormones, there is a huge connection to both external and internal environments, so spending more time outside is just so important. And on that note, the next chapter goes deep into restoring our natural biorhythms and reducing stress, which are both tightly connected to hormone balance. We discuss one hormone in particular, cortisol, and its role in the cancer process. Reading this book might feel stressful at times as you learn about all the diet and environmental factors that cause cancer, but don't despair; in the next two chapters we focus on relaxing, de-stressing, and getting the emotional areas of our terrain in balance. Deep breath, here we go!

CHAPTER 11

Stress and Circadian Rhythms

Attaining Tranquility and Reconnecting with Natural Cycles

Between stimulus and response, there is a space. In that space lies our freedom and our power to choose our response. In our response lies our growth and our happiness.

—Viktor Frankl, *Austrian neurologist, psychiatrist, Holocaust survivor, and founder of logotherapy*

The environment, through light, food, and stress, flips the switches on genes to produce hormones, which in turn flip other genes—for growth, death, or repair—on and off.

—T. S. Wiley, Lights Out: Sleep, Sugar, and Survival

Stress is the most powerful carcinogen imaginable. It increases inflammation, spikes blood sugar, and disables the immune system. Metastasis is promoted when the body or mind is stressed, and so is angiogenesis. Yet chronic stress in its many forms—emotional, physical and chemical—is the norm of modern living. A diet high in sugar causes a chronic stress response in the body, as does constant exposure to toxins. Today's persistent stress and pressures of daily life, now mostly considered "normal," are a far cry from the intermittent physical stressors experienced by our ancestors, like running from a bear or eating a poisonous plant. In truth, the sporadic stress our ancestors experienced was a foundational aspect of human evolution—a concept called *hormesis*, which also happens to be the foundational concept of homeopathic medicine. Hormesis is the idea that low exposures to an environmental stressor, such as a toxic plant, or a metabolic stressor, such as nutritional ketosis, can elicit a favorable biological response. But low-dose "good" stress is not the norm today. In 2015 the American Psychological Association reported that one in four Americans said they were highly stressed.[1] Chances are, if you are reading this book, either you or someone in your life has cancer, and that diagnosis alone is highly stressful.

Stress of any kind triggers a complex metabolic cascade that includes the production of cortisol, our primary stress hormone. Cortisol also regulates many normal bodily functions, including the sleep-wake cycle. When in excess, however, cortisol pushes several aspects of the cancer process forward, chiefly metastasis.[2] The stressors of modern living significantly deplete levels of another powerful anticancer hormone, melatonin, also considered the sleep hormone. A 2015 meta-study of melatonin concluded that melatonin not only reduces the side effects of chemotherapy but is also effective at eliminating cancer cells.[3] Unfortunately, our addiction to screens (TVs, computers, smartphones) has major suppressive effect on this chemopreventive hormone. Bright artificial lights suppress melatonin and are a Group 2B carcinogen.[4] We are living far outside our natural circadian rhythm, the natural cycle of the human clock that stems from the Earth's cycles. This imbalance, recognized long ago in Chinese medicine, is now causing a massive metabolic disruption: cancer.

From a dietary perspective, stress comes in many forms, from pesticides and artificial colors to high-sugar, high-carbohydrate, and low-fat diets. Eating foods that provoke an immune response—which for most humans means grains, legumes, dairy, and sugar—causes chronically elevated cortisol. Both our bodies and minds are under constant, chronic stress, which is just as destructive as chronic inflammation. Yet despite all this stress 55 percent of Americans didn't take their paid vacation time in 2015.[5] What is wrong with this picture?

For years medical doctors have offhandedly remarked, "Reduce your stress," to millions of Americans. But it's not working—stress is still considered one of the primary causes of heart disease, which, second to cancer, is the leading cause of death in America. Stress, sugar, and synthetic hormone and toxin exposures are slowly killing us. The good news is they are all avoidable. In this chapter, we explore the mechanics of the stress response and how stress contributes to cancer. We identify types of stressors, food-based ones in particular. We focus, too, on biorhythms, sleep, and melatonin.

Our metabolic approach focuses on supporting adrenal health with micro-nutrients and specific phytonutrients, eating seasonally, fasting, and using adaptogenic herbs. We emphasize getting back into harmony with the essential determinants of health—the primary focus of Ayurvedic and Chinese medicine for thousands of years. We encourage eating within a time frame that is in accordance with our cellular "clock." And it almost goes without saying that we promote getting outside and away from all kind of screens; this couldn't be more critical to our well-being. Being stressed out, living outside of our natural biorhythms, and not sleeping is downright carcinogenic. In fact, just one night without sleep alters the body's biological clock, causing significant changes to the immune, endocrine, and neurological systems.[6] Let's look at what happens in the body when we experience stress and how that response fuels the cancer process.

The Body's Response to Stress

You may have heard of, or personally experienced, the physical "fight-or-flight" response—the running away from a saber-toothed tiger. Today, instead of a tiger, that may look more like opening a big bill or getting into a car accident. Fight or flight is a sympathetic nervous system response. The opposing response, "rest and digest," is a response of the parasympathetic nervous system, which is activated during times of relaxation, rest, and mediation. During fight or flight, or an acute stress response, several things happen: The heart rate increases, blood pressure rises, blood vessels constrict, glucose is released by the liver, digestion is inhibited, the intestines stop moving, and erection is inhibited. All these responses are directed by stress hormones, including cortisol. Cortisol is made from cholesterol, which is the mother molecule also used to make the sex hormones. During a stressful event it becomes more important for the body to increase its respiratory rate to enable running fast then it is to reproduce; so when stress is high, sex hormone production is reduced. Think about the mother who lifted a car off her baby; a moment of superhuman powers. (This is technically called hysterical strength, a display of extreme strength beyond what is believed to be normal.) It usually occurs when people are in life-or-death situations and is an example of just how powerful stress hormones can be. After the baby is safe, Mom's parasympathetic response takes over and her blood pressure lowers, her heart rate decreases, intestinal motility increases, production of gastric secretions is increased, and sex hormones are again produced. In the Western world, however, stress levels are so high and coming from so many different places, it's as if we are trying to lift cars off babies all day long. Many of us are simply exhausted, which stems from adrenal fatigue, more technically called hypothalamic-pituitary-adrenal (HPA) axis dysregulation.

The stress response is largely directed by the HPA axis, a complex set of direct influences and feedback interactions among three endocrine glands. It is these interactions that also modulate many body systems including digestive, immune, neurological, metabolic, and reproductive. The hypothalamus, located in the brain, coordinates the autonomic nervous system and the activity of the pituitary. It also controls body temperature, thirst, and hunger, and is involved in sleep and emotional activity. The pituitary is a pea-sized gland encapsulated within a bony structure in the base of the brain like a pit. It is considered the master control gland and makes growth-triggering hormones, including thyroid-stimulating hormones.

The adrenal glands are two triangular shaped glands that sit atop the kidneys like a hat. They produce anywhere from thirty to sixty different hormones—including cortisol, progesterone, and DHEA—which influence nearly every bodily function. The adrenals also produce a small amount of sex hormone, and they take over the production of estrogen in women after menopause. Long-term stress is the leading reason why many women later in life are loaded with menopausal symptoms; their adrenals are burned out from years of stress and have no more "juice" to produce needed estrogen and progesterone. If we look at menopause from an adrenal perspective, HRT makes even less sense. We need adrenal support most of all.

When confronted with a stressful situation—whether it's a chemical exposure, or an emotional or physical trigger—the adrenal glands immediately increase the production of cortisol. Cortisol is called the stress hormone for good reason, because it influences, regulates, or modulates many of the changes that occur in the body in response to stress, including, but not limited to: blood sugar levels; fat, protein, and carbohydrate metabolism needed to maintain healthy blood glucose levels; immune responses; inflammatory actions; blood pressure; heart and blood vessel tone and contraction; central nervous system activation; and more. With all these actions, it's no wonder stress causes heart attacks! When the adrenal glands are continuously overworked and levels of cortisol become too elevated, too often it can leave one feeling chronically "wired and tired." You may know the feeling: utter exhaustion, then tucking into the covers for bed, and—hello, you're wide awake.

There are many symptoms that indicate HPA axis dysregulation and the associated metabolic imbalances that occur in response to long-term cortisol activation. These include fatigue, salt cravings, low libido, thyroid disorders, difficulty handling stress, mild or deep depression, PMS and fertility issues, becoming light-headed upon standing, poor focus, less enjoyment and happiness with life, anxiety, worsened blood sugar control, increased insulin resistance / diabetes, infertility, increased visceral fat accumulation (belly fat), decreased immunity, and cancer. Elevated cortisol has a suppressive impact on the enzyme that converts inactive thyroid hormones into active ones, significantly slowing metabolism and increasing weight gain. When women try literally everything to lose weight but cannot, the usual culprit is high stress. It is metabolically impossible to lose weight when cortisol is high, as our metabolism screeches to a halt. When the adrenal glands are in a constant state of alarm, the pituitary gland becomes sluggish from overwork. As a result, the reproductive system suffers, leading to low progesterone in women and low testosterone in men (hence the infertility epidemic). What's more, prolonged, elevated cortisol also runs down the liver's ability to detoxify discarded estrogens. Those estrogens become overly abundant and circulate back into the bloodstream in a more toxic form. You get it: Chronic stress causes bodywide mayhem—and cancer.

Stress and Cancer

Cancer incidence, progression, and mortality are directly linked to stress and circadian rest and activity cycle disruption. A chronically stressed-out lifestyle that is out of sync with circadian rhythms (not sleeping, excess screen time, little outdoor time, and eating non-nutritive food out of season) causes disturbances to the pineal gland hormone melatonin and also to cortisol, which both bump up cancer risk exponentially. Chronic stress also causes insulin resistance, increases the production of IGF-1 and inflammation, weakens the immune system, alters the gut microbiota, and drives angiogenesis and metastasis.[7] Think about it: Metastasis is like cancer's version of the fight-or-flight response. Since stress influences neurochemical, hormonal, digestive, inflammatory, and immunological functioning and these changes all influence the carcinogenic process, it is not surprising that stress fuels tumor growth and dissemination.[8]

Specifically, cortisol suppresses immune function when it is present in high amounts, causing NK cell activity to decrease by up to 50 percent.[9] Stress also induces increased permeability of the gut, allowing bacteria and antigens to cross the epithelial barrier and activate the mucosal immune response. Stress alters the composition of the microbiome by decreasing microbial diversity. From a metabolic perspective, a high cortisol level wreaks major havoc on blood sugar balance. During times of stress, cortisol can provide the body with needed glucose by tapping into stored proteins in the liver (gluconeogenesis). Elevated cortisol over the long term, however, consistently produces excess glucose, leading to increased blood sugar levels. And since cancer cells have the ability to increase their rate of glucose consumption, having high stress adds fuel to a growing cancer process (recall the Warburg effect). High stress hormone levels also cause insulin resistance, and the involvement of insulin in carcinogenesis is attributed to its role in increasing cell proliferation and suppression of apoptosis.[10] Sugar makes cancer invincible, and cortisol provides its shield.

So what are all of these stressors? Some of them might surprise you.

Types of Stressors

Over the years, we've had many patients report low stress levels, but ironically they are usually the ones with the highest amount of stress in their lives! Many of us are exposed to stressors all day long in the form of environmental and metabolic toxins, and don't even think twice about it. Stress comes in three primary forms: mental/emotional, physical/metabolic, and chemical. The stressors in the mental/emotional category are the easiest to recognize as they are associated with strong emotions like sadness, fear, or anger. Emotional stressors include: work pressure, financial worry, family-related issues, divorce, imprisonment, loss of a loved one, abuse, neglect, moving, losing a job, raising children, or writing a book. Health issues such as chronic pain, disability, and of course having cancer are stressful. Sixty-seven percent of Americans reported in 2015 that they had received a diagnosis of at least one chronic illness—that is a lot of very sick people walking around. Caring for a loved one with cancer is also incredibly stressful. Some studies have found that a cancer diagnosis can have a greater impact on family members than patients, and is associated with increased morbidity for the caregivers.[11] Certainly most of us can recognize when these emotional stressors are affecting our daily lives. Chemical stressors, on the other hand, are more likely to unnoticed.

Toxic Stressors

As we discussed at length in chapter 5, we are exposed to a slew of toxins on a daily basis. Exposure to pesticides, herbicides, preservatives, heavy metals, cleaning products, body care products, airborne chemicals, smoking, and prescription and street drugs all elicit an oxidative stress response. There are over twenty thousand pesticide products containing 620 active ingredients currently on the market. You may not realize it, but if you eat a nonorganic apple, you're also eating forty-seven different pesticides, six of which are known or probable carcinogens.[12] Conventionally raised produce causes an increased toxic load, creating oxidative stress for both the detoxification and immune systems. Toxins such as pesticides cause the formation of dangerous free radicals like ROS. Oxidative stress damages mitochondria and causes inflammation—and we know how that fuels the fires of cancer. This might seem overwhelming, but we have to start taking a very close look at the food and drinks we are consuming. Nonorganic produce is literally coated in toxic pesticides. Yes, even a salad can be a stressor. Therefore, eating wild, organic, and biodynamic foods should be considered a powerful stress-reducing activity.

The third category, physical and metabolic stress, used to be the primary type of daily stressors ancestral humans had to deal with. Historically we would encounter times without food, which would kick us into ketosis—a healthy form of protective "good" stress. We might also become dehydrated, eat the wrong plant, get fatigued when running from a mountain lion, or develop an infection. These metabolic and often short-term stressors actually give the immune system a boost by helping the adaptive immune system develop long-term memory to antigens while also cleaning out dead immune cells. Today, however, these physical and metabolic stressors have taken on a very different tone. For starters, over-exercising (think ultra marathons and endorphin junkies) cause both high oxidative stress and prolonged elevated cortisol. This type of exercise (or deliberate rush, like jumping out of an airplane) is not part of evolutionary stress. This observation dates back to the authoritative *The Yellow Emperor's Classic of Medicine*, written in China some-time around 2600 BC. To achieve health and longevity back then, the book reports that people "ate a balanced diet at regular times, arose and retired at regular hours, avoiding stressing their bodies and minds, and refrained from overindulgence of all kinds."[13] People were encouraged to cultivate the Tao, which means living a more simple and natural way of life, concepts that seem almost foreign in modern America.

By now, you get the idea that sugar and a high caloric intake cause prob-lems across every terrain element, and stress is no exception. As opposed to a lack of food, today we have an overabundance of calories. We can slug down more sugar in thirty minutes than our ancestors would consume in an entire year. Since the primary function of cortisol is to balance the effect of insulin, it's pretty simple: When insulin is chronically high, so is cortisol. If you eat more than 30 grams of sugar a day (less for kids) you are living in chronic stress, even without any other stressors present. A special note about kids: It is always better to eat less than more. Children do this natu-rally. They go through cycles of being hungry and not wanting to eat, which is an evolutionary pattern. As parents, try not to force your children to eat if they are not hungry! Especially when they are sick. In fact, a 2016 study found that intermittent fasting inhibits the development and progression of the most common type of childhood leukemia, acute lymphoblastic leuke-mia, or ALL.[14]

Second to the stress caused by our high-sugar diets, our overconsumption of allergenic foods is a huge dietary stressor. An estimated one in ten people have at least one food allergy, and one in a hundred people have celiac disease. Rates of food allergies are soaring and are also going undiagnosed. Currently some physicians believe that food allergies are the leading cause of undiagnosed symptoms, and that at least 60 percent of Americans suffer from symptoms—including hypothyroidism, behavior issues, and depression—that are associated with food allergies. Food sensitivities to gliadin, casein, soy, eggs, peanuts, artificial colors, and more place the adrenal glands in a chronic stress response. As mentioned earlier, when a food allergen is consumed the body produces histamine, an inflammation-producing compound modulated by cortisol, which also pushes metastasis. The more histamine released, the more cortisol it takes to control the inflammatory response, and the harder the adrenals have to work to produce more cortisol. The harder the adrenals have to work, the more fatigued they become, and the less cortisol they produce, allowing histamine to inflame tissues even more. Now you can see why so many people suffer greatly from seasonal allergies. If you've got the sniffles, chances are you've got high stress and it's time to look at your diet.

The primary cause of the increased frequency of food allergies appears to be the excessive, regular consumption of a limited number of foods and the high level of added preservatives, stabilizers, artificial colorings, and flavorings. This, in conjunction with the deforestation of our microbiomes. Other factors include genetics, improper digestion, poor integrity of the intestinal barrier, and eating while stressed (e.g., while driving or working). Many of our patients over the years have expressed serious resistance to taking gluten or dairy out of their diets, yet taking away this cortisol trigger can be the difference between a metastatic cancer and one that stays local and controlled. You decide.

Lastly on the food-stressor front, nothing has contributed more to adrenal fatigue than the low-fat diet. The basic biochemical fact is that both stress and sex hormones are produced from cholesterol (just Google it!). The combination of insufficient cholesterol and chronic stress makes the body unable to create sex hormones. This set of circumstances causes what's known as the *pregnenolone steal*. Pregnenolone is a steroid made from cholesterol and is the precursor to most of the steroid hormones, including the progestogens, androgens, estrogens, and cortisol. During times of stress, pregnenolone will favor producing cortisol over estrogen (remember, it's more important to save the baby than to make another one). This effect causes infertility, "early menopause" (a bogus diagnosis in our opinion), hormone imbalance, PMS, and menopause, which often drives women to HRT. Avoiding cholesterol-rich foods like eggs, lamb, and liver is not a good idea. Fat is our friend, it always has been, and always will be.

All this said, when cortisol is out of balance, it disrupts what is the most ancient and healing of human activities: sleep.

Sleep: The Elixir of Life

Sleep is fundamental to life, yet more than sixty million Americans report sleep problems such as insomnia, or awakening four hours into a night's sleep and being unable to get back to sleep for an hour or two. If this scenario sounds familiar, you are not alone. This is the most commonly reported sleep disturbance. Overall sleep duration decreased by up to two hours during the second half of the twentieth century. Today many people are in bed only five or six hours a night on a regular basis. These millions of sleep-deprived people find themselves willing to do anything to get some sleep. Sleep deprivation is so awful it is used as a torture tactic (just ask any new mom). And unfortunately, the antidote offered by Western medicine is, again, drugs. Not only is zolpidem (Ambien), the most commonly prescribed sleeping pill, addictive, but a 2012 study in the *British Medical Journal* found those who regularly take prescription sleeping pills were five times as likely to die over a period of two and a half years and to develop cancer.[15] Cancer risk is increased in those who don't sleep, and is especially higher in shift workers and also in those who often cross time zones during air travel. In 2007 IARC concluded that shift work is probably carcinogenic to humans (IARC Group 2A).

When we sleep—adults need at least eight hours a night and kids at least twelve—hormones are released, tissue growth and repair occurs, neurological pathways are regenerated, detoxification occurs, and the immune system is replenished. And, you probably guessed it, sleep affects the body's reaction to insulin. Just two nights of poor sleep can increase levels of IGF-1.[16] Sleep deprivation also causes a decrease in leptin, known as the satiety hormone, and an increase in ghrelin, or the hunger hormone. In other words, not enough sleep stimulates the appetite, and this leads to increased weight. What's more, ghrelin is associated with cancer progression, including proliferation, apoptosis, and cell invasion and migration.[17] Not sleeping is straight-up carcinogenic, so why are so many of us having a hard time getting enough Z's?

Many of the conditions related to terrain elements we've discussed in previous chapters are also major contributors to insomnia. Allergies, asthma, gastrointestinal problems such as reflux, hormone imbalance, blood sugar imbalance, toxic overload, arthritis, and chronic pain can all contribute to insomnia.[18] If you experience sleep disturbances, then paying special attention to balancing blood sugar, detoxifying, rebalancing your hormones, and reducing inflammation should be top priorities. What you will find is that following our approach not only addresses a cancer-promoting terrain, but also helps manage many other chronic conditions, disturbed sleep among them. For any and all chronic issues, *adequate sleep is paramount*. Practicing good "sleep hygiene" refers to healthy practices that encourage a complete and restful night sleep. Eating early in the evening, avoiding alcohol and other stimulants like caffeine in the evening, getting exercise, establishing a regular relaxing bedtime routine, going to bed at the same time every night, associating your bed with sleep and not work, and making your bedroom a relaxation oasis are all proven steps that support a good night's sleep. It just sounds nice, doesn't it?

Cortisol responds rapidly to our daytime food intake and, as we explained, is made worse with a diet high in sugar. It is produced in a cyclic fashion and should be highest in the morning and lowest at night. Any disruption in this rhythm results in dysfunction in the body and sleepless nights. An afternoon ice-cream cone not only causes a spike in insulin, but also in cortisol, making it harder to fall asleep. Blood glucose levels are normally lowest in the early-morning hours (why *breakfast* literally means "breaking the fast"). However, with an HPA axis imbalance, cortisol levels may not be sufficient to maintain an adequate blood glucose level during the night, causing middle-of-the-night awakenings from hunger. Low glucose signals an internal alarm (remember, glucose is the main fuel for all cells, including brain cells) that disrupts sleep so the person can wake up and refuel. Waking up in the middle of the night to eat is a signature behavior of adrenal dysregulation.

Second to imbalanced blood sugar, the primary reason behind the modern insomnia epidemic is not getting enough exposure to natural light during the day while getting way too much exposure to artificial light from TVs, computers, and cell phones. The pattern of being awake during the day when it is light and sleeping at night when it is dark is a natural part of human life, and this is totally disrupted by our modern lifestyle. The result is depressed levels of melatonin, which also happens to be one of the most powerful anticancer hormones (and natural antioxidants) the body produces. Screen time is causing its extinction. Let's take a closer look at melatonin and its role in the cancer process.

Melatonin and Cancer

Melatonin is a hormone made by the pineal gland, which is located in the brain. The pineal is generally inactive during the day, but when the sun sets and darkness descends, it switches on and begins to produce melatonin. Melatonin levels in the blood normally stay elevated for about twelve hours, or all through the night, while cortisol levels are low. Daytime levels of melatonin, by contrast, are barely detectable. However, exposure to bright indoor light and artificial light outside of normal daylight hours decreases secretion of melatonin, which is a concern when it comes to cancer. Melatonin triggers tumor suppressor genes, suppresses tumor angiogenesis, and works as a powerful anticarcinogenic antioxidant that can cross the blood-brain barrier.[19] An ample amount of melatonin secretion is also vital to the immune system. Several studies have found that at least six hours of prolactin (a reproductive hormone influenced by melatonin) secretion in the dark is required to maintain function of T cells and NK cells. However, getting six hours or less of sleep inhibits this action. It takes three and a half hours of melatonin secretion to occur before prolactin production even gets started.[20] Additional studies have found that women exposed to artificial light during nighttime hours, especially night-shift workers, experience a higher incidence of breast cancer. It is therefore not surprising that taking melatonin alone or in combination with chemotherapy improves tumor regression outcomes and reduces side effects.[21] Remember, electricity was only just invented (in the early 1800s); before that, for over two million years the only light our eyes had ever seen was sunlight and fire. Now many people see neither, and melatonin levels are declining as a result. Our genes respond to our environment, and a loss of melatonin in response to a loss of exposure to natural light is an epigenetic reaction to modern living that contributes to the cancer process.

Dr. Nasha has recommended high-dose melatonin for oncology patients for several years—dosages as high as 20–40 milligrams a day—with great success. (Quick disclaimer: Melatonin is a hormone, and melatonin supplementation should be done under medical supervision as misuse can impair the function of other hormones.) Melatonin is emerging as a very powerful and nontoxic cancer therapy. There are hundreds of whitepapers on its mechanisms. Low-dose melatonin, between 0.5 and 3 milligrams a day, impacts sleep cycles, whereas doses above 10 milligrams—especially at levels of 20–40 milligrams daily—impact circadian cycles and angiogenesis, act as a natural aromatase inhibitor, enhance many chemotherapy agents, sensitize cancer cells to radiation while protecting the healthy cells, and protect from chemotherapy toxicity.[22] Taking melatonin supplements is one approach, but the most powerful epigenetic and terrain changes happen when diet and lifestyle are balanced first. There is no magic pill! In fact, living in such extreme discordance from the natural rhythms of the Earth is one of the greatest environmental and lifestyle factors contributing to cancer-promoting imbalances in the body. In the past 250 years of human existence we have succeeded in almost completely disconnecting from our intricate relationship to the Earth, to our own great detriment.

Where We Went Wrong: Living against Our Biorhythms

Cancer, and disease in any form, is viewed as a violation of nature's laws. Natural laws (well established in Chinese and naturopathic medicine) are elements, also known as health determinants, that are required by everyone in order to live. This ancient approach to health asserts that when life is not in accordance with these natural laws, imbalances such as cancer can ensue. They include the following:

Breath and fresh air: We can live only three minutes without breathing. When many of us are stressed, our breathing becomes short and tense, impairing circulation. We are also exposed to many airborne toxins.

Clean water and hydration: Without water, we can live only three to five days. Dehydration causes an overload of toxins in the body, and many of our water sources contain carcinogens. Most Americans are dehydrated.

Sleep and normal biorhythms: Getting at least eight to ten hours of sleep between the hours of 10 p.m. and 7 a.m. is critical for several processes in the body. When sleep occurs outside those hours, it interrupts key systems. Studies have found humans can live without sleep for between eleven days and thirty months.[23]

Rest and recreation: Downtime encourages lowered cortisol levels. Play, as exemplified by children, creates happiness. Experiencing joy and happiness is critical for health.

Sunlight: Until this past century, humans derived vitamin D from the sun. For much of our existence, the majority of days were spent outside. As we have shown, vitamin D has many critical anticancer actions.

Solar, lunar, and life cycles: In the past, we changed our diets based on the time of year. We fasted and were in ketogenic states for much of the winter, with more abundance of carbohydrates in the summer. We have disrupted this system and no longer eat seasonally; enjoying pineapples in Minnesota in January is not normal!

Exposure to natural forces and nature: Exposures to various temperatures, rain, and wind are good physiological stressors. We are meant to be hot in the spring and summer when we are filled with estrogen and cold in the winter when the carbohydrates are gone and insulin and estrogen levels decline. With furnaces and air conditioners we have broken this rhythm, and now our bodies live in a perpetual summer.

Gaia theory (or Gaia principle): This theory asserts that humans interact with our organic surroundings on Earth to form a self-regulating, complex system that contributes to maintaining optimal conditions for life on the planet. This is evidenced by how our microbiome is populated and how it reacts to dietary intake.

Nutrition and digestion: Without food for forty or so days, we die. Our genome and our entire body rely on nutrients from the diet, and we have radically altered its composition.

As you can see, these health determinants are not well followed in the modern West. Where the Western model views cancer as something that "happens" to a person, naturopathic medicine recognizes the *vis medicatrix naturae*, the healing power of nature. Cancer does not exist in nature, only in humans and pets. So what is the message? That we are out of balance in one or more areas of the terrain. Think about it. When is the last time you laughed, felt truly happy, rested, recreated, slept outside, walked on the ground in bare feet, drank 60 ounces of water, went a day without looking at a screen, enjoyed a nourishing meal, or ate more than ten different vegetables in a day? When is the last time you felt hungry, wet, or cold? On average, children today spend thirty minutes or less outside every day. One in five do not typically play outside at all. This is less outdoor time than prison inmates get. We could not be more disconnected from the natural circadian rhythms of the planet: We look at computers all day, spend less time outside, stay up too late, and maintain the same ambient temperature all day. We eat a high-sugar, high-calorie diet year-round. All it takes are low levels of exposure to modern living—the noise, the toxins, the commute, the food, feeling burned out at work, getting little or disrupted sleep, financial concerns, no time to relax and play, light pollution, screen time, sugary foods, xenoestrogen exposure, never taking vacation—and *bam*! Our ancient DNA snaps while we rush to a PTA meeting.

Internal Clocks and Intermittent Fasting

Speaking of the perpetual rush of modern life, did you know that mechanical clocks were invented only in 1656? Before that, humans evolved according to daily, monthly, and annual patterns. In fact, scientists have discovered that every cell in the body is a clock. Humans—completely independent of the pocket watch—have an exquisitely accurate internal biological clock that times normal daily events such as sleep and wake-fulness. Our circadian rhythms represent an evolutionarily conserved adaptation to the environment that can be traced back to the earliest life-forms.[24] The discovery of these "clock genes" led to the realization that circadian gene expression is actually widespread throughout the body in organs and tissues. In fact, gene expression is rhythmic, guided by by environmental cues. Some genes are supposed to turn on at night, some in the daytime. The human body is truly amazing. That said, there is accumulating epidemiological and genetic evidence showing that the disruption of circadian rhythms is linked to cancer and that the abnormal metabolism seen in cancer could also be a consequence of disrupted circadian clocks.[25] Turns out, staying up until midnight eating cupcakes and watching *Dancing with the Stars* is sending a dangerously altered message to your genes, albeit entertaining.

In addition to cellular clocks, the gut microbiome is also involved in controlling our circadian rhythms. Gut microorganisms also produce metabolites in diurnal patterns, which influences the expression of circadian clock genes in organs such as the liver. Researchers from the University of Chicago Medical Center found that our microbes sense what, when, and how much food is consumed, which in turn produces "metabolic signals that feed into the regulation of circadian networks which control our metabolism," lead researcher Eugene Chang told the news magazine *The Scientist* in 2015. "Western-type diets alter these microbial signals in a way that disturbs circadian functions." Turns out, our dietary habits are the largest contributor to circadian rhythm imbalance. It was only fifteen thousand short years ago that we became capable of controlling the interactive Earth-given food supply that ensured our survival. No one species has ever had unlimited access to carbohydrate energy without regard for effort, season, competition, or natural disaster. This is why research—and lots of anecdotal evidence—keeps pointing to the benefits of intermittent fasting.

Fasting helps reset circadian rhythms. It acts as a good stressor, similar to an acute immune or inflammatory response. Fasting revs up cellular defenses against genetic damage while increasing the body's responsiveness to insulin. For example, mice that feasted on fatty foods for eight hours a day and subsequently fasted for the rest of each day did not become obese

Labs to Assess Stress and Circadian Rhythm Imbalance

One way to assess cortisol levels and circadian imbalance is to run an adrenal stress index (ASI) panel. This is a saliva test that looks at cortisol levels throughout the day along with other stress markers and gives an idea of the degree of cortisol dysregulation. Genetic assessments, in particular looking at the enzyme catechol-O-methyl-transferase (COMT), which breaks down catecholamine hormones like estrogen and also cortisol, can be very important. A polymorphism in the gene for COMT has been linked to several mental disorders and certain cancers. Fortunately, magnesium and vitamin C support those with COMT SNPs!

or show dangerously high insulin levels. From an evolutionary perspective, three meals a day is a strange modern invention; we simply eat too much too often. The volatility in our ancient ancestors' food supplies contributed to frequent fasting, something completely foreign to most people today. These evolutionary pressures selected genes that strengthened areas of the brain involved in learning and memory, which increased the odds of finding food and surviving. Periodic fasting, or at least eating within an eight-hour window during daylight hours, reduces the risk of cancer and has been found to also support weight loss. In practice, if your first meal is at 7 a.m., your last should be no later than 3 p.m. Try it.

The Metabolic Approach to Stress Reduction and Biorhythm Restoration

For starters, we absolutely need to start living in closer harmony with the natural world on physical, mental, and moral planes. It is the excess in life that is the main contributor to cancer—and that is the very definition of modern living: too much stimulation, too much food. Just look at the last thirty years. Compare an episode of *Mr. Rogers* to *PAW Patrol*. And we wonder why our children don't sleep! We are constantly bombarded with stimuli, and the antidote is natural tranquilizers. We must stop with the chronic screen time and get outside. Camping, playing outside, and, yes, taking vacations are not just fun, they are essential for the prevention and management of cancer. Small studies have found that even four days and nights spending time outside and mimicking a Paleolithic lifestyle of moderate exercise and caloric intake can significantly improve several metabolic markers, including insulin levels.[26] Sitting is now considered the next cigarette-smoking crisis: We simply are not designed to sit indoors in front of a computer, just as we are not designed to inhale genetically modified tobacco wrapped in dioxin-coated paper. Lifestyle approaches that encourage calmness, peacefulness, quiet, and serenity are imperative.

In addition to recalibrating outdoors, our approach for this terrain element focuses on restoring the health of the adrenal glands while balancing the cortisol response with specific nutrients and adaptogenic herbs. From a lifestyle perspective, we focus on eating seasonally. Lastly, one of the most interesting and novel approaches to stress therapy is to actually deliberately try to elicit it by eating chemoprotective phytonutrients. Next we explore the concept of hormesis a little further.

Hormesis and Adaptive Stress Responses

As we have described, hormesis is the adaptive response of cells and organisms to a moderate (usually intermittent) stress. It is also known as preconditioning or provoking an adaptive stress response. It is defined as a process whereby exposures to a low dose of a chemical agent or environmental factor that is damaging at higher doses induces an adaptive beneficial effect on the cell or organism. For our purposes, examples of hormesis include dietary energy restriction (fasting) and exposures to low doses of certain phytochemicals. Studies have shown that in response to these low-dose stressors, cells increase their production of protective and restorative proteins, including growth factors and phase 2 and antioxidant enzymes such as superoxide dismutase and glutathione peroxidase.[27] There is also evidence that phytochemicals exert beneficial effects by activating adaptive stress response signaling pathways. Phytochemicals such as resveratrol (found in organic red grapes and pistachios), sulforaphanes (found in cruciferous vegetables like cauliflower), curcumin (from the herb turmeric), capsaicin (from spicy peppers), and allicin (from garlic) activate these stress response pathways, which helps protect cells against stress.[28]

This phenomenon of hormesis harks back to one of the essential health determinants we just talked about, the Gaia principle. Survival advantages were conferred on plants capable of producing noxious, bitter-tasting chemicals and to the humans able to tolerate these phytochemicals and gain the plant's caloric benefit. In short, the more bitter a food, the more chemoprotective the response. The diverse amount of phytochemicals present in vegetables, spices, and tea is likely related to the acquisition of adaptive cellular stress responses and detoxification enzymes in humans that enabled us to consume plants containing potentially toxic chemicals.[29] And this tolerance of bitter taste has followed humankind from snack to sanatorium; for centuries Ayurvedic medicine (traditional Indian medicine) has recommended the use of bitter melon as a functional food to prevent and treat diabetes. It looks and tastes more like a cucumber than a cantaloupe and contains at least three active substances with antidiabetic properties, including charantin, which has been confirmed to have a blood-glucose-lowering effect. Not surprisingly, extracts from bitter melon also inhibit cancer cell growth by inducing apoptosis and cell cycle arrest.[30] More good news about bitter melon—it's low-glycemic: A whole cup of it contains less than 1 gram of sugar and 3 grams of carbohydrate. Other bitter foods discussed in previous terrain chapters, including dandelion greens, Jerusalem artichokes, and arugula, also help elicit a hormesis response.

Bitter foods are associated with the heart in Chinese medicine. They help to clear heat and keep the heart cool, and since stress is commonly associated with heart disease, bitter foods get even more props. We suggest the use of herbal bitter formulas during meals, and especially for those transitioning onto the ketogenic diet as it can support digestion. So now that we have stimulated healthy and protective stress by fasting and eating bitter foods, let's look at how we can support those overworked adrenals.

Key Adrenal Nutrients:
Vitamins C and E and Magnesium

There are three key micronutrients involved in the adrenal cascade: vitamins C and E and magnesium. We have already discussed vitamin C in detail in chapter 7, but it also has vast activity in supporting the adrenal glands. In fact, it is the most important vitamin involved in adrenal metabolism. The more cortisol is produced, the more vitamin C is used by the body, which is why people often get sick after a stressful event. Vitamin C acts as an antioxidant within the adrenal gland itself. Because vitamin C is water-soluble and used quickly by the body, it should be consumed several times a day, especially during times of high stress. Rich and diverse food sources of vitamin C include parsley, Irish moss seaweed, purslane, and borage. Borage (star-flower) is an annual herb native to the Mediterranean that tastes similar to cucumber. Both the leaves and flowers are edible, and it makes an attractive salad addition. Borage has long been used by herbalists as a restorative tonic for the adrenal glands.

Irish moss is a reddish sea vegetable that grows in the intertidal zone along the North Atlantic. The carrageenan extracted from Irish moss has been used worldwide as a thickening agent in many foods and cosmetics. While carrageenan-containing seaweeds have been used for centuries in food preparations for their gelling properties, the refined, isolated carrageenan found in modern processed foods was removed from the list of approved ingredients in organic foods in late 2016 due to the digestive issues it confers. Here we have a great example of how a whole food contains many valuable properties that interact together but when certain compounds are isolated through modern processing methods they can become toxic. In this case, carrageenan was separated from vitamin C. Yet another reason why we need to study whole foods rather food isolates. We recommend avoiding the food additive carrageenan altogether unless ingesting in the moss whole food form.

A key point is, whole sea vegetables are highly indicated for an anticancer and ketogenic diet. Nori, wakame, arame, kombu, and others have been used for centuries in Japanese and Chinese medicine in the treatment of cancer. Why? Because they have been shown to exhibit anticancer, antioxidant, anti-inflammatory, and antidiabetic activities.[31] They are highly nutrient-dense (rich in vitamins, minerals, and unsaturated fats), are low-glycemic, and exert powerful stimulation of beneficial members of the microbiota such as the *Bifidobacterium* and *Lactobacillus*. Nori wraps (used to make sushi) make the perfect keto tortilla, packing only 1 gram of carbohydrate.

Another adrenal-supportive micronutrient is vitamin E, which is a fat-soluble group of vitamins, including the tocopherols and tocotrienols. It neutralizes free-radical molecules inside the adrenal glands and elsewhere. (The manufacturing of adrenal hormones generates free radicals that can damage adrenal tissue if not controlled.) Vitamin E is also essential for six different enzymatic reactions in the adrenal cascade. The best food sources are sunflower seeds and turnip and mustard greens.

Although we discussed magnesium in chapter 8, it deserves another mention with regard to adrenal health. Magnesium acts like a spark plug for the adrenal glands and is essential to the production of such hormones as cortisol. Clams, Swiss chard, cocoa powder, and sunflower and sesame seeds are rich sources.

The Power of Adaptogenic Herbs

For thousands of years a centerpiece of the Chinese medicine approach to cancer has been the employment of herbs. Study after study says the same thing: We need more research into the powerful protective and anticancer effects of herbs, because what has already been discovered is spectacular. *Adaptogenic herbs* are a category of medicinal plants that are able to enhance a "state of nonspecific resistance" to stress. Adaptogens possess stress-protective effects including antifatigue and anti-infection; they also have restorative activities, while exerting a normalizing impact on the HPA axis.[32] Several herbs act as adaptogens, but most notable are the fabulous five: ginseng, rhodiola, holy basil, ashwaganda, and licorice root. Not only do these herbs exert anti-stress effects, they also have extremely powerful effects on many of the cancer hallmarks, including the Warburg effect. For one, rhodiola has demonstrated antidepressant effects while supporting immune function and decreasing the growth of bladder cancer.[33] The best part is that they can all be taken orally in the form of teas and tonics. We should all drink them on a daily basis!

The three primary types of ginseng—panax, American, and Siberian—are some of the most potent of all the adaptogens. Ginseng has been found to improve resistance to viral stressors and improve immune function, and has also been found in several studies to help diminish cancer-associated fatigue. The ginsenosides from panax ginseng have been found to be cytotoxic and induce apoptosis in cancer cells.[34] Amazing what can be achieved with a cup of ginseng tea.

Ayurvedic texts denote holy basil (also called tulsi) as the "the Incomparable One," a pillar of herbal medicine and a goddess incarnated in plant form. It continues as one of India's most cherished and sacred healing plants. It has been found to normalize blood sugar and enhance gastric mucosal strength. A member of the mint family, holy basil contains powerful anticancer compounds that have been found to inhibit proliferation, migration, and invasion as well as inducing apoptosis of pancreatic cancer cells.[35]

Licorice root is one of the best-known adrenal-supportive herbs. It helps increase energy and vitality and naturally balances cortisol. This herb has the ability to increase the half-life of circulating cortisol, which takes the demand to produce more off the adrenal glands. Its lignans also exhibit modulating impacts on estrogen metabolism. When estrogen levels are high, it has the ability to inhibit estrogen action, and when estrogen levels are low, it has shown the ability to enhance the estrogenic response—a hormone helper to say the least. This activity is important because the adrenally exhausted male and female often have altered estrogen metabolism, as we learned in the last chapter. This herb is best for those in later stages of adrenal exhaustion. For those with advanced adrenal fatigue, sipping on licorice root tea all day long is a great way to manage the stress response, especially if you can couple the tea with a quiet moment of breathing and mediation.

Eating Seasonally and Wild

Aside from spending a huge amount of time indoors glued to our screens, the greatest change to human biorhythms has occurred with our disconnection from eating wild foods and from eating seasonally. Until about fifteen thousand years ago, there were few, if any, permanent homes or villages. We were nomads for 99 percent of our history and, like the animals, we followed a seasonal migration pattern. When the land was devoid of desired plants and animals we moved on. Being human has allowed us to adapt to many habitats and combine different foods to create a sustainable diet. The seasons change, and so should our food sources, which is why we often take a seasonal approach to our dietary recommendations. What's interesting is that the nutrient content of both plants and animals changes with the seasons, depending on what their food sources are.[36] The Earth's wild food sources live in harmony with the natural biorhythms of the planet. Together with humans, plants and animals are products of millions of years of adaptation and evolution. Humans—and our genomes—have been eating the foods and their corresponding nutrients varying with the season for most all of our existence.

The Earth makes one complete revolution about the Sun each year. In spring (the English word meaning "to rise") dark, bitter, and leafy greens are the first foods to poke out of the ground in many areas—nature's provision of hormesis-inducing phytonutrients. In spring, plants direct nutrients to their newly sprouting shoots, buds, and leaves. Those bitter greens not only provided phytonutrient-dense carbohydrates for many humans coming out of a winterlong, primarily ketotic state, but also stimulated liver detoxification processes. Spring has always been a time of renewal, sorely needed after our livers spent the winter months producing ketones. Daylight hours are shorter in winter, so historically humans would have less time to procure food and nighttime fasting would last longer. Conversely, summer is the time of abundance. When there is more sunlight we are able to process higher amounts of glucose as we have more daylight hours of activity. In the fall we slow down, and our bodies require more calories for surviving. Plants prepare for dormancy by directing nutrients and sugars back into roots and other interior storage sites. Naturally, our ancestors would swing from a ketogenic-type diet in the winter to a higher-carbohydrate and plant-based diet in the summer.

In other words, there is no one diet for all seasons, but it should always be changing based on the seasons and what is available to you locally. Foods that travel far distances or get picked before they are ripe have a fraction of the nutrients found in local and wild plants, nutrients that are so desperately needed by our immune systems and more.[37] Nutrient depletion is a huge stress on the body, and it can lead to cancer. In today's world, we need all the nutrients we can get (not to mention needing to get our hands in the dirt and to pick wild foods to help populate our microbiomes with friendly bacteria). We encourage our patients to start tuning in to what foods are available to them on a seasonal basis, and rotating diets accordingly.

The Lessons of De-Stressing

Modern life is just all about excess. For most of our existence, humans had no possessions. We walked everywhere, and extra stuff, well, was just considered extra baggage. Today we have huge homes, huge cars, and supersized portions. All this modern living—and don't get us wrong, we have houses and cars, too—is bringing significant stress to our minds and bodies. Cancer really is a messenger, telling us that we are not living and eating in accordance with natural laws. And even with all the comforts and sweet tastes modern life has to offer, many people are sad, anxious, depressed, and lonely. Sadly, rates of depression have been skyrocketing, especially among children. After accidents and cancer, suicide is the third-leading cause of death in people ages fifteen to twenty-four, and approximately 20 percent of teens experience depression. Depression affects almost all cancer patients at one point or another, making it hard to stay positive and find the energy to endure months and years of treatments, tests, and side effects.

Depression makes even the happiest of people think that life isn't worth experiencing. Energy vanishes, and what was once was pleasurable now elicits no feeling. Our modern diet and lifestyle are like a big old shot of Novocaine: They make many of us feel totally numb. Just as we've lost touch with the essential determinants of health, many people have lost feeling, connection, and purpose. Chronic stress—especially dietary stress—is a major cause of this. We will explore many of these factors in the next chapter about mental and emotional well-being. State of mind is everything and, as you will learn, has just as big an impact on your terrain as your genes.

But don't worry, there are a slew of good-mood foods, mind-body medicine approaches, and cannabinoids that act like a pinch in the arm. These can lift those that find themselves in the shadows of despair into the warm sunshine of all life has to offer, whether you have cancer or not. The power of the mind to prevent and overcome cancer is the strongest tool you have. Let's learn how to sharpen it.

CHAPTER 12

Mental and Emotional Well-Being

Cultivating the Most Powerful Medicine of All

When an illness is part of your spiritual journey, no medical intervention can heal you until your spirit has begun to make the changes that the illness was designed to inspire.

—Caroline Myss, Anatomy of the Spirit

Everything is energy and that's all there is to it. Match the frequency of the reality you want and you cannot help but get that reality. It can be no other way. This is NOT philosophy. This is physics. —Albert Einstein

Second to food, emotions and thought patterns are our primary epigenetic modifiers. Our mind really can change our matter, for better or worse. But we are not completely responsible for our thought patterns: Research has found that infants exposed to stress, lack of emotional nurturing, or overactive stress responses can transmit these epigenetic marks to future descendants—including the trait of maternal nurturing.[1] So yes, you can partially "blame" your parents for how you feel, but you also have the ability to completely reprogram negative thought patterns. We cannot blame others for our lives or our diseases. But you can harness the power of positive thinking to improve your response to treatments, or even achieve the spontaneous regression or remission that occurs in over 20 percent of all cancer cases without therapy.[2] The book *Mind Over Medicine* by Dr. Lissa Rankin tells us that almost 80 percent of patients taking a placebo ("the sugar pill") heal themselves through using only the power of the mind. Mind over medicine is right. Ever since the 1600s, when mathematician and philosopher René Descartes invoked the paradigm of separating mind and body, we've been trying to glue the two back together. You cannot truly heal the body without the help of your mind.

This terrain element, mental and emotional health, is typically the most difficult for people to address. The simple "How are you feeling?" or "Are you happy?" questions can actually cut pretty deep for some. We've noticed that during our retreats, consultations, and webinars, when we talk about the mental and emotional sphere some patients tend to check out. Often these are the ones who do absolutely everything else right. They're engaged in taking supplements diligently, exercising regularly, and modifying their diets. Yet their labs, symptoms, and progression of disease suggest something else is going on—they progress. When a patient completely disengages from discussion of the mind-body connection, it's like a huge spotlight shining on a closed door. It usually means the person must partake in some sort of total emotional transformation for healing to occur. For many of us, that can be scarier than cancer.

But dealing—or not dealing—with emotional health can mean the difference between a vertical change and a horizontal change. Emotional "dis-ease" is a major speed bump for anyone seeking optimal health. At some point along your journey, you may find that certain disease markers are refusing to change, or some physical symptoms just won't leave the building. You plateau. Or perhaps after a lengthy remission you experience a recurrence. What's going on? Very likely there is a mind-body factor at play. Maybe you are stuck in a relationship, unhappy in your job, struggling with addiction, or have an unresolved relationship or past trauma you never worked through. If you don't work on this stuff, it will undermine even the most intelligent Western and holistic treatment strategies.

As scary as a cancer diagnosis feels, it is an invitation to total transformation. Not just in diet, herbal treatments, and water filtration systems, but in one's entire way of being. Making all these external adjustments is like only rearranging the furniture. They will be fruitless, or at least stunted, if the subconscious is not explored. If only external changes are made, the old self has simply been provided with new tools to play its games: An old habit of overworking might reappear as long hours researching the diagnosis on the internet. New dietary changes may become new fuel for past tensions in the family. Exercise may occur fairly regularly for a few weeks, but then a sedentary lifestyle returns because life is "too busy with practitioner appointments." When unhealthy mental and behavioral patterns do not change, rarely will the progression of cancer. Dr. Nasha has seen this thousands and thousands of times.

A cancer diagnosis, even if it feels shocking, is sometimes not surprising. Psychologist Lawrence LeShan, author of *Cancer as a Turning Point*, found that there is often a significant trigger, or "final blow," to the system that precedes a diagnosis, often occurring six months to two years earlier. It is widely believed that cancer begins as an energetic imbalance years before it is ever psychically detected. Chronic heightened emotional states create a perfect breeding ground for illness, as we learned in the last chapter. And in fact there is a whole field of study, *psychoneuroimmunology*, that examines how the body's stress response and emotions of anxiety, fear, guilt, anger, and sadness weaken the immune system, interfere with healing, and even cause disease. It was founded by Dr. Candace Pert, a molecular biologist and author of the groundbreaking book *Molecules of Emotion*. Pert discovered that certain proteins and immune system cytokines facilitate and integrate communication between the brain and the body. Simply stated, she concluded that our bodies reflect our thoughts. A concept confirmed by others.

The German physician Ryke Geerd Hamer has asserted that cancer involves a specific area of the brain that controls a conflict-related organ or tissue. His controversial yet well-studied theory is that cancer originates from an unexpected shock experience, such as the loss of a loved one or a divorce. Dr. Bernie Siegel, author of *The Art of Healing: Uncovering Your Inner Wisdom and Potential for Self-Healing*, found that the drawings his cancer patients created of their disease and treatments revealed how they would respond to therapy. He believed the drawings uncovered beliefs and attitudes that positively or negatively affected healing and treatment outcomes. Dr. O. Carl Simonton was an internationally acclaimed oncologist and author of *Getting Well Again*. His pioneering insights and research in the field of psychosocial oncology found that by using imagery and belief systems, terminal cancer patients could not only improve their quality and quantity of life, but also achieve remission.

Our point here is that we are not the first people to connect thought patterns to a cancer prognosis. What you choose to focus on becomes your reality. If you haven't yet watched the documentary "The Connection: Mind Your Body," now is the time. When highly acclaimed scientists, researchers, and doctors say that mind-body medicine practices such as meditation are just as powerful as chemotherapy, radiation, and surgery, we have to listen. Our cells certainly are. In this chapter we talk about factors that impact emotions, such as imbalanced neurotransmitters, genetic SNPs, the gut-brain connection, and, of course, food. We will explain cravings and what they mean from the perspective of Chinese medicine. Our rebalancing approach focuses on connecting with communities and getting to know ourselves. We discuss the indispensible role of B vitamins for both brain and mitochondrial health. We also discuss the emerging science exploring the incredible powers of cannabinoids for both depression and cancer. This chapter is literally the heart of our metabolic approach. Enhancing the other nine terrain elements just does not work if our mind does not believe it will. We have to fully trust to triumph.

Factors That Impact Emotions

While your upbringing may have imprinted negative thought patterns into your mind, there are also other factors that can contribute to mental or emotional duress. You may have had a great childhood, but later in life started feeling flat. You may also be extremely happy and well balanced, but want to prevent depression and use the emotional tools we explain in this chapter to further enhance your healing journey. Paying attention to emotional health is critical for all of us, always. As we learned in the last chapter, stress is everywhere. So is depression. Why? In many ways we are more "connected" than ever and constantly fixated on FOMO (Fear of Missing Out), and yet this data-rich age has left many of us even lonelier, more isolated, and more anxious than ever. Mood disorders are at an all-time high, with 18.8 million Americans afflicted with depression and 19 million with anxiety—that means roughly one in ten Americans suffers with a depression or anxiety disorder.

Depression is now the leading cause of disability worldwide and brings in over $50 billion a year to the pharmaceutical industry. Yet no matter how mild or severe the depression or anxiety is, or whether it is driven by chemistry or by circumstance, the standard-of-care treatment is, you guessed it, prescription medication. Yet the current pharmacologically focused model has achieved only modest benefits in addressing a worldwide burden of poor mental health.

Meanwhile, evidence from nutritional psychiatry research into the relationships among dietary quality, nutritional deficiencies, and mental health is snowballing.[3] What we are learning is that depression—like cancer—doesn't just happen; rather it is the result of modern diets. Western medicine is failing to ask *why* we are so depressed, even though there are many known precipitating factors to consider—most of which we've already covered in this book. Affect any one of the Terrain Ten and you affect the mind and emotions. Food allergies and sensitivities, digestive insufficiencies, oxidative stress, mitochondrial dysfunction, emotional stress, hormone imbalance, toxins, nutrient deficiencies, prescription medications, inflammation, infections, chronic screen addictions, and most of all a separation from the essential determinants of health—all of these impact our emotions.

We may think we're "connected" when we consider old friends made new again on social media sites, but this "connection" is to elements of modern living that are in complete discord with our evolution. Facebook, reality TV, and video games are scrambling our emotional terrains like eggs on a griddle. People aren't talking to one another anymore, they are looking at a screen. And if we don't start looking up, our happiness will continue going down. In fact, a recent survey found that as many as one in five people say they feel depressed as a result of using social media. You get it. So now let's learn about what controls happiness on a biological level: neurotransmitters.

Neurotransmitters: The Molecules of Happiness

Neurotransmitters are a lot like hormones; they are chemical messengers that transmit signals from one neuron to the next. Neurons are nerve cells that carry messages between the brain and other parts of the body and are the basic units of the nervous system (both the parasympathetic and the sympathetic branches). Two primary neurotransmitters related to happiness are dopamine and serotonin. Serotonin helps control functions such as mood, appetite, and sleep. People with depression often have lower-than-normal levels of serotonin, which is why the antidepressants most commonly prescribed are selective serotonin reuptake inhibitors (SSRIs), fluoxetine (Prozac), for example. SSRIs block the reabsorption (reuptake) of serotonin in the brain, making more serotonin available in the body. The brain makes serotonin from the essential amino acid tryptophan (famous for its sedative effects following a turkey dinner). Serotonin is also the precursor for melatonin, the body's natural "sleeping pill." Tryptophan makes serotonin; serotonin makes melatonin. No dietary protein, no serotonin, so adding elk meat and pastured eggs into the diet can be helpful for emotional well-being.

Dopamine controls the flow of information to parts of the brain and is linked to thought, emotion, memory and the reward systems. Problems in producing dopamine can also result in movement disorders, such as Parkinson's. Dopamine-deficient depression is characterized by a low-energy, demotivated state and is also linked to addictions. Sugar ingestion releases dopamine, which is why we literally get addicted to it; like cocaine, it elicits a feeling of bliss.[4] But over time, just as with our adrenal glands and cortisol, chronic dopamine activation eventually leads to fatigue and depression. The good news is that low dopamine levels can be circumvented (as one example, the polyphenol in green tea helps increase dopamine levels). When it comes to mood, there are also our genes to consider. SNPs in genes that control our neurotransmitters can have a big impact on whether we spend more time smiling or frowning. Nutrition therapy can rescue this, but first you need to know what SNPs you have.

The Genetics of Emotions

In addition to affecting many actions of the immune system, low vitamin D levels can also lead to depression. Levels of serotonin rise with exposure to bright natural light and (like vitamin D) fall with decreased sun exposure, which is why many people experience seasonal depressive disorder. Vitamin D regulates the conversion of tryptophan into serotonin.[5] So you could be eating turkey all day long, but if you have low levels of vitamin D (which up to 90 percent of Americans do) and a SNP in your vitamin D receptor, then you are probably not making much serotonin. Folks with the MTHFR SNP (discussed in chapter 3) are also at higher risk of serious and chronic psychiatric illness because they produce less dopamine.[6] Many studies, going back to the 1960s, show an elevated incidence of folate deficiency in patients with depression and low dopamine. Recall that a MTHFR SNP inhibits the use of this vital nutrient.[7]

A SNP in the gene for the enzyme monoamine oxidase, MAOA, can impact the rate at which the body breaks down the neurotransmitters serotonin and dopamine. MAOA is dubbed the worrier or warrior gene, and knowing how it is functioning explains why antidepressant drugs will work or backfire. In the brain, the COMT enzyme also helps break down neurotransmitters and directs the routes by which dopamine travels throughout the brain. Variations in the COMT gene are associated with mental illnesses such as bipolar disorder, panic disorder, anxiety, obsessive-compulsive disorder, eating disorders, and attention-deficit hyperactivity disorder.[8]

You can see that genetic assessment may hold the key to unlocking the doors to depression, addiction, and other emotional and cognitive disorders. Antidepressants don't make depression go away. Just ask anyone who has tried to come off them without nutritional support. Discovering on a genetic level why depression is occurring can help provide the proper tools to alleviate it on an epigenetic level using deep nutrition. This is obviously important because our genes can impact personality traits, and there is evidence that these, too, can contribute to cancer.

The Type C Personality

Just as unhealthy diet and lifestyle patterns can lead to cancer, detrimental personality traits have also been linked to its development. Biobehavioral oncologists have identified the habit of holding on to toxic emotions such as anger or hate at the top of the list. Additional characteristics have been grouped in what's known as the type C personality, and include:

- Being overly conscientious and responsible
- Carrying others' burdens

- Poorly defined personal boundaries
- Wanting to please other people
- Needing approval
- Internalizing toxic emotions, such as anger, resentment, and hostility, and difficulty expressing them
- Having a low threshold for stress[9]

So how does one retire this personality? By expressing one's emotions, searching for purpose, and creating new dreams and reasons to live. By being assertive and no longer compromising. You've heard the safety talk on the airplane: Put on your own oxygen mask first before tending to others. Stop worrying about what others think. Practice being vulnerable. Be who you are. Let go of relationships that no longer push you to grow. Know that death is not the only way out of challenging situations. Dr. Brené Brown's work exploring worthiness, vulnerability, and courage can offer wonderful tools to help rediscover the authentic self. Her book *Daring Greatly* is a must-read for anyone who identifies with these patterns and traits.

The most common setbacks Dr. Nasha has observed in her patients over the years include not having the right support system, not being truly able to speak their truth, not living their authentic self for fear of hurting or disappointing another, or concern for what others may think. If this resonates with you, then know you are not alone, and know that you can change. If this is jogging any thoughts or emotions for you, start writing them down and getting them out. Emotional detox creates emotional freedom.

Every person has their own story—the collection of happy and sad events that over time can pick up momentum and begin to cause physical and psychological distress if not properly channeled. Thousands of years of Chinese medical wisdom has identified further emotion-cancer connections. For example, breast cancer commonly stems from issues with mother or child, ovarian cancer from sexual abuse or betrayal in a relationship, lung cancer from a tragic loss. Even if you've been lucky enough to have led a stress-free life, the diagnosis and treatment of cancer alone often induces post-traumatic stress disorder (PTSD) in both patient and caregivers. Cancer patients can feel powerless and without hope at some point on their journey, and certainly this can lead to depression. All this underscores the critical importance of working on old and new traumas and emotional imbalances. Feeling disempowered can actually accelerate tumor progression and promote recurrence.[10] Some estimates state that 70 percent of all patients diagnosed with cancer will have a recurrence. We reason that in some cases emotional discord is the reason why.

We hope that diving into what may feel uncomfortable may help set the groundwork and provide the motivation to open every closed door that may be inhibiting your recovery. Diet on track: check. Supplement program dialed in: check. Environmental overhaul: check. Great medical team: check. Running all your labs to stay on top of things: check. Now it is time to dive into the final frontier: your thoughts. As Saint Isaac of Nineveh said, "Dive into yourself and in your soul you will discover the stairs by which to ascend." But before we go up we're going to go down, right down into the belly of another system that controls our emotions: our gut.

A Second Brain

Dr. Michael Gershon's groundbreaking work and his book *The Second Brain*, published in 1999, pioneered the concept of a gut-brain axis. Statements like "gut feeling" or "the thought of that makes me sick to my stomach" are just two examples of how easily we relate emotion to physical reaction. The gut-brain axis (GBA) is a bidirectional line of communication that links the emotional and cognitive centers of the brain with intestinal functions. Exciting advances in research have found that the gut microbiota can profoundly influence these lines of communication. What's more, studies have shown that bacterial colonization of the gut is central to development and maturation of the nervous system.[11] Think back to chapter 6 when we talked about threats to our microbiome, such as antibiotics: It turns out they are also threats to our happiness. When we start connecting the dots among terrain elements, it comes as no surprise that clinical trials have shown that supplementation with probiotics decreases depression scores by 50 percent and improves anxiety scores by 55 percent.[12]

Since an estimated 50 percent of dopamine and approximately 90 percent of serotonin originate in the intestine, it should come as no surprise not only that "you are what you eat" but also that "you think and feel what you eat."

If we slurp down daily doses of wheat, processed foods, sugar, glyphosate, NSAIDs, and inflammatory fats then our microbiome is drastically altered, and this directly influences serotonin levels. Depression has also been associated with elevated levels of lipopolysaccharides (LPS), nutrient-binding, inflammatory toxins produced by gut bacteria in response to poor diet. Gut inflammation has also been implicated in the progressive nature of neurodegenerative diseases, such as Parkinson's.[13] The evidence of the modern diet working against us is everywhere, and when our bellies are full of toxic food, so are our minds.

Toxic Food: A2 Dairy

Take a highly emotional personal experience and mix it with atrocious eating habits and you have a recipe for a mood disorder. Hopefully you have learned how our genes and guts can predispose our thoughts and that depression is not "all in the head," as many of us were taught to believe. Two particular food groups are believed by many experts besides ourselves—including neurologist Dr. David Perlmutter, author of *Grain Brain* and *Brain Maker*—to sabotage brain health. Grains and dairy—daily staples for many Americans—may undermine the body's ability to heal as they activate an array of immune reactions and gut-brain axis inflammation. By now we've talked a lot about wheat gluten and all grains as vehicles for immune and blood sugar disorders, and it applies here, too. Gluten has been identified as a primary cause of both depression and schizophrenia. Multiple studies have found "a drastic reduction, if not full remission" of schizophrenic symptoms after initiation of gluten withdrawal.[14] Have we said it enough? Get grains out of the diet!

While some people can eat dairy, for those with mood disorders it is best to remove it from the diet for a three-month period (it takes that long to clear it from your system) to see if the symptoms or disease markers improve. As you recall from chapter 3, casein is the primary protein found in cow's milk. The protein comes in two forms, A1 or A2, depending on the breed of the cow. The A2 protein is more prevalent in milk from Jersey, Guernsey, and Normande breeds. But the Holstein—which produces A1 casein—happens to produce quite a bit more milk. More milk means more money to the farmer, and today over 90 percent of cows in commercial use are Holstein.

What Is Gluten, and Why Should We Avoid It?

Gluten—the substance that makes bread rise and gives a chewy, elastic texture to baked goods and many processed foods—is a protein made by combining two smaller proteins, gliadin and glutenin. Wheat contains the most gluten of all grains, and is about 10–15 percent protein. The remainder is starch. The more closely a grain is related to wheat, the higher the gluten content. Such grains include rye, barley, bulgur, durum, kamut, semolina, triticale (a wheat-rye hybrid), and spelt. Soaking and sprouting grains begins the enzymatic action that breaks down the gluten into peptides, making it easier to digest, but does *not* eradicate the gluten content. Even sprouted grain breads like spelt or Ezekiel still contain gluten, and just one slice can contain over 15 grams of carbohydrate.

A review paper in *The New England Journal of Medicine* lists fifty-five diseases that are believed to be caused by eating gluten, including osteoporosis, irritable bowel disease, inflammatory bowel disease, anemia, cancer, fatigue, canker sores, rheumatoid arthritis, lupus, multiple sclerosis, and almost all other autoimmune diseases.[15] Gluten is also linked to many psychiatric and neurological diseases, including anxiety, depression, schizophrenia, dementia, migraines, epilepsy, and neuropathy (nerve damage). It has also been associated with autism, heart disease, and infertility. Gluten sensitivities can affect both adults and children and are most commonly seen in Caucasians of European, mainly Irish, descent.

For more direction on following a gluten-free diet, we recommend working with a nutrition therapist. There are also online resources, including glutenfreedomproject.com, a site that Jess helped develop.

The problem is that many people can digest the A2 but not the A1 form, as explained by Keith Woodford, a professor and author of the book *Devil in the Milk: Illness, Health, and the Politics of A1 and A2 Milk*. Woodford found more than a hundred studies linking the A1 protein to diseases, including type 1 diabetes. When A1 casein, not the A2 variety, is digested it triggers the release of beta-casomorphin-7, an opioid with a structure similar to that of morphine, and which has also been linked to prostate cancer.[16] Beta-casomorphin-7 has the ability to stimulate angiogenesis by activating opiate pathways.[17] Yet another plug to get to know your food and know your farmer: Ask your local cheesemakers what kind of cows they get their milk from. Your health could be riding on it.

Beside gluten and dairy, there are also nutrient deficiencies that are not only linked to depression but further depleted by the use of psychiatric and other drugs, deficiencies in COQ10, magnesium, omega-3 fatty acids, melatonin, vitamin B_2, vitamin D, vitamin B_6, vitamin B_{12}, and folate, for example. We've mentioned most of these in relation to other terrain areas and metabolic pathways and will talk more about the B_6 vitamin at the end. For now, hopefully it is becoming clear that the most common cause of mental health problems is malnourishment, eating toxic foods, and our genome. Conventional treatment only compounds terrain destruction by failing to recognize the root cause of the imbalance in the first place—which is almost always poor diet.

The tricky part is that many of us know that the foods we are eating are bad, but keep going back. You avoid sugar for a while then one bad day at the office and you are right back at it. Why? Because food addictions are real, and cravings stem from unresolved emotional imbalances. Let's take a closer look at cravings and what they are really trying to tell us.

The Real Message behind Cravings

What do we reach for when we are hormonal, stressed, exhausted, sad, mad, lonely, or in pain? Comfort food! And why does the idea of comfort food typically not lead us to a nice head of broccoli? Because what we crave during those emotional moments is actually a clue to what elements of our terrain are out of balance. Cravings are internal cues to neglected terrain elements. But, sadly, we have even been taught to ignore or suppress our inner alarms. We use acetaminophen for a fever, ibuprofen for a headache, allopurinol for gout, fluoxetine for depression: Do those medicines alleviate the symptoms?

Sure. But do they improve the terrain, correct the imbalance, or remove the obstacle to cure? Not a bit.

Rather than expressing emotions, we tend to stuff them back inside with food or alcohol, which our minds interpret as "comfort" and "fulfillment." For example, a common craving we hear about is for crunchy foods. Crunchy foods are loud, and therefore often a cry for either needing attention or wanting to snap back at someone but feeling restrained. So we crunch away on chips or crackers. To reunite our mind and our body and start the deep healing process, we must first recognize the two are one. Much like physical pain is a signal to pay attention to the body, mental pain also stems from imbalances within the body. Certainly sometimes our food cravings are legitimate—we may need some extra protein if we've been under stress, or more salt if we're dehydrated. More commonly, however, our cravings are triggered by suppressed emotional events or trauma.

In the Chinese medical system, relationship to foods, flavors, organ systems, emotions, seasons, cycles, and the elements of nature are all entwined and illuminate patterns between health and "dis-ease." There are five flavors in Chinese medicine: bitter, sour, sweet, spicy, and salty. The organs heart, liver, spleen, lung, kidney are linked to these five flavors, and a particular craving correlates to an organ-emotion imbalance that needs attention and correction. An imbalance can be anatomical, physiological, biochemical, psychological, mental, or emotional, and foods and herbs based on these flavor categories can restore harmony.

Sweet Cravings

Sweet cravings include all things carbohydrate, so not only soda and candy bars, but breads, pastas, chips, fruit, and potatoes. These cravings signify a low-energy state. Craving sugar tells us our mitochondria are suffering. They are begging for fuel to produce more ATP (the molecules that act as the body's energy currency). Yes, sugar can make ATP, but it is less efficient and results in fewer ATP molecules than if your body used fat as the primary fuel. Sugar is that quick blast that takes you high and then just as quickly drops you low, causing you to seek more to keep the high going even while the fatigue is sustained.

What's interesting about fat is that it has no organ system, element, or flavor association, but the craving for fat signals another type of message. Fat can take on any one of the five flavors, ice cream for the sweet, or fried chicken for the salty. Fat can also take on the flavors of sour (kefir), bitter (dark leafy greens sautéed in lard), or spicy (chipotle mayonnaise). When we reach for fatty fried foods or "fake fats" like hydrogenated-oil-drenched chips, processed peanut butter, or soybean mayonnaise, we attempt to satisfy an inner longing that is not being met. Overindulging in fake fat stagnates digestion and the release of bile from the liver, causing symptoms of bloating, upper right quadrant pain, and sluggishness. What begins as an inner longing, in essence, then becomes a big gas bubble leading to a further sense of lack of worth and disconnect from self and others. Sometimes those cravings come masked in "healthy" fats such as nuts and seeds. We find a lot of folks dive headfirst into "nutville" when starting on a low-glycemic or ketogenic diet. We can overdo it, and the pattern will repeat itself. Instead, we need to explore why we must eat half a jar of nut butter a day to feel "full." It is doubtful that this is a true nutritional deficiency. What do *you* long for?

The main emotion associated with sugar cravings is one of disconnect. Our very first taste when we enter the world is sweetness: the galactose in our mother's milk. It is no accident that we all have a sweet tooth, as that early connection between mother and child is a sacred one. But imagine if that connection was lost or damaged in some way: Perhaps Mom was unable to breastfeed, or she was terribly malnourished and her terrain imbalances laid the groundwork for yours, or there was an abusive person in your life and Mom didn't save you. Any of these things can lead to a long-term behavior pattern of self-soothing and medicating with sugar. For people who have experienced trauma on any level, sugar is often the only thing that may have brought them moments of pleasure. But those moments, sadly, don't last, and the trauma becomes deeply embedded in our biology unless it is addressed on an emotional level. One addiction replaces the other. Recovering alcoholics often turn to sugar, nicotine, and other dopamine-stimulating activities as their brain has not been rewired, only rearranged. This is a horizontal shift. The deeper work goes vertical, and to make the shift that truly heals the patterns once and for all takes deep work through such processes as cognitive behavioral therapy, eye movement desensitization and reprocessing, tension and trauma releasing exercise, mindfulness-based stress reduction, biofeedback, psychotherapy, and more. The excellent book *The Body Keeps the Score* by physician Bessel van der Kolk delves deeply into trauma concepts and how to heal from them.

In traditional Chinese medicine, the sweet flavor is associated with the organs of the spleen and stomach and the element of earth. This relates to how we take in, transform, transport, and absorb information in the form of food, thought, air, and water. It is associated with mothering, nurturing, groundedness—all things you think of when you think of earth. Having a difficult relationship with one's mother, not nourishing and nurturing oneself, traveling a lot (up in the air, not on the earth), overthinking or being a worrywart are many examples of what can damage the spleen and stomach meridian. Cravings for sugar signal that the spleen is weak and the sweet tooth reigns. And to take it one step (or in this case, one organ) further, when the liver gets involved because of all the sugar it can act like a bully, putting even more pressure on the spleen, which then leads to symptoms of fatigue, edema, irregular bowel habits, and weight gain. Emotional and mental stagnation, wrongful eating, and poor sleep patterns impact the liver's metabolic and energetic processes, leading to feelings of frustration, irritability, and anger, waking between 1 a.m. and 3 a.m., tendon issues, and knee pain, to name just a few. We often reach for alcohol to soothe that emotional stagnation and stress, which further taxes the liver and depletes the spleen. It becomes a vicious cycle, but one that can be broken.

Seeking other activities and foods that satisfy the search for sweetness in your life is where to focus. Herbs such as gynostemma, licorice, tulsi, cinnamon, and vanilla all have a naturally sweet taste and can be drunk as teas or added to smoothies. A food that offers a natural sweet flavor is coconut in all of its forms, and it's also completely keto-friendly. Dr. Nasha's rule of thumb for patients craving sweet: Start with a big glass of water. Wait fifteen minutes. If you are still wanting sweet, have fat first in the form of a heaping teaspoon of coconut oil with cinnamon, a few macadamia nuts, a hard-boiled egg, or a piece of jerky. Wait another fifteen minutes. If you are still craving sweet, then perhaps go for it (and by that we mean a piece of dark chocolate [85 percent cocoa or higher] or ¼ cup of dark berries). Then go for a walk so as not to start a binge. Exercise regulates the sweet tooth by releasing endorphins. But most important, find the sweetness in your life—with nature, loved ones, or within yourself—not within a bag of M&M's. For more ideas about this, the book *Nourishing Wisdom* by Marc David has been a classic in the emotional nutrition world for over fifteen years.

Salt Cravings

Got a hankering for salt? This craving is associated with issues involving the kidneys, the adrenal glands, and water balance. It is very much influenced by the presence of stress, especially chronic stress, which leads to depleted adrenals that then stop making aldosterone, a hormone that retains sodium in the body. The adrenal glands' main duty is to squeeze out stress hormones in response to signals from our inner and outer environment. The element of water quenches those flames and restores peace and trust. The kidney energy in Chinese medicine is the water element, because the kidney acts like our own built-in water filter. When the feelings of fear and anxiety overwhelm us, it depletes our kidney both energetically and physiologically, and may result in symptoms such as lower back pain, anxiety, intense thirst, hypersensitivity, coldness, poor memory, impotence, prematurely graying hair, and frequent urination.

The craving for salt, which, from a Chinese medicine perspective, helps dissolve stagnation in the body, will help us retain some water to bathe our cells and tissues and fortify the adrenals. However, excess salt—especially the synthetic iodized version—leads to rigidity in both the mind and the body. So striking a balance of fluidity is important. Don't fear salt, as many of us have been taught—it is important to our diet; but quality is key. Choose Himalayan, Celtic, or Real Salt—*not* iodized or bleached. For most of us, there is no need to limit salt, especially if following a ketogenic diet (which actually requires *more* minerals such as sodium, potassium, magnesium, and zinc). Add a teaspoon of sea salt and a teaspoon of baking powder to a quart of water daily as a kidney cleanse. Coconut aminos are another great source of quality sodium, as are bone broths. They offer an array of minerals that will stabilize the electrolytes and restore kidney balance without the toxicity of a chip.

Sour Cravings

The flavor of sour, which calms the body and mind, is believed to move liver energy—such as the emotions of rage and depression—out of the body. It is represented as the element of wood. Much of modern living pokes sticks at this ever-so-important organ, our giant filter, and with all we throw at it, from foods to environmental toxins, it is congested and it is not happy! The liver meridian is in charge of our emotions, so when hepatic congestion mounts we can be driven to irrational behavior pretty quickly. Road rage, violence, tension: Look around today and you see a lot of this in our culture. When the liver is balanced it keeps our body detoxed and helps us overcome stagnant emotions. Sour flavors can be obtained in things like apple cider vinegar, ume plum vinegar, lemon, and fermented pickles. Perhaps next time you have an altercation, stop, breathe, and take a shot of apple cider vinegar or—Dr. Nasha's favorite post-workout or sauna—a glug of raw fermented pickle juice.

Spicy Cravings

And last but not least, the flavor of spicy, which clears cold and wind from the body and is associated to the lung energy. The lung is associated with grief and loss and the element of metal. Dysfunction can show up as allergy

Assessing Emotions with Lab Tests

Low thyroid function can be a primary cause of depression, anxiety, and fatigue. A thyroid panel that also checks thyroid antibodies is always a good idea. By now you know that we highly recommend a genetic assessment to see about SNPs like MTHFR or the vitamin D receptor, especially when it comes to mood imbalances. Finally, because of the high prevalence of celiac disease and its relation to depression, we suggest talking to your doctor about testing for that. We've found that Cyrex Laboratories offers the most comprehensive celiac test we've seen to date.

symptoms, cough, body aches, lack of sweating, and difficulty breathing when out of balance. Many of us when we are sick will reach for a big bowl of spicy soup loaded with ginger, garlic, pepper, and spring onions—all of which are "lung foods" in Chinese medicine. Exploring your own food cravings in times of stress will give you clues about what is the primary driver of your mental-emotional dance and how it relates to the rest of the terrain. For millennia, Ayurvedic and Chinese medical doctors have correlated mood, food, organ systems, and electrical conductance or resistance with terrain imbalances. This perspective offers another way to uncover unconscious beliefs and mechanisms that are most often directing the play of your life.

Taking a Metabolic Mind-Body Approach

One question we love to ask people is, *What makes you tick?* In our modern, busy, stressful, and social-media-infused lives, many people have gotten away from the activities and people that they really enjoy. But think about it: What would you do if you had a whole day with nothing you *had* to do? What hobbies do you enjoy? What brings your life meaning and purpose? Cancer is an opportunity to find it, to find your tribe, your passion, your truth, and to dive in with both feet. A cancer diagnosis can help you get really clear, really fast, on what is most important to you.

A common theme for people approaching the end of life is that they wished they had spent more time with the people they loved. As they step closer to the abyss, everything they had thought mattered dissolves, and they are left with love. Dr. Nasha has witnessed hundreds of people take the launch from their physical form to their spirit form, which has left her with a sense of peace and a lack of fear. Love is the antidote to fear. Fear keeps you from loving yourself and others and energetically predisposes us to autoimmunity. But love overcomes fear. When the chemicals of love are released throughout our body, we feel deeply connected to self and other, safe, trusting, and able to face any adversity. We have to rethink the approach we have taken for many decades of "fighting," "battling," and "killing" the cancer. Because when we do that, we are actually fighting ourselves, because the cancer *is* us. Learning to listen to what cancer is trying to teach you is often the most potent medicine there is. Cancer is a cry for self-love, for connection, and for nourishment.

As you dive deeper into your inner work, books such as Kelly Brogan's *A Mind of Your Own*, Lawrence LeShan's *Cancer as a Turning Point*, Bruce Lipton's *Biology of Belief*, and Leigh Fortson's *Embrace, Release, Heal* will help shed some light on suppressed issues, beliefs, and perceptions that may be blocking your ability to nourish yourself. And don't neglect the importance of connection that can be nurtured by meditation, prayer, and support groups. Speak up for yourself and don't sit back. Studies have found that the patients who are actively engaged in their care, ask all the questions, get second and even third opinions, are vocal about their needs and concerns, and have a great support system have longer survival and recovery rates than those who are passive in the process. We have also seen where cancer becomes a person's identity. Please don't let this happen. You are so much more than your disease, so don't let it consume your life completely, despite the intense schedule of appointments. Take time to breathe, to smile, hell, even to laugh, and to feel the sun on your face. Because, as they say, it's not over until the fat lady sings, so enjoy it. Here are a few other suggestions that can help you achieve mental and emotional wellness.

B Vitamins for Brain: Mitochondrial Requirement and Nature's Valium

We've already talked about the role other B vitamins, including B_{12} and folate, play in the health of the terrain. And there is a reason the Bs keep coming up. They help the body convert carbohydrates to glucose and metabolize fats and protein. They also help the body respond to stress and are involved in preventing cellular stress. All eight of them play essential roles in maintaining mitochondrial function, and mitochondria are compromised by a deficiency of any of them.[18] What this means is that damage to metabolism and mitochondrial function occurs in the absence of B vitamins. There is evidence that mitochondrial dysfunction is associated with abnormal brain function and mood disorders like depression.[19] Therefore, depression, like cancer, is a metabolic mitochondrial disease that can only be successfully overcome with one approach: a therapeutic diet.

In addition to being essential for metabolism, individual B vitamins have also been identified for their role in neurotransmitter production. Vitamin

B$_6$ is required for the production of dopamine, serotonin, and an amino acid neurotransmitter called gamma-aminobutyric acid (GABA). GABA promotes relaxation and reduces stress and anxiety. Widely touted as the "anxiety amino acid," GABA is our body's version of Valium. And to get that effect, rather than popping a pill you can eat foods high in vitamin B$_6$ including skipjack tuna, chicken, bell peppers, turnip greens, shiitake mushrooms, and spinach.

Don't Forget to Exercise: Movement Improves Moods

Exercise may be the most powerful natural mood-boosting factor available. Many clinical studies have clearly indicated that exercise has profound anti-depressive effects in addition to improving mitochrondrial function. These studies confirm that increased participation in exercise, sports, and other physical activities is strongly associated with decreased symptoms of anxiety, depression, and malaise. This effect can be attributed to an increase in endor-phins, which are directly correlated with mood. In fact, some researchers are finding that exercise may be even more effective than drug therapy for depression. Focusing more on restorative workouts, such as walks in nature, yoga, tai chi, and qigong, can help tremendously with mood balance.

Cannabinoids

Don't worry, we wouldn't even consider missing the incredibly important endocannabinoid system and its impact on the terrain. In fact, by the time we come out with a second edition of *The Metabolic Approach to Cancer*, the endocannabinoid system (ECS) will likely be a terrain element all its own! The ECS is a group of cannabinoid receptors located in the brain, nervous systems, and immune systems of all mammals. Cannabinoids are compounds that can activate two types of receptors within the ECS: CB1 receptors, which are located within the nervous system, brain, and nerve endings; and CB2 receptors, located primarily within the immune system. Targeting the ECS has been found to have anti-inflammatory, anticachexia, metabolic, pain management, antiseizure, and sleep-promoting effects. (Several of these are side effects of cancer or cancer therapies.) On a biological level, cannabinoids exert the induction of apoptosis in tumor cells and show an antimetastatic effect through inhibition of angiogenesis and tumor cell migration.[20]

The cannabis plant has been a source of fiber, food, oil, and medicine since prehistoric times. There are over 480 natural components found within the *Cannabis sativa* plant, also known as marijuana, and over 100 have been classified as cannabinoids.[21] The most well-known and -researched of these is delta-9-tetrahydrocannabinol, better known as THC. THC activates the CB1 site and is what causes the psychoactive (high) symptoms most associated with cannabis use. Clinically, it is most notable for its pain modulation and antinausea effects without the side effects associated with narcotics. And, more important, it does not seem to have the same proliferative effect as opiates. The opioid drugs used to relieve pain in postoperative and in chronic cancer patients have actually been found in multiple studies to stimulate the growth and spread of tumors.[22]

But there's a whole lot more medical benefit to cannabis than THC, which is a good thing, as many people are rightfully deterred from the psychoactive side effects. Enter cannabidiol (CBD), which is the second most common cannabinoid and has little to no psychotropic activity, but does have rather powerful anti-inflammatory ones. The CB2 receptors in the immune system, with the highest concentration in the spleen, are the ones that are activated by CBD. CBD has been found to potently and selectively inhibit the growth of different cancers, including breast, brain, lung, and colon.[23] The studies proving its efficacy as a cancer treatment and benefits for relieving side effects number in the thousands.

Cannabis was used in medicine for thousands of years prior to achieving its unfounded illicit-substance status in the early 1900s.[24] The suppression of marijuana as medicine is a perfect example of how the profit-focused Western model attempted to discredit natural compounds at the turn of the century in favor of moneymaking, patentable drugs. Of note: At the publication of this book there is an ongoing battle with the FDA trying to classify CBD as a Schedule I drug, putting it in same category as illicit drugs and suggesting it has no medical value, despite the thousands of studies and decades of research stating otherwise. We must remember that the medicinal use of natural products—compounds derived from natural sources—precedes recorded human history and dates back at least sixty thousand years.[25] Plants used for all of human existence have helped keep us alive, while synthetic drugs are slowly killing us with side effects and nutrient depletion. You decide.

You might now be wondering how cannabis pertains to a chapter on mental health, so let us explain. There is a growing body of evidence and clinical experience relating many of our modern mental and emotional woes to a deficient ECS. When patients are clinically endocannabinoid-deficient (yes, this is a thing), we see symptoms from fibromyalgia to migraines, anxiety to depression and sleep disturbances, which are often exacerbated by chronic stress and sugar consumption.[26] For psychological imbalances, CBD-dominant remedies can offer the most benefit for anxiety, depression, and insomnia. But it bears mentioning that just as we each have our unique microbiome and epigenetic fingerprints, so do we each have an entirely unique endocannabinoid fingerprint. This means finding the correct ratio may take some experimentation and guidance from a clinical cannabis expert. Project CBD can be a helpful resource.

The higher the CBD content and the lower the THC, the less psychoactive (meaning, the less "high" you will feel), and most folks with cancer-related anxiety or depression disorders will benefit more from the CBD-only formulas. If pain modulation or appetite support is required, a very small amount of THC may be warranted. Medical research into the immunomodulating effect of CBD is exploding, and by the time you are reading this book, we may know more than we do at the time of its writing. For example, stay tuned to the research on cannabichromene, which exerts nonpsychoactive, anti-inflammatory, and pain-relieving properties. This is particularly exciting!

Keep a Food-Mood Journal

Awareness is everything, and a journal of your foods and moods can help you make lots of connections between what you eat and why you eat. Logging what you ate; the time of day; why you ate (hungry, tired, bored); what you noted about your digestion (gas, bloating, cramping, nothing); bowel changes (undigested foods, loose stools or constipation, hemorrhoids); sleep pattern (night sweats, difficulty falling or staying asleep); energy level (want to take a nap right after you eat, or feel anxious after); physical symptoms (joint pain, headaches, skin breakouts); and also how you feel and think. Were you more or less mentally sharp? Did you feel a sense of peace and contentment, or were you feeling anxious and unsettled? Did that glyphosate-drenched bowl of cereal leave you feeling bloated, fatigued, and unsatisfied, driving you to eat more carbohydrates within an hour? Did that hearty homemade chicken soup loaded with garden-fresh vegetables soothe your body aches and warm your core while leaving you feeling content? You will start to hear your cells again. You will start to honor and listen to what they are trying to tell you.

Watching these patterns over a few weeks offers a lot of valuable data. You will start to link the physical and the emotional symptoms over time as well. They go hand in hand. In your food and mood journal, in addition to what you are eating, note the following as well: What's going on at home? Do you feel supported? Are you a caregiver for loved ones while trying to take care of yourself? Is there childhood trauma in your background or in your parents' background? Do you have a meditation or spiritual practice? Are you living your purpose? How these questions are manifested or suppressed often shows up in our relationship to food and mood. The process of keeping a journal helps to release stored emotion and bring awareness to what you are feeling, and can reveal if you are self-medicating with food or alcohol.

Cultivate an Emotional Connection to Food

Ayurvedic medicine asserts that the state of mind in which one plants, tends to, harvests, and prepares the food is paramount to how one takes in the nutrients and utilizes them for health and vitality. Connect with your local farmers, grow your own food, cultivate bliss when you cook. We highly suggest reconnecting with the whole process that it takes for the food on your plate to get there. It's all about connection. By following the dietary suggestions we have made throughout this book, your emotions will naturally start to come into balance. Of course we are not promising a magic solution, but over the years so many of our patients have been able to be weaned off their antidepressants once they stopped eating gluten alone (but remember, always check with your primary care provider as this needs to be done in tandem with specific nutrition support!). Put simply: Food controls mood.

Perhaps you are wondering what to do next: go to the grocery store or schedule a therapy session. We know. There is a lot of information to synthesize and digest. Just take it one stress-free step at a time. After reading this chapter you might realize that it's the emotional work you need to focus on first. When we ask our patients if they had to guess what caused their cancer, most of them can point to an emotional or stressful event. We encourage you to lean into this process.

In the next and final chapter, we bring everything together into the kitchen, giving you the steps and the strategies we've been using with our patients for years. Plus, there are ten recipes that correlate to the foods discussed in each of the terrain chapters to help get you started. So let's go to the kitchen, the heart of the metabolic approach to cancer where this approach moves from concept to cuisine.

CHAPTER 13

Connecting with the Terrain Ten in the Kitchen

The food you eat can be either the safest and most powerful form of medicine or the slowest form of poison.

—ANN WIGMORE, *health advocate and founder of the original Hippocrates Health Institute in Boston*

One cannot think well, love well, sleep well, if one has not dined well.

—VIRGINIA WOOLF

By now, some people's heads many be spinning from all the information covered in this book. And if you can believe it, we didn't cover *half* of all the material and other approaches that correlate with the Terrain Ten, so some of you may also have lingering questions. This is all normal. Feedback after many of our retreats has been that there was just so much information that participants needed to go home and absorb it all. And that is just what we want you to do. But we also want to give some tools and recipes to help with the integration and implementation process. Maybe you are ready to dive into everything we've suggested right away, or maybe you'd rather take it one step at a time. Whatever approach feels best for you, do that. There is no right or wrong; it is what seems right inside your own heart and does not cause stress!

Now, if you are ready to start dabbling with what we've outlined so far, then it's time to get into the kitchen, also known as your home pharmacy. In the kitchen, you can prepare your daily medicines—because that is what food is, as Hippocrates said. Our goal has always been to empower and educate patients—and those around them—to start making positive changes to their diet. But, of course, it also has to taste good and the process of making it has to feel joyful. All that said, in this closing chapter we outline some strategies to help get you started, and some key principles to help you successfully follow the dietary approaches we've recommended throughout this book. At the end of the chapter we've designed ten recipes, one for each terrain chapter, so you can start to play with some of them. In the end, you are your own best doctor, and by eating well you will feel well. For now, starting this new diet journey begins with taking the first steps, so here are some practical tips to getting rolling.

Getting Started

The most important thing is not to think of a new diet as a job or as tedious; make it fun. Take a ketogenic-diet cooking class; start a dinner club or a recipe exchange. Figure out what will make these changes a positive experience for you. If dietary changes make you miserable, then they won't work— your mind has to be in the game. Of course many people will find it really motivating when they feel better, look better, and also when their lab results improve. Dr. Nasha runs monthly labs for individuals with active cancer in order to monitor their responses to changes. Testing your blood glucose and ketones daily is also important if you are following a ketogenic diet, and can be motivational. However, if testing feels overwhelming—which it does for some—then skip it! By letting others know your goals and asking for support you'll be less likely to succumb to pressures. This whole process works best if everyone in your house is on board. It takes a village, so cultivate a positive support system.

Many people will want to help by making food for you and your caregivers, so we recommend sending out an email or a letter letting these kindhearted people know what foods to focus on, which ones to avoid, and send several recipes along to help guide them (use the ones at the end of this chapter!). When people spend a lot of time preparing a meal with love and thought for someone going through cancer, it is really hard not to eat it. So set everyone up for success ahead of time by letting them know what foods are a part of your therapeutic nutrition plan.

Next, it's time to make your nutrition plan, and to clean out and stock your kitchen full of healing foods.

The Seven P's

Don't forget the seven P's: Prior, Proper, Planning, Prevents, Piss, Poor, Performance. You have to have a plan, or you will find yourself hungry, grumpy, and heading for the next drive-through. Meal planning, or at least making a plan for your day, is not only helpful, it's essential, especially when just getting started. They say it takes three months to create new habits, so give yourself some time! Start with sitting down once a week with a notepad and writing out what you will have for dinner six nights of the week. Knowing you can make enough leftovers for lunch is a great planning stratgy. Most people generally eat the same one or two things for breakfast, but be sure to rotate them seasonally. You can create a shopping list based on your menu plan. Once a week or month sit down with your favorite ketogenic and Paleo cookbooks and flag recipes you'd like to try. When they are flagged, recipes are easier to find.

We suggest subscribing to a couple of different food and cooking magazines, or start searching for "keto recipes" or "Paleo blogs" online. But don't spend too much time on the computer: thirty minutes max. We love *Paleo Magazine* for the great recipes and also for the lifestyle tips that can help make you feel like you are not alone out there with this new diet. You can make folders for different meals, create files on your computer, or Pin it. Whatever works best for your style. Either way, new recipes help bring creativity. Once you've got a plan, it's time to make your kitchen into a foodie haven!

Clean and Stock: The Kitchen Detox

Set aside an afternoon or a couple of hours to dive into your fridge, freezer, and pantry. Then determine where purged foods will go (soup kitchens, friends, donations, garbage, et cetera) and get boxes or bags for each destination. We suggest pulling all the food out, then cleaning the entire area

Remove These Foods
from Your Fridge and Freezer

Soda and sugary drinks: This includes fruit juices, vitamin waters, alcoholic beverages and mixers, soda, diet soda and more. Sugary drinks are the number one cause of weight gain, and the hidden sugar consumption that leads to diabetes and fuels cancer cells.

Nonorganic/non-grass-fed meat and dairy products: All animal and animal by-products should be clean (that is, organic and grass-fed, wild-caught, pasture-raised, free of hormones, antibiotics, nitrates, et cetera). Clean out processed meats such as bacon or sausage that are made with artificial nitrates.

Processed foods: This includes ready-made biscuits, bagels, pizzas, dinners, bread, or anything that is in a ready-made package that contains more than five ingredients or any ingredients you can't pronounce. Condiments that contain gluten, soy, corn, MSG, sugar, or preservatives have to go. Read labels on all condiments and refer to the list below for ingredients to avoid.

Processed dairy and eggs: Dairy products that are not organic can contain rBGH, which is linked to cancer (this includes cottage cheese and yogurt). Eggs that are not organic and pasture-raised contain higher amounts of omega-6 fatty acids (the inflammatory fats). Remove artificial eggs and all butter substitutes.

Nonorganic produce items: Fruits and vegetables, especially those from the "dirty dozen" list, should always be organic.

with a nontoxic cleaner. Keep a notepad close by to make a list of what foods need to be replaced (for example, ketchup containing HFCS will need to be replaced with a sugarless version). Read labels on everything that has a label and follow these two rules: (1) Avoid any store-bought, packaged food with more than five ingredients; and (2) if you can't pronounce it, don't know what it is, or it is not food (it's a chemical, preservative, additive, et cetera), chuck it.

Remove These Foods from Your Pantry

Refined flour products / packaged foods: This includes baking items like white flour, potato starch, corn starch, white rice flour, et cetera. Also any boxed cereals, pastas, crackers, cookies, et cetera. The rule applies that if a food has sugar, more than five ingredients, and/or any that you can't pronounce, it goes bye-bye.

Gluten and grains: Discard anything that contains wheat, barley, rye, spelt, oats, corn, bulgur, white rice, millet, amaranth, corn, quinoa, et cetera (including pastas, cookies, and breads).

Sugar and sugary foods: Supplies of white sugar, brown sugar, agave, corn syrup, cane syrup, processed honey, cookies, candy, pastries, snack bars, granola bars, and sugary cereals all need to go. Any product that contains added sugar on the label (naturally occurring sugar is that found in fruit) should be purged.

Beans and soy products: Unless it is organic and fermented, soy is a GM food, contains lectins, and can have unwanted immune effects. Beans in general are high in starch and can be difficult to digest due to their lectin content.

Inflammatory oils: These include common cooking oils like nonorganic canola (it's usually GM), vegetable, corn, soy, safflower, and cooking oil sprays.

Setting Up a Nontoxic Kitchen

The idea for this step is to create a kitchen space that is not only easy to use and well stocked, but also free of toxins. So once you've gotten all the unhealthy foods out, it's time to take a closer look at your systems, gadgets, storage options, and products. Food storage containers and products including plastic, such as Tupperware, plastic bags, and plastic wrap, can contain endocrine-disrupting chemicals like BPA and other compounds that are carcinogenic. Consider switching to glass jars for food storage,

TABLE 13.1. INGREDIENTS TO AVOID

Ingredient	Where Found and Adverse Effects
Artificial sweeteners (i.e., saccharin, aspartame, acesulfame potassium, and sucralose)	Found in yogurts, soda, sugar-free products, gum, diet products, and more. These have major adverse effects on the kidneys, liver, and brain. Responsible for 95 percent of adverse effects from food reported to FDA annually. Cause headaches, IBS, anxiety, seizures, and more.
Artificial colors	Found in candy, cereal, soft drinks, sports drinks, mac and cheese, pastries, etc. Including blue #1, red dye #3, and yellow #6. Artifical colors are associated with increased tumor risk, thyroid cancer, and behavioral disorders.
Artificial emulsifiers	Substances that stabilize an emulsion, in particular a food additive used to stabilize processed foods. Examples include: mono- and diglycerides, soy lecithin.
Artificial flavors	Found in many packaged foods and pre-prepared dishes. Artificial flavors are chemical mixtures that mimic a natural flavor, and can be made of hundreds of different chemical (or ester) combinations.
Benzoate preservatives (e.g., BHT, BHA, TBHQ)	Preservatives found in cereals, chewing gum, potato chips, etc. Affect the neurological system, alter behavior, and have the potential to cause cancer.
High-fructose corn syrup (HFCS)	Found in condiments such as ketchup, salad dressings, and processed foods such as frosting. HFCS is a major contributor to diabetes and weight gain. Causes massive insulin spikes.

using reusable bags for produce, and using aluminum foil rather than plastic wrap.

Next look under your sink at the cleaning products. As we discussed in chapter 5, cleaning products can be some of the most toxic products in your

Ingredient	Where Found and Adverse Effects
Monosodium glutamate (MSG)	An amino acid used to enhance flavor in soups, salad dressings, chips, frozen entrées, and restaurant foods. Causes cell damage or death, headaches, vision issues, fatigue, and more.
Natural flavors	Found in many packaged foods, even those in health food stores. May include beef and dairy by-products and MSG. Foods labeled "natural" are not subject to government controls.
Partially hydrogenated oils, trans fats, refined vegetable oils	Used to enhance and extend the shelf life of food products and are among the most dangerous substances you can consume. Found in chips, fried foods, packaged foods, crackers, etc. Cause increased risk for heart disease, interfere with hormone balance, cause weight gain, inflammation, and more.
Potassium bromate	An oxidizing agent used as a food additive, mainly in breadmaking. It is carcinogenic and has neurodisruptive effects.
Sodium benzoate	A type of preservative commonly used in fruit pies, jams, beverages, and condiments. When combined with vitamin C and heated, it is a known carcinogen.
Sodium nitrate and sodum nitrites	Used as a preservative and flavoring in bacon, ham, hot dogs, luncheon meats, and other processed meats. These are highly carcinogenic once they enter the human digestive system.
Sugar / cane sugar / cane juice / any added sweetener	Found in processed foods, fruit juices, pastries, protein bars, condiments, etc. Foods that have any type of added sugar are major contributors to weight gain, diabetes, cancer, heart disease, and more.

home. Ingredients including DEA, TEA, and 1,4-dioxane in cleaners contribute to cancer and hormone disruption. Most household cleaning needs can be met safely and inexpensively with a sturdy scrubber sponge and simple ingredients like water, liquid castile soap (such as Dr. Bronner's), vinegar, lemon juice, essential oils, and baking soda for scrubbing grease and grime. At least look for products that indicate that they are plant-based and biodegradable.

Your pots and pans are next. Nonstick surfaces and metal pans (such as aluminum pans) coated with a synthetic polymer called polytetrafluoro-etheylene (PTFE, also known as Teflon) are highly toxic. Toxic fumes from the chemicals released from these pots and pans at high temperatures are associated with smaller birth weight and size in newborn babies, elevated cholesterol levels, abnormal thyroid hormone levels, liver inflammation, and weakened immune defense against disease. We suggest using cast iron or stainless steel cookware.

Your drinking and cooking water is important to assess. Over one hundred chemicals have been identified in public drinking water, including antibiotics, other antimicrobials, estrogenic steroids, antidepressants, calcium channel blockers, chemotherapy drugs, and more. We suggest a point-of-use-activated carbon filter system or reverse osmosis for the home. One should be used on showerheads as well. Also, most plastic water bottles contain BPA, so switch to steel or glass. Test your well water annually for heavy metals and minerals.

Having the right kitchen appliances and gadgets will make cooking and prep that much easier. Kitchen gadgets we suggest include:

- Food processor (for mixing, grating, slicing, and shredding)
- High-powered blender (such as a Vitamix or Ninja; basically a juicer that will keep the pulp for extra fiber and with which you can make nut milks, nut butters, and more)
- Dehydrator (great for making nut-and-seed granola and breads and drying surplus vegetables)
- Crock-Pot (makes cooking dinner a breeze; just throw ingredients in and by dinner soup is ready!)
- Recycling and compost setup (For the sake of our planet, please make space in your kitchen, garage, or storage area to sort glass, cans, plastic, and paper. Many cities will pick these items up for you. A small compost bin on the kitchen counter can be used to collect organic produce scraps, coffee grounds, organic teas, eggshells, and can enhance the nutrient density of the produce items you grow in your garden.)

Stocking Your Fridge, Freezer, and Pantry

When you hit the grocery store, the key is to stock up on fresh and frozen organic vegetables, low-sugar fruit, and fresh herbs. These foods should make up the majority of your diet and the contents of your fridge. Ideally you will stock the fridge with cruciferous vegetables (broccoli, brussels sprouts, cabbage), dark leafy greens (kale, spinach, collards), onions (garlic, leeks, chives), and other vegetable families. Organic berries and green apples are great low-glycemic fruits. What's next on the list are organic, grass-fed meats, wild fish, pastured chicken and eggs, game meats, preservative-free shellfish, and nitrate-free organic bacon and sausage. Pre-prepared bone broths are great to have on hand and can be fresh or frozen.

Fermented foods and clean condiments (including sauerkraut; kimchi; pickles; gluten-free, sugar-free, preservative-free, and organic mustards, ketchup, salsas, and berry jams; coconut aminos; olives; Paleo mayo; horseradish; capers; and sun-dried tomatoes) are all great staples to have on board. Nuts, seeds, and their associated flours, milks, and oils should also be kept stocked. Extra nuts and seeds should be stored in glass jars in the freezer to preserve freshness. Pecans, walnuts, macadamia nuts, Brazil nuts, almonds, chia seeds, and flaxseeds are all great to have on hand. Olive, coconut, avocado, and MCT oils make fast, easy, and low-sugar salad dressings when combined with apple cider vinegar, chopped garlic, and herbs. Healthy beverages to keep stocked include sparkling water in glass containers, homemade iced green tea, kombucha, homemade kefir, and homemade nut milks with added herbs, such as turmeric.

In your pantry, stock canned full-fat coconut milk (without carrageenan), sustainably harvested tuna and sardines, sugar-free pasta sauce (glass jars are best), and olives. Dried herbs, mushrooms, spices, and teas are also important to have at home. The spice cabinet is the most healing part of the home. Dried teas, basil, oregano, turmeric, cumin, curry, coriander, bay leaves, thyme, rosemary, cinnamon, nutmeg, cayenne, tarragon, and others are the flavors you'll need! (Refill your bottles and buy in bulk to save money.) Crucial baking supplies include: baking soda, vanilla, cocoa nibs, nut flours, and shredded coconut. Sea vegetables include nori, wakame, arame, and seaweed snacks. These make great additions to soups. As you can see, there are so many low-glycemic and ketogenic-diet-friendly foods to bring into your house! So now that you are cleaned out and stocked with a nutrient-dense food supply, let's summarize the principles for following the most effective and potent anticancer diet ever developed.

Summary of Principles of the Metabolic Approach and Diet

Within each chapter we have discussed many foods to incorporate into your diet and many to avoid. The key recommendation running through most of the chapters is to implement a *low-glycemic, ketogenic-type diet that also incorporates intermittent fasting*. There is so much therapeutic benefit obtained from not eating. But for starters, the number one secret to success when you change your diet is to focus on the foods you *should* be eating, not the ones that you should avoid. That mind-set will only set you up to feel deprived, left out, and uninspired with your new diet. Rather, we want you to think of yourself as an ambassador for your health and an inspiration to others. You've learned about a powerful new therapy that can prevent or help manage cancer: food. Remember, there is no one-size-fits-all anticancer diet anymore. Each individual has a unique genetic code, a different cancer, and a different terrain. This is what makes our approach unparalleled.

There are three core principles to following this approach: low-glycemic; high-quality; and seasonal, diverse, and phytonutrient-dense foods. Since getting off sugar is akin to coming off a drug, we spend some extra time on it in our three-tiered approach for those who need to take things step by step. So roll up your sleeves and get started. Here is what you need to focus on.

A Tiered Approach to Starting a Low-Glycemic Diet

The number one priority for this approach is to remove from your diet all sources of sugar and carbohydrates, aside from vegetables and low-sugar fruits. We always recommend following a ketogenic diet for those with active cancer to help halt the process. (Refer back to chapter 4 for more details on diving into the ketogenic diet.) Meanwhile, for those who need to take things step by step, or for those who feel overwhelmed—we have created a three-tiered process that leads comfortably toward the ketogenic diet. It doesn't matter which step you are ready to take first to reduce the amount of sugar and starch in your diet—every bite matters.

The first tier involves cutting the "whites"—white sugar and white flour (which should be a step adopted by everyone, no matter what).

The second tier involves removing gluten-containing grains because of the major negative impact they have on blood sugar, our genes, the immune system, inflammation, and mood balance. Not to mention that eating two pieces of whole wheat bread is equivalent to eating 2 tablespoons of sugar.[1]

The third tier removes all grains, legumes, and other high-starch foods and replaces them with vegetables. This is the tier that gets people into a low-glycemic, plant-dense, therapeutic, and Paleo way of eating. This is a great place to land for those in remission, those with early-stage cancers, and those looking to prevent the occurrence of cancer. It's how Dr. Nasha and Jess advocate eating to everyone, and how they themselves eat. Look through these three tiers to determine which is the best starting point for you, or if you are ready to dive into the ketogenic diet.

Tier 1: Kicking the Whites

If you are just starting out with diet changes, have been eating a standard American diet, have a blood sugar disorder, or feel like you have low motivation and willpower for diet changes, then this is your zone. If removing things from your diet feels too restrictive, then we suggest first integrating the "crowd-out method" where you increasingly eat more vegetables (which will already make a positive impact on your terrain) while eliminating space for less healthy foods. You can revisit the sugar monster later, but always remember: Nothing is impossible. In this first tier, Jess has folks start out by tracking their sugar intake for three days—no diet change required. Read all labels and keep a running tally of how much sugar you eat and drink in a day. This includes sugar in your coffee and fruit.

Once you have a baseline for how much sugar you are eating, begin to decrease the amount by 10–20 percent every three to seven days. So if you are eating 150 grams of sugar a day, within seven days you want it down to 120 grams. Eventually, you want your sugar intake to be 20–40 grams a day or lower. By slowly decreasing the amount of sugar you may avoid the unpleasant effects of carbohydrate withdrawal, which can include fatigue, headaches, irritability, and other unpleasant symptoms. Once you get through the withdrawal period, which can last three weeks or more, you won't really miss sugar. Yes, really. We've heard it from patients over and over again. Your taste buds will change, and things that used to taste good will seem way too sweet to eat. Start by avoiding anything that contains white flour and white sugar (such as candy, cake, cookies, ice cream, and soda). Here are a few more tips for kicking the sugar habit:

Don't keep sugar-laden foods at home. Just like alcoholics cannot keep alcohol in the house, you cannot keep sugar in the house. The temptation is too great. Only keep enough for one serving. If guests bring sugar-rich foods over for a party, make sure they leave with them.

Remove corn from your diet. Since so much of the sugar in processed food comes from a corn base it's best to avoid corn as well. We've worked with people who are coming off sugar who report eating whole cans of corn, but were unsure where that craving came from. Chances are that if you've been eating a lot of sugar you are probably also allergic to corn.

Protein, protein, and more protein. Protein helps keep blood sugar levels stable thereby reducing cravings. Protein also helps to form the enzymes we need for digestion and gut healing as well as neurotransmitters such as serotonin. Eggs for breakfast are great, or—for those who are sensitive to eggs—do as they do in Eastern countries and have bone broth and kimchi for breakfast. If that sounds a little too extreme, think about meat and vegetables for breakfast, or a nut-and-seed granola (recipe at the end of this chapter).

Tier 2: Remove Gluten-Containing Grains

After you feel like you are really on top of Tier 1 and ready to integrate more sugar-lowering changes into your diet, then you are ready for Tier 2. The important thing to remember here is that this is not a "diet" in the traditional

TABLE 13.2. TIER 1 FOOD SUBSTITUTES

High-Sugar Food	Tasty Substitute
Coffee drinks with syrups, creamers, and/or sugars	Organic coffee with full-fat canned coconut milk (carrageenan free), vanilla extract, and a pinch of cinnamon
Doughnut or pastry	Almond-flour muffins or coconut-flour pancakes
Candy bar	Strawberries with sweetened cocoa nibs and coconut whipped cream
Ice cream	Smoothie with unsweetened almond milk, berries, Brazil nuts, ice, monk fruit sweetener, and whey protein powder

Note: In addition, we recommend reading *The Blood Sugar Solution*, by Dr. Mark Hyman, and *Nourishing Traditions*, by Sally Fallon.

sense of the word. You are making these changes forever, so you want to set yourself up for success, and for sustainability. Often people ask how long they have to stay gluten and sugar free. The answer is *forever*. So don't move on to Tier 2 until you feel like you are ready.

Now that you have learned how to look out for sugar, the next step is addressing the amount of carbohydrates in the form of grains in your diet, especially gluten-containing grains. Gluten-free diets are not fad diets, and consumption of modern wheat is incredibly destructive to our terrain, as you have discovered throughout this book.

The Dos and Don'ts of a Gluten-Free Diet

Getting started can seem overwhelming. People will say, "But gluten is in *everything*!" We can assure you that gluten is *not* in everything, as evidenced earlier in the shopping in this chapter. For starters, take a grocery store tour. Many health food stores offer store tours where you can learn about (and sample!) many gluten-free foods. Next, it's important to start cooking. This is the centerpiece to making diet changes. Learning how to cook will make it easier to follow the diet. Consider taking a cooking class or hiring a personal chef who can show you some basics. Then, calling on your awareness is important: Identify times of day, social situations, and specific comfort foods where you crave gluten-containing foods and replace those with new habits and routines. Reprogram.

Keep your mind-set away from deprivation and more toward abundance, health, and creativity. Communicate that you are gluten free because you *want* to be, not because you *have* to be. It's a health choice, much like exercising or eating organically. Let this be an opportunity for you to become an educator, not a victim, and welcome to an exciting new world of food! When you shop, read the labels on everything! Gluten can be found in many unexpected places (like in mustard, soy sauce, and processed meats). If you are unsure of an ingredient, contact the food manufacturer to confirm if a product you like is gluten-free or not.

Now for the don'ts, which, for newcomers to this approach, means *don't skip meals*. When blood sugar levels drop, cravings for high-carbohydrate foods increase. Think about eating six small meals a day when starting out. Next, don't assume that because it's gluten-free it's healthy. There are many, many sugary, processed, GMO gluten-free foods out there. Finally, don't become overwhelmed or afraid of food. There are hundreds of things to eat that don't contain gluten. Fruits, vegetables, meats, fish, nuts, and seeds are *all* gluten free!

Eating Out

For most people starting out with diet changes, knowing what to order when eating out can seem overwhelming, but don't despair. If all else fails, have a snack before eating out and enjoy some tea and a mini fast while enjoying the company of your friends and family. You don't have to eat to enjoy time with others, and connecting with other people as opposed to isolating yourself will help your terrain! The first step to eating out is getting to know what ingredients are likely to contain hidden gluten (many sauces, soy sauce, or anything that's breaded, for example) and not ordering those. We also suggest looking at the menu online ahead and calling the restaurant around 4 p.m. (if you are going out to dinner, that's before people have arrived and you're likely to get a manager who can confirm what can be made free of gluten).

Explain your dietary needs before you order and ask the waiter to check with the chef whether something contains gluten or how it is prepared. (Many times one of us has asked the waiter something like if there is a dedicated fryer

TABLE 13.3. TIER 2 FOOD SUBSTITUTES

Gluten-Containing Food	Tasty Substitute
Cereal or oatmeal	Nut-and-seed granola (recipe later in the chapter)
Bagel or toast	Coconut- or almond-flour tortillas (try the Siete brand) or nori wraps
Pizza	Pizza crusts can be made using nut and seed flours and even cauliflower and cheese! We also like mini pizzas made on eggplant crusts.
Pasta	Try spaghetti squash or zucchini as noodles or think about adding sweet potatoes or pumpkin instead.

Note: In addition to this list, we recommend reading *Wheat Belly*, by Dr. William Davis, and *Grain Brain*, by Dr. David Perlmutter.

for french fries and they insist there is, only to discover that there is not when they actually check with the kitchen.) Speak to the manager before you order if it seems your waiter doesn't quite get it. Then, have confidence. Don't be afraid to ask for modifications to your selections. For example, ask for rice, polenta, potatoes, or a vegetable instead of pasta or couscous. It's hard, but try not to feel embarrassed or high-maintenance when requesting your food be gluten free. Your waiter doesn't have to sit in the chemo chair, you do. So speak up.

Tier 3: Paleo-Type, Low-Glycemic, and Nutrient-Dense

The jump from Tier 2 to Tier 3 means moving from a modern diet to a diet more genetically in line with our ancestry and our genetics. It removes all foods that have been introduced since the advent of agriculture. This phase is where we really start to see therapeutic benefits—not just for cancer, but for all chronic illnesses. Here we take out all grains, both gluten containing and gluten free, as well as all beans (lentils, chickpeas, black beans), all refined sugar, dairy, and all processed foods in general. This is a whole food, plant-based diet that includes quality proteins and healthy fats. This is the diet we try to get all our patients eating and then move to a ketogenic diet if they don't completely respond here.

This phase is very rich in vegetables. In fact, we recommend at least ten different types of vegetables *every* day, including at least two dark leafy greens like spinach or kale, two cruciferous vegetables like broccoli and cabbage, two servings of garlic, onions, or shallots, two servings of mushrooms, one fermented vegetable, and one other that can include dark berries, eggplant, artichoke, bell peppers, asparagus, tomatoes, and so forth. The key thing to note about Tier 3 is that the only form of carbohydrate comes from vegetables or low-glycemic fruit, such as berries, bitter melon, and green apples.

This phase of the diet is also very high in fiber. Most people will lose weight on this diet. While this may alarm family members, you now know that there is a big difference between dangerous metabolic weight loss (cachexia) and therapeutic weight loss. There are some phenomenal cookbooks out there that can help get you started, including the *21-Day Sugar Detox*, by Diane Sanfilippo, and *Good Morning Paleo*, by Jane Barthelemy. There are lots of tricks and tips for getting started on a Paleo-type diet. First off, the key is to get creative with vegetables: Cauliflower makes great rice; spaghetti squash and zucchini make amazing noodles. Vegetables should be the main event. Salad is the base for proteins. Dip artichoke leaves in a meat and liver sauce. And speaking of sauce, that is where the secret is. Fish and vegetables can seem plain after a while, but zesting things up with a dill sauce or a red wine mushroom sauce makes dishes come to life. We encourage people to think about different cuisines, such as tacos on a cabbage leaf, lasagna layered with summer squash, or an Asian stir-fry with sprouts. It's also worth noting that having ethnic variety adds diverse flavor profiles to your dishes to prevent burnout.

Start going to farmers markets and growing your own vegetables to get the freshest and most flavorful and most nutrient-dense varieties. When children grow their own vegetables they are much more likely to eat them, not to mention it's a wonderful outdoor family activity. Next, if you are not following an autoimmune diet, try cooking with nut flours. You can make muffins, breads, pancakes, and all sorts of baked goods using almond, hazelnut, chestnut, sunflower, and coconut flours. Nuts and seeds also make great crusts for fish and chicken dishes. When making nut- or seed-flour baked goods, experiment with natural, low-glycemic sweeteners such as fresh stevia leaf, monk fruit sweetener, chicory root, green applesauce, or local or manuka honey. Desserts are for special occasions like holidays and birthdays, and these sweeteners are low in sugar and full of taste, with even a bit of therapeutic benefit.

Once people spend some time here in Tier 3 land, making the switch to a ketogenic diet is often not so daunting. It involves paring down vegetables to get daily carbohydrate intake somewhere close to 20 grams or less, while increasing fats to close to 120 grams in some cases. (Refer back to chapter 4 for more information.)

When it comes to managing cancer, the most therapeutic diet is a ketogenic one. We have explained in just about every terrain chapter how a ketogenic diet acts to: lower blood sugar, improve immune function, decrease inflammation, decrease metastases, and reset circadian patterns. Our hope is that now you have the tools and motivation to get started.

Focus on Food Quality

The second core principle to taking a metabolic approach to cancer is to start choosing organic, sustainably raised (biodynamic) plants, animals, and animal by-products. Yes, we know that making the switch to organic may seem expensive. Between 1985 and 2000 the price of fruits and vegetables doubled and fish increased 30 percent, while sugars and sweets decreased by 25 percent and soda became 66 percent cheaper. It is horrifying how subsidies have made broccoli more expensive than a Dr Pepper! Nevertheless, what we tell people is that it sometimes takes looking at your budget and asking yourself questions like, "Which is more important, medicinal foods or new clothes every month?" It can necessitate a review of your priorities (oddly, it is sometimes the most well-off people who have a hard time spending more money on food). Just as a reference point, however, Jess spends more money per month on groceries than on her mortgage.

As we've discussed throughout this book, conventionally raised animals are too toxic to eat. They are fed hormones, antibiotics, and genetically modified diets that increase their content of inflammatory omega-6 fatty acids. Not the best choice. Looking for 100 percent pasture-raised and wild-caught animals, or hunting your own, is how we suggest finding animal products. Animal by-products such as eggs and raw cheeses (if dairy is a part of your program) should come from those same animals. (Remember that if your ferritin levels are high, you want to avoid red meat. Your bio-individualized diet might differ in many ways from someone else's. It depends on your particular genetics and lab studies.)

We know that eating vegetables and low-glycemic fruit helps prevent cancer. Over two hundred epidemiological studies have found a consistent association between the low consumption of fruits and vegetables and cancer. When key micro- and phytonutrients are not present in the diet, DNA repair and immune functioning are impaired. Yet we also know that exposure to the pesticides used in the growing of these plants causes cancer. In 2012, the American Academy of Pediatrics issued a statement urging children to reduce exposure to pesticides because of substantial increased risk of brain tumors and acute lymphocytic leukemia, reduction in IQ, and abnormal behaviors associated with attention-deficit/hyperactivity disorder and autism.[2]

However, despite the documented adverse health effects of pesticides, their use has increased almost 25 percent in recent decades. An estimated one billion pounds of pesticides are applied annually to US farms, forests, lawns, gardens, and golf courses. Our continual low-dose exposure to these toxins increases the risk of genetic mutations, depletes our immune functioning, causes inflammation, and elicits an oxidative stress response in the body. Choosing organic or biodynamically raised produce items could not be more critical when it comes to the cancer crisis.

Seasonal, Diverse, Phytonutrient-Dense, and Properly Prepared

Think about changing your diet with the seasons. This is beneficial from both a preventive and a reharmonizing standpoint. Start by visiting your local farmers market to see what foods are abundant in your area. As the bumper sticker says, "Know your farmer, know your food." In summer think about focusing on fish, eggs, vegetables, and fruit. In fall, eat red meat (it's hunting season) and poultry, along with herbs and cruciferous vegetables that are still growing in the garden. Winter is ketogenic and fasting time. This can be challenging for many people during the holidays with the cravings for sweet foods, but eating sweets is the opposite of what we should be doing! We highly encourage you to start new family traditions that are not steeped in sugar. In spring, it's time for renewal, and focusing on bitter greens to support the body's purging of the fatty foods of the winter can also help detoxify the body.

You may have noticed that there were several foods that were mentioned in just about every chapter as having the most powerful terrain actions: onions, garlic, turmeric, wild fish, mushrooms, green tea, broccoli, parsley, and dark leafy greens. (Try to have these every day.) As you get into the groove of eating seasonally, know that the micro- and phytonutrient content of all these foods is higher when they are in season. Also, many benefits of these foods are negated if they are cooked to high temperatures. We never bake over 300°F and also never sauté using high heat.

Now we will summarize each chapter and provide a corresponding recipe for you so that you can start improving your terrain with the most powerful natural medicine there is: food. To create these recipes, we incorporated foods from other chapters to make incredibly powerful, phytonutrient-dense and ketogenic-friendly recipes. Enjoy!

Epigenetics

In the first of the ten terrain chapters we talked a lot about the importance of balanced amino acids, folate, and cruciferous vegetables. These food sources are critical for many aspects of genetic health, including DNA synthesis and methylation, the epigenetic process that helps regulate healthy gene expression. Other recipes include bone broths and other sources of complete proteins, but here we have created a salad that incorporates many of the superfoods shown to affect several cancer hallmarks. Normally this Middle Eastern dish uses bulgur wheat, but since a main recommendation of this book is to get back to eating a pre-agricultural diet, we use the cruciferous vegetable cauliflower in lieu of the grain. Parsley, the starring herb in this recipe, contains the highly powerful phytonutrient apigenin. In fact, every ingredient in this recipe has been mentioned as having anticancer properties! We made this at one of our retreats and it was a huge hit.

Cauliflower Tabbouleh with Sunflower Seeds and Parsley

½ head cauliflower,
  coarsely chopped

3 tablespoons cold-pressed
  extra-virgin olive oil

1 teaspoon sea salt

2 cups flat-leaf parsley leaves,
  chopped

1 cup epazote or mint, chopped

2 scallions, sliced

2 garlic cloves, pressed and
  coarsely chopped

3 teaspoons grated lemon zest

3 tablespoons fresh lemon juice

3 tablespoons turmeric

3 tablespoons MCT oil

¼ teaspoon crushed red
  pepper flakes

1 cup cherry tomatoes,
  quartered

1 cup raw sunflower seeds

1 teaspoon black pepper

Sea salt for seasoning

Grate the cauliflower so it appears ricelike. Transfer it to a large bowl and toss with the olive oil and salt. In a food processor pulse parsley, epazote, scallions, garlic, lemon zest, lemon juice, turmeric, and MCT oil until herbs are coarsely chopped. Combine mixture with the cauliflower and stir in red pepper flakes. Add tomatoes, sunflower seeds, and black pepper and gently toss to coat. Season with sea salt if necessary.

Blood Sugar

In this chapter we focused on the details of the ketogenic diet and how to steer your body away from subsisting on glucose and toward thriving on ketones. Close to 75 percent of a ketogenic diet should come from fatty foods—oils, nuts and seeds, fatty fish, avocados, coconut, and so on. Over the years, we have found that the hardest thing for many of our cereal- and toast-loving clients seems to be finding a ketogenic breakfast option they enjoy. The solution: cinnamon keto granola. This granola is lavished with the highest fat and most phytonutrient-dense nuts and seeds, and cinnamon is added for its benefits in regulating blood sugar. This recipe can be made in bulk and it also makes a great snack to keep in the car, both of which add to the appeal of this recipe.

Jack's Cinnamon Keto Granola

¼ cup pine nuts

¼ cup pecans, chopped

¼ cup Brazil nuts,
   chopped or sliced

1 tablespoon vanilla extract

¼ cup MCT oil

3 tablespoons cinnamon

2 tablespoons fresh ground flax

Soak nuts overnight if possible, but not required. If soaked, then rinse well.

Place the pecans and Brazil nuts into a bowl and mix with MCT oil, cinnamon, and vanilla extract. Preheat oven to 285°F (140°C). Place the mixture on a baking tray and spread into a very thin layer. Bake for 35–45 minutes, stirring every 5–10 minutes until nuts are crisp. Remove from heat and mix in the pine nuts and ground flax (freshly ground in a coffee grinder)—both of which oxidize in any type of heat. Let cool and enjoy with some coconut cream and a few blueberries.

Toxins

In chapter 5, we spoke about the power of fasting and sauna for detoxifying the body of carcinogens. Several other foods and herbs were highlighted for their detoxifying abilities, including milk thistle and dandelion greens. When we talked about how phase 1 and 2 detox work, the importance of protein also was illuminated. This recipe uses a light fish bone broth as a stock to provide the protein needed by the liver and adds powerful greens and broccoli sprouts.

Spring Green Soup

2 tablespoons cold-pressed
   extra-virgin olive oil

2 shallots or small red onions, chopped

5 cups fish or organic chicken bone
   broth (visit Wise Choice Market
   website to order fish broth)

1 cup chopped dandelion greens

1 cup chopped beet greens

2 tablespoons fresh or dried thyme

1 avocado, pitted and diced

Sea salt and black pepper, to taste

½ cup broccoli sprouts

Heat the olive oil in a soup pot. Add the shallots or onions. Cook, stirring occasionally, for 5–7 minutes until soft. Add the broth. Bring to just below a boil, then reduce heat to medium-low and cook for 5 minutes. Remove from heat and stir in the greens and thyme until wilted. Allow the soup to stand, uncovered, for 10 minutes. Pour the soup into a blender, add the avocado, and puree until thick and creamy. Season the soup with salt and pepper to taste. Top with sprouts and serve.

Microbiome

As we learned in chapter 6, our microbiome is a critical element of our immune system's functioning and also influences several other aspects of our terrain. Modern diets are consistently found to be low in fiber, the best food for our microbes. This recipe is a fiber-rich microbe-friendly breakfast (or lunch with a salad).

Asparagus and Leek Frittata

1 whole medium leek, sliced

1 cup whole asparagus, chopped

4 tablespoons MCT oil

½ cup red onions

¾ cup macadamia nuts

¼ cup fresh basil leaves

1 tablespoon fresh or dried turmeric

10 eggs from pasture-raised hens

Sea salt and black pepper

Preheat oven to 300°F (150°C). Sauté the leeks and asparagus in MCT oil until soft. In a food processor, blend the onions and macadamia nuts, then pulse in fresh basil and turmeric. Gently whisk the eggs in a mixing bowl. Spread the nut mixture then the asparagus and leeks across the bottom of a well-greased 8-inch pie pan, forming a layered crust. Cover with eggs. Season with salt and pepper to taste. Bake for 45–55 minutes or until the middle doesn't jiggle. Serve with a watercress salad or fermented salsa.

Immune System

When we think of being sick, there is one dish that always comes to mind: chicken soup. Our take on it uses organic chicken bone broth alongside powerful immune-boosting mushrooms, seaweed, radishes, and garlic. Remember that fasting is also a powerful tool for the immune system—but there is no recipe for that! Sipping broth and green tea are also great immune-boosting strategies.

Mama Mia Mushroom Chicken Immune Soup

2 tablespoons coconut oil

1 shallot, chopped

12 garlic cloves, minced

2 cups medicinal mushrooms
(combination of shiitake, maitake, and lion's mane), chopped

2–3 tablespoons fresh
grated ginger

1 daikon radish, sliced thin

4 cups organic chicken bone broth

½ cup wakame seaweed

Juice and zest of 1 lemon

Heat the coconut oil in a soup pot. Add the shallots and garlic to the coconut oil, and allow to soften while you chop the mushrooms. Add mushrooms to the garlic and shallots. Sauté them gently while you chop the ginger and daikon radish. When everything has softened, 10 to 15 minutes, add the bone broth and wakame. Bring to a simmer and cook about 10 minutes more. Squeeze lemon juice and sprinkle lemon zest on top and enjoy.

Inflammation and Oxidation

A primary focus of the inflammation chapter was to learn how to balance types of fatty acids by increasing foods high in omega-3 fatty acids, such as wild fish like sardines and salmon, while reducing omega-6 fatty acids, typically in the form of vegetable oils. It has been a challenge for us to get patients to eat sardines, but when they are prepared in a salad like this they taste very similar to tuna! Adding the quercetin-rich capers helps on the anti-oxidant front, making this a very powerful—and delicious—meal.

Sardine Salad with Capers

2 4.4-oz cans wild sardines
  packed in water
¼ cup capers
2 tablespoons freshly grated or
  prepared horseradish
  (i.e. Bubbies brand, in water
  and vinegar)

¼ cup kalamata olives, diced
⅓ cup Paleo or homemade
  mayonnaise
2 tablespoons dried dill
¼ cup onion, diced
2 sheets nori or whole red
  lettuce leaves

Drain the sardines and mix all ingredients together in a mixing bowl. Serve wrapped in red lettuce or inside a nori sheet.

Angiogenesis, Circulation, and Metastasis

In chapter 9 we learned the benefits of green tea. Strive to drink several cups of it a day. This recipe is a nutritional powerhouse meal with the fusion of two highly potent anticancer foods: green tea and wild fish. Poaching salmon or chicken in green tea is commonplace throughout Asia. Coconut aminos is a tasty and gluten-free soy sauce alternative, and the toasted sesame oil gives this dish a distinctly Asian flavor. Adding cilantro and broccoli spouts provides some detoxifying elements.

Eastern Green Tea Poached Fish

6 cloves elephant garlic,
  crushed
4 slices fresh ginger
  (½ inch thick)
4 lime slices
1 teaspoon toasted sesame oil
2 tablespoons coconut aminos
2 cups slightly warm matcha
  green tea

1 tablespoon extra-virgin
  olive oil
2 4-oz. wild-caught salmon
  or halibut filets
Sea salt and black pepper
  to taste
¼ cup chopped cilantro
¼ cup chopped fresh basil
¼ cup broccoli sprouts

Add the garlic, ginger, lime, sesame oil, and aminos to the warm tea and mix gently. In a large skillet, heat the olive oil over low heat. Add the salmon and cook for about 5 minutes, or until it is beginning to soften. Flip and add the tea mixture to skillet. Reduce the heat, cover, and simmer gently for 8–10 minutes, or until the center of the salmon flakes easily. Remove the salmon from the skillet. Salt and pepper to taste. Drizzle the liquid mix over salmon and garnish with cilantro, basil, and sprouts.

Hormone Balance

As we discovered in the hormone chapter, many things contribute to estrogen dominance in both men and women, and it is a fuel for all cancers. Seed cycling is one way to help support the body's hormone balance.[3] The concept of seed cycling is the integration into the diet of different seeds during various times of the month to capitalize on the oils, vitamins, and nutrients. The seeds commonly used in this seed rotation are flaxseeds and pumpkin seeds in the first fifteen days of the month (phase 1), and sesame and sunflower seeds in the latter half of the month (phase 2).

Seed Cycle Pesto Nori Nut Wraps

PESTO, PHASE 1

⅓ cup flaxseeds

⅓ cup raw pepitas (pumpkin seeds)

2 cups loosely packed fresh basil leaves

1 cup loosely packed arugula

1 garlic clove

1 tablespoon fresh lemon juice

¼ cup olive oil

½ teaspoon sea salt

Black pepper, to taste

PESTO, PHASE 2

½ cup raw sunflower seeds

½ cup raw sesame seeds

2 cloves garlic, peel intact

2 cups packed chopped kale leaves

1 cup packed fresh basil leaves

½–1 teaspoon red pepper flakes

⅓–½ cup extra-virgin olive oil

Salt and pepper to taste

Nori sheets, for wrapping

Blend the pesto ingredients together. Scoop ¼ cup of the pesto and spread onto a nori wrap. Wrap like a burrito and enjoy!

Stress and Circadian Rhythms

Stress is a highly prevalent aspect of modern living that impacts the terrain on many levels. In addition to getting outdoor time, eating within an eight-hour window of daylight is highly beneficial. Adaptogenic herbs help support restoration of the highly overworked adrenal glands. Teas and tonics that have few to no calories, sugar, or carbohydrates are excellent things to sip during fasting days. This is one of our favorites. It's our ketogenic-diet take on the Master Cleanse, which is an unhealthy sugar blast of maple syrup. An herbal tonic is used to help restore, tone, and invigorate the HPA axis and is prepared with a selected assortment of adaptogenic herbs.

Adaptogenic Tea Tonic for Fasting

1 ounce dried ginseng

1 ounce dried rhodiola

1 ounce dried holy basil

1 ounce dried astragalus

2 tablespoons apple cider vinegar

2 teaspoons liquid bitters (found at health food stores in the digestive health section)

1 quart boiling water

Place all dried herbs into separate tea bags. Add the tea bags, the vinegar, and the bitters into the pot of boiling water, taking care not to let the tea bags break or spill. Let steep overnight. Remove the bags of herbs and pour into a glass container and refrigerate. Sip as desired for 36 hours.

Mental and Emotional Well-Being

We all want something sweet from time to time; it's human nature. But moderation is key. Cocoa, the magical elixir that produces chocolate, has many anticancer actions, including acting as a powerful antioxidant. If you are craving something sweet, a small slice of this does the trick. Adding spice to chocolate gives it a wonderful anti-angiogenic kick, too, and lavender contains essential oils (linalool and linalyl) that encourage the natural release of tension. A flavor explosion and also low in sugar!

Chocolate Chili Lavender Cake

⅔ cup granulated monk
   fruit sweetener
8 drops lavender essential oil
½ teaspoon ground cayenne pepper
½ teaspoon cinnamon
½ teaspoon gelatin powder

10 ounces coconut oil,
   plus additional for coating
   the pan
1½ cups cocoa powder
8 eggs from pastured hens
Pinch of sea salt

Heat oven to 285°F (140°C). Mix all the ingredients together in a food processor. Coat an 8-inch pie pan with coconut oil and transfer the mixture into the pan. Bake for 45 minutes or until the filling doesn't jiggle. Remove from oven, let cool slightly, and slice. Top with fresh berries or whipped coconut cream.

Acknowledgments

We want to wish every one of our readers the best of luck on their healing journey. There are over thirty collective years of experience and research that went into this book both to help prevent cancer and to improve the quality of life with it. We are thrilled by the possibilities the new field of oncology nutrition therapy has to offer. Thank you for reading, and thank you to all the people who have supported and encouraged us on this journey.

From Jess: I would like to thank my husband, Dave, for all the help creating the time, space, and encouragement needed to write this book. It would not be possible without you. I'd also like to thank my family (Susan, Abey, Sean, Brooke, Tom, Kit, and Jim) and friends for your support even if some of you weren't sure exactly what *metabolic* or *ketogenic* meant. Makenna, thanks for being an incredible editor and book doula; it was a painful and beautiful birthing experience and you made it happen! I am forever grateful to my dear old dad who passed away while this book was being written and to whom it is dedicated. There are no words to describe the experience of writing a book about cancer while at the bedside of someone you love who is dying from it. Thank you for showing me what it means to stay motivated and positive in the face of a dismal diagnosis.

Nasha, thank you for all your years of experience, wisdom, and dedication to cultivating this terrain-based approach. I will forever admire your courage to speak the truth, your incredible intelligence, and the support and motivation you gave me to keep writing while in the throes of my father's dying and death process. I also have so much gratitude for the researchers who have dedicated time to exploring the role food plays in health. Please, please keep going. To all my clients who have implemented these metabolic approaches: Every remission brings me much hope and affirmation. Finally, thanks to my daughter, Pepper. I know I missed many nights putting you to sleep, many Saturdays playing, but I did this for you. Thank you for giving me a reason to try to make the world a cancer-free place for you and the next generations.

From Dr. Nasha: It is difficult to acknowledge just a handful of people who have contributed to my life and the writing of this book in a significant way. I do not exaggerate when I say that every human experience touches me and imprints on me in some way. I thrive in community. I am touched by acts of kindness. I feel that a smile, the simplest of gestures, can change one's day. I have an uncanny ability to remember faces, even years later—a checker at a grocery store, a person on an airplane, a fellow attendee at a conference. If we had even a brush of eye contact or communication, I take a little piece of that experience with me. Even the challenging moments as they mirror back some form of me. That being said, there are clearly moments in my life where someone has changed the trajectory and offered me a new path. Those paths may not have been clear-cut or easy—some of those paths required me to do a *lot* of bushwhacking! But man, did they offer up their own healing, self-exploration, deeper connection, and inspiration to keep trekking.

To my beloved redheaded warrior, Steve Ottersberg. What twenty-two-year-old man would decide to fall in love with a woman with one foot out of this world? I thank you for doing so and for always having my back; you know this story better than anyone, as you have lived it with me for over twenty-five years. To Louise Edwards, my mentor, who carries the flame of naturopathic medicine in every cell of her body and who was my safe haven in the years when medical school tried to smolder that flame out of me, I am forever grateful. Thank you to so many amazing healers, teachers, and mentors in the field of medicine who feed my brain and inspire my lifelong-learner tendencies like no other. To my patients both—those who are thriving and those who have launched their next adventure—I am overwhelmed with gratitude for the years we have shared, for your stories I hold sacred, for the amazing things you have taught me, and for the gift to be part of your world in some of the most intimate moments of your lives. To my dear friends who have watched over me for years, worried I would burn out my own candle with all the passion and fire I contain—your ability to root me, nourish me, laugh and cry with me, sustains that passion. To my mom who someday may actually take some of my advice☺, for raising me to be a fierce woman who does not shy away from being the outlier—always. And finally, to Cancer, for without you, I would not be writing this book. Embarking on this path of learning has convinced me to continually explore my own Terrain Ten issues to keep them in check so I may live a long, vital, optimal-health life.

Blessings everyone!

NASHA AND JESS
Durango, Colorado
Janaury 2017

Resources

Recommended Doctors and Clinics
Supporting Terrain-Centric Integrative Oncology Care

These resources offer more endorsements, recommendations, referrals, and resources that are in alignment with the integrative oncology model.

FON (Force of Nature) Consulting: list of doctors and clinics trained in integrative oncology care. fonconsulting.com

Nutrition Therapy Institute. www.ntischool.com

Ojai Cares. ojaicares.org

Oncology Association of Naturopathic Physicians (OncANP). www.oncanp.org

Optimal Terrain Consulting: list of preferred providers that have completed mistletoe training. optimalterrainconsulting.com

Physicians' Association for Anthroposophic Medicine: list of doctors and clinics trained in integrative care. paam.wildapricot.org

Remission Nutrition. www.remissionnutrition.com

Society for Integrative Oncology (SIO). integrativeonc.org

Wallace, Jeanne. www.nutritional-solutions.net

Organizations Promoting Terrain-Centric Integrative Oncology Care

4Wholeness: integrative oncology care in breast cancer. www.4wholeness.com

American Academy of Environmental Medicine. www.aaemonline.org

American Association of Naturopathic Physicians (AANP). www.naturopathic.org

American Holistic Medical Association (AHMA). www.holisticmedicine.org

The Angiogenesis Foundation: cancer-fighting foods based on the work of Dr. William Li. www.angio.org

The Annie Appleseed Project. annieappleseedproject.org

Believe Big: Christian organization with a list of doctors using mistletoe therapy. www.BelieveBig.org

Commonweal. www.commonweal.org

Environmental Working Group (EWG). www.ewg.org

FON (Force of Nature) Consulting. fonconsulting.com

Healing Journeys: a resource for cancer patients. www.healingjourneys.com

International Academy of Biological Dentistry and Medicine (IABDM). iabdm.org

International Academy of Oral Medicine and Toxicology (IAOMT). iaomt.org

International Organization of Integrative Cancer Physicians (IOICP). www.ioicp.com

iTHRIVE Plan. www.iThrivePlan.com

Life Extension. "Innovative Doctors and Health Practitioners."
    health.lifeextension.com/innovativedoctors
Oncology Association of Naturopathic Physicians (OncANP).
    naturopathic physicians specializing in integrative oncology. www.oncanp.org
The Organic Center. "Publication Archive." www.organic-center.org/scientific-resources
    /publication-archive
Price Pottenger. price-pottenger.org
Society for Integrative Oncology (SIO). integrativeonc.org
The Weston A. Price Foundation (WAPF). www.westonaprice.org

Food Resources

Bulletproof Coffee: coffee and other nutrient-dense foods and supplements. www.bulletproof.com
Cali'Flour Foods: premade keto friendly pizza crusts. www.califlourfoods.com
Dry Farm Wines: great wine club resource that sources organic, biodynamic, low-sulfite,
    low-sugar wines from around the world; coined the "keto-friendly" wine company.
    www.dryfarmwines.com
Eat Wild: Jo Robinson's comparisons of nutritional density in foods today, and offering
    better options. www.eatwild.com/products/index.html
Hunter Gatherer Foods: pili nuts—the perfect keto snack. www.eatpilinuts.com
Local Harvest: directory of farmers markets, family farms, and resources nationwide.
    www.localharvest.org
Thrive Market: online resource delivering organic, healthy foods to your door at a
    discounted price. thrivemarket.com
US Wellness Meats: a wonderful resource for organic, grass-fed, and grass-finished meat,
    poultry, and dairy products along with bone broths and other healthy foods able to ship
    nationwide; also a wonderful newsletter and resources to educate on food politics and
    food as medicine. grasslandbeef.com
USDA National Farmers' Market Directory: up-to-date list of farmers markets around the
    United States that highlight local, regional, seasonal, and organic foods. www.ams
    .usda.gov/local-food-directories/farmersmarkets
Wise Choice Market: great resource providing nationwide delivery of real food such as bone
    broths; raw, cultured vegetables; and wild seafood. www.wisechoicemarket.com

Recommended Books and Journals about Integrative Oncology Care

JOURNALS

Cancer Defeated. www.cancerdefeated.com
Cancer Strategies Journal. cancerstrategiesjournal.com
Naturopathic Doctor News and Review (NDNR). ndnr.com
Natural Medicine Journal. www.naturalmedicinejournal.com
Townsend Letter: The Examiner of Alternative Medicine. www.townsendletter.com

BOOKS

*The 30-Day Ketogenic Cleanse: Reset Your Metabolism with 160 Tasty Whole-Food Recipes and
    Fitness Plans* by Maria Emmerich (Victory Belt Publishing, 2016)

Anticancer: A New Way of Life by David Servan-Schreiber (Viking Press, 2009)

Beating Cancer with Nutrition: Clinically Proven and Easy-to-Follow Strategies to Dramatically Improve Quality and Quantity of Life and Changes for a Complete Remission by Patrick Quillin and Noreen Quillin (Nutrition Times Press, 1998)

Beyond the Magic Bullet: The Anti-Cancer Cocktail by Raymond Chang, MD (Square One Publishers, 2012)

The Big Fat Surprise: Why Butter, Meat, and Cheese Belong in a Healthy Diet by Nina Teicholz (Simon & Schuster, 2014)

Cancer as a Metabolic Disease: On the Origin, Management, and Prevention of Cancer by Thomas Seyfried (Wiley, 2012)

Cancer as a Turning Point: A Handbook for People with Cancer, Their Families, and Health Professionals by Lawrence LeShan (Dutton, 1989)

Cancer Free! Are You Sure? by Jenny Hrbacek (New Voice Publications, 2015)

The Cantin Ketogenic Diet: For Cancer, Type I Diabetes, and Other Ailments by Elaine Cantin (Elaine Cantin, 2012)

The Case against Sugar by Gary Taubes (Knopf, 2016)

The Complete Guide to Fasting: Heal Your Body through Intermittent, Alternate-Day, and Extended Fasting by Dr. Jason Fung and Jimmy Moore (Victory Belt Publishing, 2016)

Death by Food Pyramid: How Shoddy Science, Sketchy Politics, and Shady Special Interests Have Ruined Our Health by Denise Minger (Primal Blueprint Publishing, 2013)

Deep Nutrition: Why Your Genes Need Traditional Food by Catherine Shanahan (Flatiron Books, 2017)

Defeat Cancer: 15 Doctors of Integrative and Naturopathic Medicine Tell You How by Connie Strasheim (BioMed Publishing Group, 2011)

The Definitive Guide to Cancer: An Integrative Approach to Prevention, Treatment, and Healing by Lise Alschuler and Karolyn Gazella (Celestial Arts, 2010)

The Definitive Guide to Thriving after Cancer: A Five-Step Integrative Plan to Reduce the Risk of Recurrence and Build Lifelong Health by Lise Alschuler and Karolyn Gazella (Ten Speed Press, 2013)

Dying to Be Me: My Journey from Cancer, to Near Death, to True Healing by Anita Moorjani (Hay House, 2012)

Eating on the Wild Side: The Missing Link to Optimum Health by Jo Robinson (Little, Brown and Company, 2013)

Embrace, Release, Heal: An Empowering Guide to Thinking about, Talking about, and Treating Cancer by Leigh Fortson (Sounds True, 2011)

The Emperor of All Maladies: A Biography of Cancer by Siddhartha Mukherjee (Scribner, 2010)

Fat Chance: Beating the Odds against Sugar, Processed Food, Obesity, and Disease by Robert Lustig (Hudson Street Press, 2013)

Fat for Fuel: A Revolutionary Diet to Combat Cancer, Boost Brain Power, and Increase Your Energy by Dr. Joseph Mercola (Hay House, Inc., 2017)

Fight Cancer with a Ketogenic Diet: Using a Low-Carb, Fat-Burning Diet as Metabolic Therapy by Ellen Davis, MS (Gutsy Badger Publishing, 2017)

Five to Thrive: Your Cutting-Edge Cancer Prevention Plan by Lise Alschuler and Karolyn Gazella (Active Interest Media)

Folks, This Ain't Normal: A Farmer's Advice for Happier Hens, Healthier People, and a Better World by Joel Salatin (Center Street, 2011)

The Gene: An Intimate History by Siddhartha Mukherjee (Scribner, 2016). Really, all of
   Siddhartha Mukherjee's books.
Healing Spices: How to Use 50 Everyday and Exotic Spices to Boost Health and Beat Disease
   by Bharat Aggarwal (Sterling Publications, 2011)
Honest Medicine: Effective, Time-Tested, Inexpensive Treatments for Life-Threatening Diseases,
   Including Multiple Sclerosis, Epilepsy, Liver Disease, Lupus, Rheumatoid Arthritis, and Other
   Diseases by Julia Schopick (Innovative Health Publications, 2011)
The Journey through Cancer: Healing and Transforming the Whole Person by Jeremy Geffen
   (Three Rivers Press, 2006)
Keto Clarity: Your Definitive Guide to the Benefits of a Low-Carb, High-Fat Diet by Jimmy Moore
   with Eric C. Westman, MD (Victory Belt Publishing, 2014)
Keto for Cancer: The Ketogenic Diet as a Targeted Nutritional Strategy by Miriam Kalamian
   (Chelsea Green Publishing, 2017)
Ketogenic Diet and Metabolic Therapies: Expanded Roles in Health and Disease edited by Susan A.
   Masino (Oxford University Press, 2016)
The Ketogenic Kitchen: Low Carb. High Fat. Extraordinary Health by Domini Kemp and Patricia
   Daly (Chelsea Green Publishing, 2016)
Knockout: Interviews with Doctors Who Are Curing Cancer—And How to Prevent Getting It in the
   First Place by Suzanne Somers (Crown Publishers, 2009)
Life over Cancer: The Block Center Program for Integrative Cancer Treatment by Keith Block
   (Bantam Dell, 2009)
Lights Out: Sleep, Sugar, and Survival by T. S. Wiley (Pocket Books, 2000)
Living Downstream: An Ecologist Looks at Cancer and the Environment by Sandra Steingraber
   (Addison-Wesley Publishing, 1997)
Naturopathic Oncology: An Encyclopedic Guide for Patients and Physicians, 3rd ed, by Neil
   McKinney (Creative Guy Publishing, 2010)
Nourishing Traditions: The Cookbook That Challenges Politically Correct Nutrition and the Diet
   Dictocrats by Sally Fallon (New Trends Publications, 2001)
Outliving Cancer: The Better, Smarter Way to Treat Your Cancer by Robert Nagourney (Basic
   Health Publications, 2013)
Pottenger's Prophecy: How Food Resets Genes for Wellness or Illness by Gray Graham, Deborah
   Kesten, and Larry Scherwitz (White River Press, 2010)
Questioning Chemotherapy by Ralph Moss (Equinox Press, 1995)
Radical Remission: Surviving Cancer against All Odds by Kelly Turner (Harper One, 2014)
The Secret History of the War on Cancer by Devra Davis (Basic Books, 2009)
Textbook of Naturopathic Integrative Oncology by Dr. Jody E. Noé, MS, ND (CCNM Press, 2011)
Tripping over the Truth: How the Metabolic Theory of Cancer Is Overturning One of Medicine's
   Most Entrenched Paradigms by Travis Christofferson (Chelsea Green Publishing, 2017)
The Wild Wisdom of Weeds: 13 Essential Plants for Human Survival by Katrina Blair (Chelsea
   Green Publishing, 2014)

TEDTalks and Documentaries about Terrain-Centric Integrative Oncology

"Can We Eat to Starve Cancer?" by William Li (February 2010). *TEDTalks*: angiogenesis.
   www.ted.com/talks/william_li

The Connection: documentary on the connection of mind and body. theconnection.tv

"The Dangers of Willful Blindness" by Margaret Heffernan (March 2013). *TEDTalks*: about wanting to find the answers, but when you do, you don't want to change in order to deal with the findings. www.ted.com/talks/margaret_heffernan_the_dangers_of _willful_blindness

"Experiments That Point to a New Understanding of Cancer" by Mina Bissell (June 2012). *TEDTalks*: extracellular matrix. www.ted.com/talks/mina_bissell_experiments_that _point_to_a_new_understanding_of_cancer

"Meet the Future of Cancer Research" by Eva Verte (February 2005). *TEDTalks*. www.ted .com/talks/eva_vertes_looks_to_the_future_of_medicine

"Minding Your Mitochondria" by Terry Wahl (July 13, 2015). *TedTalks*: MD who cured herself of multiple sclerosis through diet. terrywahls.com/tedxiowacity-minding -your-mitochondria-with-dr-terry-wahls

"A New Strategy in the War on Cancer" by David Agus (October 2009). *TEDTalks*: how we are focusing on the wrong thing: the cancer cells instead of the terrain. www.ted.com /talks/david_agus_a_new_strategy_in_the_war_on_cancer

Websites, Blogs, and Additional Media Outlets about Integrative Oncology News and Research

Cancer Free University: Jenny Hrbacek's new website where she interviews thought leaders in Integrative Oncology. www.CancerFreeUniversity.com

Cancer Wellness TV: a patient resource for integrative cancer support. www.cwellness.com

Elaine Cantin: ketogenic coach; resource site. www.elainecantin.com

Dominic D'Agostino: researcher in all things ketogenic. www.ketonutrition.org

Ellen Davis: ketogenic resource site. www.ketogenic-diet-resource.com

dminder: app for tracking sun exposure and getting recommendations on exposure for optimal health. dminder.ontometrics.com

Elite HRV (Heart Rate Variability): instant biofeedback about how diet, lifestyle, stress, exercise, sleep, and more impact you and your health. www.elitehrv.com

Alison Gannett: ketogenic coach. www.alisongannett.com

Green Med Info: references on natural medicine. www.greenmedinfo.com

Heart Math: great mindfulness-based app. www.heartmath.com

Miriam Kalamian: ketogenic coach. www.dietarytherapies.com

Klose Training: lymphedema certification. klosetraining.com

LDN Research Trust: great research resource on application of low-dose naltrexone, along with other integrative therapies. www.ldnresearchtrust.org

MyFitnessPal: tool for measuring your actual macronutrient intake; helps folks assess the truth about what they are eating daily. www.myfitnesspal.com

Noteable Labs: tissue assay testing to choose more appropriate and individualized treatment. www.notablelabs.com

Oncology Rehab: lymphedema support. www.oncologyrehab.net

Radical Remission Project: workshops, website, and blog. www.radicalremission.com

Science Daily: huge resource for research coming out daily; option to focus on the oncology and cancer articles. www.sciencedaily.com

Notes

Introduction: The Cancer Crisis

1. Akulapalli Sudhakar, "History of Cancer, Ancient and Modern Treatment Methods," *Journal of Cancer Science and Therapy* 1, no. 2 (December 1, 2009): 1–4, doi:10.4172 /1948-5956.100000e2.

2. N. Howlader et al., eds., "SEER Cancer Statistics Review, 1975–2011," National Cancer Institute, Bethesda, MD, last updated December 17, 2014, http://seer.cancer.gov/csr /1975_2011. Based on November 2013 SEER data.

3. M. C. King, J. H. Marks, and J. B. Mandell, "Breast and Ovarian Cancer Risks Due to Inherited Mutations in BRCA1 and BRCA2," *Science* 302, no. 5645 (October 24, 2003): 643–46, doi:10.1126/science.1088759.

4. J. J. Mangano, "A Rise in the Incidence of Childhood Cancer in the United States," *International Journal of Health Services* 29, no. 2 (1999): 393–408, https://www.ncbi.nlm .nih.gov/pubmed/10379458.

5. Melissa Jenco, "AAP Responds to Study Showing Link between Cell Phone Radiation, Tumors in Rats," *AAP News*, May 27, 2016, http://www.aappublications.org/news/2016 /05/27/Cancer052716.

6. Dave Levitan, "Adolescent / Young Adult Cancer Survivors Have Significantly Increased CVD Risk," *Cancer Network*, March 10, 2016, http://www.cancernetwork.com/cancer -complications/adolescent-young-adult-cancer-survivors-have-significantly-increased -cvd-risk.

7. Preetha Anand, Ajaikumar B. Kunnumakara, Chitra Sundaram, Kuzhuvelil B. Hariku-mar, Sheeja T. Tharakan, Oiki S. Lai, Bokyung Sung, and Bharat B. Aggarwal, "Cancer Is a Preventable Disease That Requires Major Lifestyle Changes," *Pharmaceutical Research* 25, no. 9 (September 2008): 2097–116, doi:10.1007/s11095-008-9661-9.

8. Neil McKinney, *Naturopathic Oncology: An Encyclopedic Guide for Patients and Physicians* (Victoria, Canada: Liaison Press, 2016).

9. Douglas Hanahan and Robert A. Weinberg, "Hallmarks of Cancer: The Next Genera-tion," *Cell* 144, no. 5 (March 4, 2011): 646–74, doi:10.1016/j.cell.2011.02.013.

10. Timothy J. Key, Arthur Schatzkin, Walter C. Willett, Naomi E. Allen, Elizabeth A. Spencer, and Rith C. Travis, "Diet, Nutrition and the Prevention of Cancer," *Public Health Nutrition* 7, no. 1A (February 2004): 187–200, doi:10.1079/PHN2003588.

11. Mei-Sing Ong and Kenneth D. Mandi, "New Guidelines for Breast Cancer Screening," *Health Affairs* 35, no. 1 (January 2016): 180, doi:10.1377/hlthaff.2015.1513.

12. "Developments in Cancer Treatments, Market Dynamics, Patient Access and Value: Global Oncology Trend Report 2015," QuintilesIMS Institute, http://www.imshealth.com /en/thought-leadership/quintilesims-institute/reports/global-oncology-trend-2015.

13. K. Robin Yabroff, Emily C. Dowling, Gery P. Guy, Matthew P. Banegas, Amy Davidoff, Xuesong Han, Katherine S. Virgo, et al., "Financial Hardship Associated with Cancer in the United States: Findings from a Population-Based Sample of Adult Cancer Survivors," *Journal of Clinical Oncology* 34, no. 3 (January 20, 2016): 259–67, doi:10.1200/JCO.2015.62.0468.

14. "FDA News Release: FDA Commissioner Announces Avastin Decision," US Food and Drug Administration, November 18, 2011, last updated March 12, 2014, http://www.fda .gov/NewsEvents/Newsroom/PressAnnouncements/ucm280536.htm.

15. Vishal Ranpura, Sanjaykumar Hapani, and Shenhong Wu, "Treatment-Related Mortality with Bevacizumab in Cancer Patients," *JAMA* 305, no. 5 (February 3, 2011): 487–94, doi:10.1001/jama.2011.51.

16. "Nutrition for the Person with Cancer during Treatment," *American Cancer Society*, accessed November 20, 2016. https://www.cancer.org/treatment/survivorship -during-and-after-treatment/staying-active/nutrition/nutrition-during-treatment.html.

Chapter 1: The Solution Is a Metabolic Approach

1. Bharat B.Aggarwal and Shishir Shishodia, "Molecular Targets of Dietary Agents for Prevention and Therapy of Cancer," *Biochemical Pharmacology* 71, no. 10 (May 14, 2006): 1397–421, doi:10.1016/j.bcp.2006.02.009.

2. Keith I. Block, Charlotte Gyllenhaal, Leroy Lowe, Amedeo Amedei, A. R. M. Ruhul Amin, Amr Amin, Katia Aquilano, et al., "Designing a Broad-Spectrum Integrative Approach for Cancer Prevention and Treatment," *Seminars in Cancer Biology* 35, supplement (December 2015): s276–304, doi:10.1016/j.semcancer.2015.09.007.

3. Song Wu, Scott Powers, Wei Zhu, and Yusuf A. Hannun, "Substantial Contribution of Extrinsic Risk Factors to Cancer Development," *Nature* 529, no. 7584 (January 7, 2016): 43–47, doi:10.1038/nature16166.

4. Soroush Niknamian, Vahid Hosseini Djenab, Sora Niknamian, and Mina Nazari Kamal, "The Prime Cause, Prevention and Treatment of Cancer," *International Science and Investigation Journal* 5, no. 5 (December 2016): 102–24, http://isijournal.info/journals /index.php/ISIJ/article/view/246.

Chapter 3: Genetics, Epigenetics, and Nutrigenomics

1. D. P. Labbé , G. Zadra, E. M. Ebot, L. A. Mucci, P. W. Kantoff, M. Loda, and M. Brown, "Role of Diet in Prostate Cancer: The Epigenetic Link," *Oncogene* 34, no. 36 (September 3, 2015): 4683–91, doi:10.1038/onc.2014.422.

2. Preetha Anand, Ajaikumar B. Kunnumakara, Chitra Sundaram, Kuzhuvelil B. Harikumar, Sheeja T. Tharakan, Oiki S. Lai, Bokyung Sung, and Bharat B. Aggarwal, "Cancer Is a Preventable Disease That Requires Major Lifestyle Changes," *Pharmaceutical Research* 25, no. 9 (September 2008): 2097–116, doi:10.1007/s11095-008-9661-9; Thomas N. Seyfried, Roberto E. Flores, Angela M. Poff, and Dominic P. D'Agostino, "Cancer as a Metabolic Disease: Implications for Novel Therapeutics," *Carcinogenesis* 35, no. 3 (December 2013): 515–27, doi:10.1093/carcin/bgt480.

3. Gordana Supic, Maja Jagodic, and Zvonko Magic, "Epigenetics: A New Link between Nutrition and Cancer," *Nutrition and Cancer* 65, no. 6 (August 2, 2013): 781–92, doi:10.1080 /01635581.2013.805794.

4. NIH, "What Are Single Nucleotide Polymorphisms (SNPs)?" Genetics Home Reference, https://ghr.nlm.nih.gov/primer/genomicresearch/snp.

5. Mojgan Hosseini, Massoud Houshmand, and Ahmad Ebrahimi, "MTHFR Polymorphisms and Breast Cancer Risk," *Archives of Medical Science* 7, no. 1 (February 2011): 134–37, doi:10.5114/aoms.2011.20618.

6. Hannah Landecker, "Food as Exposure: Nutritional Epigenetics and the New Metabolism," *Biosocieties* 6, no. 2 (June 2011): 167–94, doi:10.1057/biosoc.2011.1.

7. Cindy D. Davis and Eric O. Uthus, "DNA Methylation, Cancer Susceptibility, and Nutrient Interactions," *Experimental Biology and Medicine* 229 (November 2004): 988–95, http://journals.sagepub.com/doi/abs/10.1177/153537020422901002.

8. Maddalena Rossi, Alberto Amaretti, and Stefano Raimondi, "Folate Production by Probiotic Bacteria," *Nutrients* 3, no.1 (January 2011): 118–34, doi:10.3390/nu3010118.

9. D. P. Bezerra, J. F. Marinho Filho, A. P. Alves, C. Pessoa, M. O. de Moraes, O. D. Pessoa, M. C. Torres, E. R. Silveira, F. A. Viana, and L. V. Costa-Lotufo, "Antitumor Activity of the Essential Oil from the Leaves of *Croton regelianus* and Its Component Ascaridole," *Chemistry and Biodiversity* 6, no. 8 (August 2009): 1224–31, doi:10.1002/cbdv.200800253.

10. Edith Perez and Joanne Mortimer, *Journal of Clinical Oncology* 32, no. 30 (October 20, 2014).

11. Benjamin F. Voight, Sridhar Kudaravalli, Xiaoquan Wen, and Jonathan K. Pritchard, "A Map of Recent Positive Selection in the Human Genome," *PLOS Biology* 4, no. 3 (March 7, 2006): 446–58, doi:10.1371/journal.pbio.0040072.

12. Daniel Lieberma, *The Story of the Human Body: Evolution, Health, and Disease* (New York: Pantheon Books, 2013).

13. Jared M. Diamond, *Guns, Germs, and Steel* (New York: Spark Publications, 2003).

14. The Norwegian University of Science and Technology (NTNU), "Feed Your Genes: How Our Genes Respond to the Foods We Eat," *ScienceDaily*, September 20, 2011, http://www.sciencedaily.com/releases/2011/09/110919073845.htm.

15. Angela Harras, *Cancer Rates and Risks*, 4th ed. (Washington, DC: National Institutes of Health, 1996), NIH Publication no. 96-691.

16. Patrick J. Stover, "Influence of Human Genetic Variation on Nutritional Requirements," *American Journal of Clinical Nutrition* 83, no. 2, supplement (February 2006): 436s–42.

17. M. Lorenzi, D. F. Montisano, S. Toledo, A. Barrieux, "High Glucose Induces DNA Damage in Cultured Human Endothelial Cells," *Journal of Clinical Investigation* 77, no. 1 (January 1986): 322–25, doi:10.1172/JCI112295.

18. Haibo Liu and Anthony P. Heaney, "Refined Fructose and Cancer," *Expert Opinion on Therapeutic Targets* 15, no. 9 (September 2011): 1049–59, doi:10.1517/14728222.2011.588208; Eiji Furuta, Hiroshi Okuda, Aya Kobayashi, and Kounosuke Watabe, "Metabolic Genes in Cancer: Their Roles in Tumor Progression and Clinical Implications," *Biochimica et biophysica acta (BBA)* 1805, no. 2 (April 2010): 141–52, doi:10.1016/j.bbcan.2010.01.005.

19. Ali M.Ardekani and Sepideh Jabbari, "Nutrigenomics and Cancer," *Avicenna Journal of Medical Biotechnology* 1, no. 1 (April–June 2009): 9–17, http://www.ncbi.nlm.nih.gov/pmc/articles/PMC3558114.

20. Gray Graham, Deborah Kesten, and Larry Scherwitz, *Pottenger's Prophecy: How Food Resets Genes for Wellness or Illness* (Amherst, MA: White River Press, 2011).

21. Gijs A. Kleter, Ad A. C. M. Peijnenburg, and Henk J. M. Aarts, "Health Considerations Regarding Horizontal Transfer of Microbial Transgenes Present in Genetically Modified Crops," *Journal of Biomedicine and Biotechnology* 2005, no. 4 (2005): 326–52, doi:10.1155/jbb.2005.326.

22. "New Cancer Cases Rise Globally, but Death Rates Are Declining in Many Countries," Institute for Health Metrics and Evaluation, accessed November 3, 2016, http://www.healthdata.org/news-release/new-cancer-cases-rise-globally-death-rates-are-declining-many-countries.

23. Anthony Samsel and Stephanie Seneff, "Glyphosate, Pathways to Modern Diseases II: Celiac Sprue and Gluten Intolerance," *Interdisciplinary Toxicology* 6, no. 4 (December 2013): 159–84, doi:10.2478/intox-2013-0026.

24. Leah Schinasi and Maria E. Leon, "Non-Hodgkin Lymphoma and Occupational Exposure to Agricultural Pesticide Chemical Groups and Active Ingredients: A Systematic Review and Meta-Analysis," *International Journal of Environmental Research and Public Health* 11, no.4 (April 23, 2014): 4449–527, doi:10.3390/ijerph110404449.

25. Sándor Spisák, Norbert Solymosi, Péter Ittzés, András Bodor, Dániel Kondor, Gábor Vattay, Barbara K. Barták, et al., "Complete Genes May Pass from Food to Human Blood," *PLOS ONE* 8, no. 7 (July 30, 2013): e69805, doi:10.1371/journal.pone.0069805.

26. Chris D. Meletis and Kimberly Wilkes, "Mitochondria: Overlooking These Small Organelles Can Have Huge Clinical Consequences in Treating Virtually Every Disease," *Townsend Letter*, June 2015, http://www.townsendletter.com/June2015/mito0615.html.

27. "GM Crops List," International Service for the Acquisition of Agri-Biotech Applications, accessed November 3, 2016, http://www.isaaa.org/gmapprovaldatabase/cropslist.

28. Kelsey L. Tinkum, Kristina M. Stemler, Lynn S. White, Andrew J. Loza, Sabrina Jeter-Jones, Basia M. Michalski, Catherine Kuzmicki, et al., "Fasting Protects Mice from Lethal DNA Damage by Promoting Small Intestinal Epithelial Stem Cell Survival," *Proceedings of the National Academy of Sciences of the United States of America* 112, no. 51 (December 22, 2015): e7148–54, doi:10.1073/pnas.1509249112.

29. Michael T. Murray, *How to Prevent and Treat Cancer with Natural Medicine* (New York: Riverhead Books, 2002).

30. Kumar S. D. Kothapalli, Kaixiong Ye, Maithili S. Gadgil, Susan E. Carlson, Kimberly O. O'Brien, Ji Yao Zhang, Hui Gyu Park, et al., "Positive Selection on a Regulatory Insertion-Deletion Polymorphism in FADS2 Influences Apparent Endogenous Synthesis of Arachidonic Acid," *Molecular Biology and Evolution* 33, no. 7 (July 2016): 1726–39, doi:10.1093/molbev/msw049.

31. Rima Obeid, "The Metabolic Burden of Methyl Donor Deficiency with Focus on the Betaine Homocysteine Methyltransferase Pathway," *Nutrients* 5, no. 9 (September 9, 2013): 3481–95, doi:10.3390/nu5093481.

32. Stuart A. S. Craig, "Betaine in Human Nutrition," *American Journal of Clinical Nutrition* 80, no. 3 (September 2004): 539–49, http://ajcn.nutrition.org/content/80/3/539.full.

33. H. Pellanda, "Betaine Homocysteine Methyltransferase (BHMT)–Dependent Remethylation Pathway in Human Healthy and Tumoral Liver," *Clinical Chemistry and Laboratory Medicine* 51, no. 3 (March 1, 2013): 617–21, doi:10.1515/cclm-2012-0689.

34. Ana Lúcia Vargas Arigony, Iuri Marques de Oliveira, Miriana Machado, Diana Lilian Bordin, Lothar Bergter, Daniel Prá, and João Antonio Pêgas Henriques, "The Influence

of Micronutrients in Cell Culture: A Reflection on Viability and Genomic Stability," *BioMed Research International* 2013 (May 2013): 1–22, doi:10.1155/2013/597282.

35. Keith Block, C. Gyllenhaal, L. Lowe, A. Amedei, A. R. Amin, A. Amin, K. Aquillano, et al., "Designing a Broad-Spectrum Integrative Approach for Cancer Prevention and Treatment." *Seminars in Cancer Biology 35*, supplement (December 2015): s276–304, doi:10.1016/j.semcancer.2015.09.007.

36. Avinash M. Topè and Phyllis F. Rogers, "Evaluation of Protective Effects of Sulforaphane on DNA Damage Caused by Exposure to Low Levels of Pesticide Mixture Using Comet Assay," *Journal of Environmental Science and Health, Part B* 44, no. 7 (September 4, 2009): 657–62, doi:10.1080/03601230903163624.

37. Yolanda Lorenzo, Aamia Azqueta, Luisa Luna, Félix Bonilla, Gemma Dominguez, and Andrew R. Collins, "The Carotenoid β-Cryptoxanthin Stimulates the Repair of DNA Oxidation Damage in Addition to Acting as an Antioxidant in Human Cells," *Carcinogenesis* 30, no. 2 (December 4, 2008): 308–14, doi:10.1093/carcin/bgn270.

38. Pesticide Action Network, "Sweet Bell Peppers," What's on My Food?, accessed November 3, 2016, http://whatsonmyfood.org/food.jsp?food=PP.

Chapter 4: Sugar, Cancer, and the Ketogenic Diet

1. Lise Alschuler and Karolyn A. Gazella, *The Definitive Guide to Cancer: An Integrative Approach to Prevention, Treatment, and Healing* (New York: Celestial Arts, 2010).

2. Wanxing Duan, Xin Shen, Jianjun Lei, Quinhong Xu, Yongtian Yu, Rong Li, Erxi Wu, and Qingyong Ma, "Hyperglycemia, a Neglected Factor during Cancer Progression," *BioMed Research International* 2014, no. 4176 (February 2014): 1–10, doi:10.1155/2014/461917.

3. Joseph E. Pizzorno and Michael T. Murray, *Textbook of Natural Medicine* (St. Louis, MO: Churchill Livingstone Elsevier, 2006).

4. Rachel K. Johnson, Lawrence J. Appel, Michael Brands, Barbara V. Howard, Michael Lefevre, Robert H. Lustig, Frank Sacks, et al., "Dietary Sugars Intake and Cardiovascular Health: A Scientific Statement from the American Heart Association," *Circulation* 120, no. 11 (August 24, 2009): 1011–20, doi:10.1161/CIRCULATIONAHA.109.192627.

5. George A. Bray, Samara Joy Nielsen, and Barry M. Popkin, "Consumption of High-Fructose Corn Syrup in Beverages May Play a Role in the Epidemic of Obesity," *American Journal of Clinical Nutrition* 79, no. 4 (April 2004): 537–43, http://ajcn.nutrition.org/content/79/4/537.abstract.

6. Zhong Q. Wang, Aamir R. Zuberi, Xian H. Zhang, Jacalyn Macgowan, Jianhua Qin, Xin Ye, Leslie Son, Qinglin Wu, Kun Lian, and William T. Cefalu, "Effects of Dietary Fibers on Weight Gain, Carbohydrate Metabolism, and Gastric Ghrelin Gene Expression in Mice Fed a High-Fat Diet," *Metabolism* 56, no. 12 (December 2007): 1635–42, doi:10.1016/j.metabol.2007.07.004.

7. NIH, "Lactose Intolerance," *Genetics Home Reference*, accessed November 20, 2016, https://ghr.nlm.nih.gov/condition/lactose-intolerance.

8. Susanna Larsson, Leif Bergkvist, and Alicja Wolk, "Milk and Lactose Intakes and Ovarian Cancer Risk in the Swedish Mammography Cohort," *American Journal of Clicnical Nutrition* 80, no. 5 (November 2004): 1353–57, http://ajcn.nutrition.org/content/80/5/1353.full.

9. Andrew Curry, "Archaeology: The Milk Revolution," *Nature* 500, no. 7460 (July 31, 2013): 20–22, doi:10.1038/500020a.

10. Kei Nakajima, Tohru Nemoto, Toshitaka Muneyuki, Masafumi Kakei, Hiroshi Fuchigami, and Hiromi Munakata, "Low Serum Amylase in Association with Metabolic Syndrome and Diabetes: A Community-Based Study," *Cardiovascular Diabetology* 10 (April 17, 2011): 34, doi:10.1186/1475-2840-10-34.

11. Pinna Rolfes and Whitney Rolfes, *Understanding Normal and Clinical Nutrition* (Brooks Cole, 2011).

12. NIH, "Overweight and Obesity Statistics," US Department of Health and Human Services, accessed January 12, 2017, https://www.niddk.nih.gov/health-information /health-statistics/Documents/stat904z.pdf.

13. Edward Giovannucci, David M. Harlan, Michael C. Archer, Richard M. Bergenstal, Susan M. Gapstur, Laurel A. Habel, Michael Pollak, Judith G. Regensteiner, and Douglas Yee, "Diabetes and Cancer: A Consensus Report," *Diabetes Care* 33, no. 7 (July 2010): 1674–85, doi:10.2337/dc10-0666.

14. Rainer J. Klement and Ulrike Kämmerer, "Is There a Role for Carbohydrate Restriction in the Treatment and Prevention of Cancer?" *Nutrition and Metabolism* 8 (2011): 75, doi:10.1186/1743-7075-8-75.

15. Yasuhito Onodera, Jin-Min Nam, and Mina J. Bissell, "Increased Sugar Uptake Promotes Oncogenesis via EPAC/RAP1 and O-GlcNAc Pathways," *Journal of Clinical Investigation* 124, no. 1 (January 2, 2014): 367–84, doi:10.1172/jci63146.

16. Yong Wu, Joy Lin, Landon G. Piluso, and Xuan Liu, "High Glucose Inhibits p53 Function via Thr55 Phosphorylation," *FASEB Journal* 24, no. 1, supplement 503.5 (April 2010), http://www.fasebj.org/content/24/1_Supplement/503.5.abstract.

17. S. A. Bustin and P. J. Jenkins, "The Growth Hormone-Insulin-Like Growth Factor-I Axis and Colorectal Cancer," *Trends in Molecular Medicine* 7, no. 10 (October 2001): 447–54, doi:10.1016/S1471-4914(01)02104-9.

18. Surendra K. Shukla, Teklab Gebregiworgis, Vinee Purohit, Nina V. Chaika, Venugopal Gunda, Prakash Radhakrishnan, Kamiya Mehla, et al., "Metabolic Reprogramming Induced by Ketone Bodies Diminishes Pancreatic Cancer Cachexia," *Cancer and Metabolism* 2 (September 1, 2014): 18, doi:10.1186/2049-3002-2-18.

19. Neil McKinney, *Naturopathic Oncology: An Encyclopedic Guide for Patients and Physicians* (Richmond, BC: Creative Guy Publishing, 2010).

20. Ibid.

21. Wei-Xing Zong, Joshua D. Rabinowitz, and Eileen White, "Mitochondria and Cancer," *Molecular Cell* 61, no. 5 (March 3, 2016): 667–76, doi:10.1016/j.molcel.2016.02.011.

22. Charles W. Schmidt, "Unraveling Environmental Effects on Mitochondria," *Environmental Health Perspectives* 118, no. 7 (July 2010): A292–97, http://www.ncbi.nlm.nih.gov/pmc /articles/PMC2920932.

23. Susana Romero-Garcia, María Maximina B. Moreno-Altamirano, Heriberto Prado-Garcia, and Francisco Javier Sánchez-García, "Lactate Contribution to the Tumor Microenvironment: Mechanisms, Effects on Immune Cells and Therapeutic Relevance," *Frontiers in Immunology* 7 (February 16, 2016): 52, doi:10.3389 /fimmu.2016.00052.

24. Thomas N. Seyfried, Roberto E. Flores, Angela M. Poff, and Dominic P. D'Agostino, "Cancer as a Metabolic Disease: Implications for Novel Therapeutics," *Carcinogenesis* 35, no. 3 (December 2013): 515–27, doi:10.1093/carcin/bgt480.

25. Bryan G. Allen, Sudershan K. Bhatia, Carryn M. Anderson, Julie M. Eichenberger-Gilmore, Zita A. Sibenaller, Kranti A. Mapuskar, Joshua D. Schoenfeld, John M. Buatti, Douglas R. Spitz, and Melissa A. Fath, "Ketogenic Diets as an Adjuvant Cancer Therapy: History and Potential Mechanism," *Redox Biology* 2 (August 7, 2014): 963–70, doi:10.1016/j.redox.2014.08.002.

26. Stephen D. Hursting, Sarah M. Dunlap, Nikki A. Ford, Marcie J. Hursting, and Laura M. Lashinger, "Calorie Restriction and Cancer Prevention: A Mechanistic Perspective," *Cancer and Metabolism* 1 (March 7, 2013): 10, doi:10.1186/2049-3002-1-10.

Chapter 5: Carcinogens, Cancer, and Detoxification

1. Anne Platt McGinn, "POPs Culture," *World Watch Magazine* 13, no. 2 (March/April 2000), http://www.worldwatch.org/node/485.

2. Xiaomei Ma, Patricia A. Buffler, Robert B. Gunier, Gary Dahl, Martyn T. Smith, Kyndaron Reinier, and Peggy Reynolds, "Critical Windows of Exposure to Household Pesticides and Risk of Childhood Leukemia," *Environmental Health Perspectives* 110, no. 9 (September 2002): 955–60, https://www.ncbi.nlm.nih.gov/pmc/articles/PMC1240997.

3. Michael T. Murray and Joseph E. Pizzorno, *Encyclopedia of Natural Medicine* (Rocklin, CA: Prima Publishing, 1998).

4. Ellen K. Silbergeld, Daniele Mandrioli, and Carl F. Cranor, "Regulating Chemicals: Law, Science, and the Unbearable Burdens of Regulation," *Annual Review of Public Health* 36 (March 2015): 175–195, doi:10.1146/annurev-publhealth-031914-122654.

5. M. T. Smith, K. Z. Guyton, C. F. Gibbons, J. M. Fritz, C. J. Portier, I. Rusyn, D. M. DeMarini, et al., "Key Characteristics of Carcinogens as a Basis for Organizing Data on Mechanisms of Carcinogens," *Environmental Health Perspectives* 124, no. 6 (June 2016): 713–21, doi:10.1289/ehp.1509912.

6. Sharon Ruth Skolnick, "Exposing Airports' Poison Circles," *Earth Island Journal* 15, no. 4 (Winter 2000–2001), http://www.areco.org/ExpAir.pdf.

7. Maria E. Morales, Revecca S. Derbes, Catherine M. Ade, Jonathan C. Ortego, Jeremy Stark, Prescott L. Deininger, and Astrid M. Roy-Engel, "Heavy Metal Exposure Influences Double Strand Break DNA Repair Outcomes," *PLOS ONE* 11, no. 3 (March 11, 2016): e0151367, doi:10.1371/journal.pone.0151367.

8. "Casings," FAO Corporate Document Repository, accessed November 21, 2016, http://www.fao.org/docrep/010/ai407e/AI407E20.htm.

9. Gary D. Friedman, Natalia Udaltsova, James Chan, Charles P. Quesenberry, and Laurel A. Habel, "Screening Pharmaceuticals for Possible Carcinogenic Effects: Initial Positive Results for Drugs Not Previously Screened," *Cancer Causes and Control* 20, no. 10 (December 2009): 1821–35, doi:10.1007/s10552-009-9375-2.

10. John Neustadt and Steve R. Pieczenik, "Medication-Induced Mitochondrial Damage and Disease," *Molecular Nutrition and Food Research* 52, no. 7 (July 2008): 780–88, doi:10.1002/mnfr.200700075.

11. Henry Delincée and Beatrice-Louise Pool-Zobel, "Genotoxic Properties of 2-Dodecyl-cyclobutanone, a Compound Formed on Irradiation of Food Containing Fat," *Radiation Physics and Chemistry* 52, no. 1 (June 1998): 39–42, doi:10.1016/S0969-806X(98)00070-X.

12. Mathieu Boniol, Philippe Autier, Peter Boyle, and Sara Gandini, "Cutaneous Melanoma Attributable to Sunbed Use: Systematic Review and Meta-Analysis," *BMJ* 345 (July 24, 2012): e4757, doi:10.1136/bmj.e4757.

13. William E. Sumner, Leonidas G. Koniaris, Sarah E. Snell, Seth Spector, Jodeen Powell, Eli Avisar, Frederick Moffat, Alan S. Livingstone, and Dido Franceschi, "Results of 23,810 Cases of Ductal Carcinoma-in-Situ," *Annals of Surgical Oncology* 14, no. 5 (May 2007): 1638–43, doi:10.1245/s10434-006-9316-1.

14. Joseph E. Pizzorno, and Michael T. Murray, *Textbook of Natural Medicine* (St. Louis, MO: Churchill Livingstone Elsevier, 2006).

15. John C. Cline, "Nutritional Aspects of Detoxification in Clinical Practice," *Alternative Therapies in Health and Medicine*, May/June 2015, https://issuu.com/presspad/docs/i14004.

16. Katrina Blair, *The Wild Wisdom of Weeds: 13 Essential Plants for Human Survival* (White River Junction, VT: Chelsea Green Publishing, 2014).

17. Vasil Georgiev Georgiev, Jost Weber, Eva-Maria Kneschke, Petko Nedyalkov Denev, Thomas Bley, and Atanas Ivanov Pavlov, "Antioxidant Activity and Phenolic Content of Betalain Extracts from Intact Plants and Hairy Root Cultures of the Red Beetroot *Beta vulgaris* cv. Detroit Dark Red," *Plant Foods for Human Nutrition* 65, no. 2 (June 2010): 105–11, doi:10.1007/s11130-010-0156-6.

18. M. N. Gould, "Cancer Chemoprevention and Therapy by Monoterpenes," *Environmental Health Perspectives* 105, supplement 4 (June 1997): 977–79, http://www.ncbi.nlm.nih.gov/pmc/articles/PMC1470060.

19. Emey Suhana Mohd Azamai, Suhaniza Sulaiman, Shafina Hanim Mohd Habib, Mee Lee Looi, Srijit Das, Nor Aini Abdul Hamid, Wan Zurinah Wan Ngah, and Yasmin Anum Mohd Yusof, "*Chlorella vulgaris* Triggers Apoptosis in Hepatocarcinogenesis-Induced Rats," *Journal of Zhejiang University Science B*, 10, no. 1 (January 2009): 14–21, doi:10.1631/jzus.B0820168.

20. Patricia A. Egner, Jin-Bing Wang, Yuan-Rong Zhu, Bau-Chu Zhang, Yan Wu, Qi-Nan Zhang, Geng-Sun Qian, et al., "Chlorophyllin Intervention Reduces Aflatoxin-DNA Adducts in Individuals at High Risk for Liver Cancer," *Proceedings of the National Academy of Science of the United States of America* 98, no. 25 (December 4, 2001): 14601–6, doi:10.1073/pnas.251536898.

21. Stefania Miccadei, Donato Di Venere, Angela Cardinali, Ferdinando Romano, Alessandra Durazzo, Maria Stella Foddai, Rocco Fraioli, Sohrab Mobarhan, and Giuseppe Maiani, "Antioxidative and Apoptotic Properties of Polyphenolic Extracts from Edible Part of Artichoke (*Cynara scolymus* L.) on Cultured Rat Hepatocytes and on Human Hepatoma Cells," *Nutrition and Cancer* 60, no. 2 (March 2008): 276–83, doi:10.1080/01635580801891583.

22. Lizzia Raffaghello, Changhan Lee, Fernando M. Safdie, Min Wei, Federica Madia, Giovanna Bianchi, and Valter D. Longo, "Starvation-Dependent Differential Stress Resistance Protects Normal but Not Cancer Cells against High-Dose Chemotherapy,"

Proceedings of the National Academy of Sciences of the United States of America 105, no. 24 (June 17, 2008): 8215–20, doi:10.1073/pnas.0708100105.

23. Stephen D. Hursting, Jackie A. Lavigne, David Berrigan, Susan N. Perkins, and J. Carl Barrett, "Calorie Restriction, Aging, and Cancer Prevention: Mechanisms of Action and Applicability to Humans," *Annual Review of Medicine* 54 (February 2003): 131–52, doi:10.1146/annurev.med.54.101601.152156.

Chapter 6: The Mighty Microbiome

1. Scott J. Bultman, "Emerging Roles of the Microbiome in Cancer," *Carcinogenesis* 35, no. 2 (February 2014): 249–55, doi:10.1093/carcin/bgt392.

2. Fredrik Bäckhed, Ruth E. Ley, Justin L. Sonnenburg, Daniel A. Peterson, and Jeffery I. Gordon, "Host-Bacterial Mutualism in the Human Intestine," *Science* 307, no. 5717 (March 25, 2005): 1915–20, doi:10.1126/science.1104816.

3. Ian F. N. Hung and Benjamin C. Y. Wong, "Assessing the Risks and Benefits of Treating *Helicobacter pylori* Infection," *Therapeutic Advances in Gastroenterology* 2, no. 3 (May 2009): 141–47, doi:10.1177/1756283x08100279.

4. Tina J. Hieken, Jun Chen, Tanya L. Hoskin, Marina Walther-Antonio, Stephen Johnson, Sheri Ramaker, Jian Xiao, et al., "The Microbiome of Aseptically Collected Human Breast Tissue in Benign and Malignant Disease," *Scientific Reports* 6 (August 3, 2016): 30751, doi:10.1038/srep30751.

5. Josef Neu and Jona Rushing, "Cesarean Versus Vaginal Delivery: Long-Term Infant Outcomes and the Hygiene Hypothesis," *Clinics in Perinatology* 38, no. 2 (June 2011): 321–31, doi:10.1016/j.clp.2011.03.008.

6. Bidisha Paul, Stephen Barnes, Wendy Demark-Wahnefried, Casey Morrow, Carolina Salvador, Christine Skibola, and Trygve O. Tollefsbol, "Influences of Diet and the Gut Microbiome on Epigenetic Modulation in Cancer and Other Diseases," *Clinical Epigenetics* 7, no. 1 (October 16, 2015): 112, doi:10.1186/s13148-015-0144-7.

7. Laura B. Bindels and Jean-Paul Thissen, "Nutrition in Cancer Patients with Cachexia: A Role for the Gut Microbiota?" *Clinical Nutrition Experimental* 6 (April 2016): 74–82, doi:10.1016/j.yclnex.2015.11.001.

8. "Microbes in the Human Body," The Marshall Protocol Knowledge Base, accessed August 21, 2016, http://mpkb.org/home/pathogenesis/microbiota.

9. Maureen P. Corry, "The Cost of Having a Baby in the United States," *Childbirth Connections*, May 9, 2013, http://www.medscape.com/viewarticle/803426_2.

10. Meredith Betz, "C-Section Trends Out of Control in South Florida," *Nonprofit Quarterly*, October 12, 2015, https://nonprofitquarterly.org/2015/10/12/c-section-trends-out-of-control-in-south-florida.

11. Neu and Rushing, "Cesarean Versus Vaginal Delivery: Long-Term Infant Outcomes and the Hygiene Hypothesis."

12. Alison Stuebe, "The Risks of Not Breastfeeding for Mothers and Infants," *Reviews in Obstetrics and Gynecology* 2, no. 4 (Fall 2009): 222–31, http://www.ncbi.nlm.nih.gov/pmc/articles/PMC2812877.

13. Antonio M. Persico and Valerio Napolioni, "Urinary P-Cresol in Autism Spectrum Disorder," *Neurotoxicology and Teratology* 36 (March 2013): 82–90, doi:10.1016/j.ntt.2012.09.002.

14. Gordon E. Schutze, Rodney E. Willoughby, Michael T. Brady, Carrie L. Byington, H. Dele Davies, Kathryn M. Edwards, Mary P. Glode, et al., "Clostridium Difficile Infection in Infants and Children," *Pediatrics* 131, no. 1 (January 1, 2013): 196–200, doi:10.1542/peds.2012-2992.

15. Anthony Samsel and Stephanie Seneff, "Glyphosate, Pathways to Modern Diseases II: Celiac Sprue and Gluten Intolerance," *Interdisciplinary Toxicology* 6, no. 4 (December 2013): 159–84, doi:10.2478/intox-2013-0026.

16. Benoit Chassaing, Omry Koren, Julia K. Goodrich, Angela C. Poole, Shanthi Srinivasan, Ruth E. Ley, and Andrew T. Gewirtz, "Dietary Emulsifiers Impact the Mouse Gut Microbiota Promoting Colitis and Metabolic Syndrome," *Nature* 519, no. 7541 (March 5, 2015): 92–96, doi:10.1038/nature14232.

17. Sameer Kalghatgi, Catherine S. Spina, James C. Costello, Marc Liesa, J. Ruben Morones-Ramirez, Shimyn Slomovic, Anthony Molina, Orian S. Shirihai, and James J. Collins, "Bactericidal Antibiotics Induce Mitochondrial Dysfunction and Oxidative Damage in Mammalian Cells," *Science Translational Medicine* 5, no. 192 (July 3, 2013): 192ra85, doi:10.1126/scitranslmed.3006055.

18. Jo Robinson, *Eating on the Wild Side: The Missing Link to Optimum Health* (New York: Little, Brown and Company, 2013).

19. Surajit Karmakar, Subhasree Roy Choudhury, Naren L. Banik, and Swapan K. Ray, "Molecular Mechanisms of Anti-Cancer Action of Garlic Compounds in Neuroblastoma," *Anti-Cancer Agents in Medicinal Chemistry* 11, no. 4 (May 2011): 398–407, doi:10.2174/187152011795677553.

20. Bharat B. Aggarwal and Debora Yost, *Healing Spices: How to Use 50 Everyday and Exotic Spices to Boost Health and Beat Disease* (New York: Sterling Publishing, 2011).

21. Georgetown University Medical Center, "Oregano Oil May Protect Against Drug-Resistant Bacteria, Georgetown Researcher Finds," *ScienceDaily*, October 11, 2001, https://www.sciencedaily.com/releases/2001/10/011011065609.htm.

22. Sue C. Chao, D. Gary Young, and Craig J. Oberg, "Effect of a Diffused Essential Oil Blend on Bacterial Bioaerosols," *Journal of Essential Oil Research* 10, no. 5 (September 1998): 517–23, doi:10.1080/10412905.1998.9700958.

23. Zhanguo Gao, Jun Yin, Jin Zhang, Robert E. Ward, Roy J. Martin, Michael Lefevre, William T. Cefalu, and Jianping Ye, "Butyrate Improves Insulin Sensitivity and Increases Energy Expenditure in Mice," *Diabetes* 58, no. 7 (July 2009): 1509–17, doi:10.2337/db08-1637.

24. Sunisa Siripongvutikorn, Ruttiya Asksonthong, and Worapong Usawakesmanee, "Evaluation of Harmful Heavy Metal (Hg, Pb and Cd) Reduction Using *Halomonas elongata* and *Tetragenococcus halophilus* for Protein Hydrolysate Product," *Functional Foods in Health and Disease* 6, no. 4 (April 27, 2016): 195–205, http://ffhdj.com/index.php/ffhd/article/view/240.

25. J. Beuth, H. L. Ko, K. Oette, G. Pulverer, K. Roszkowski, and G. Uhlenbruck, "Inhibition of Liver Metastasis in Mice by Blocking Hepatocyte Lectins with Arabinogalactan Infusions and D-Galactose," *Journal of Cancer Research and Clinical Oncology* 113, no. 1 (February 1987): 51–55, doi:10.1007/BF00389966.

26. Hyunnho Cho, Hana Jung, Heejae Lee, Hae Chang Yi, Ho-kyung Kwak, and Keum Taek Hwang, "Chemopreventive Activity of Ellagitannins and Their Derivatives from Black Raspberry Seeds on HT-29 Colon Cancer Cells," *Food and Function* 6, no. 5 (May 2015): 1675–83, doi:10.1039/c5fo00274e.

Chapter 7: Immune Function

1. Adit A. Ginde, Mark C. Liu, and Carlos A. Camargo, "Demographic Differences and Trends of Vitamin D Insufficiency in the US Population, 1988–2004," *Archives of Internal Medicine* 169, no. 6 (March 23, 2009): 626–32, doi:10.1001/archinternmed.2008.604.

2. Marina Rode von Essen, Martin Kongsbak, Peter Scherling, Klaus Olgaard, Niels Ødum, and Carsten Geisler, "Vitamin D Controls T Cell Antigen Receptor Signaling and Activation of Human T Cells," *Nature Immunology* 11 (2010): 334–49, doi:10.1038/ni.1851.

3. A. Katharina Simon, Georg A. Hollander, and Andrew McMichael, "Evolution of the Immune System in Humans from Infancy to Old Age," *Proceedings of the Royal Society B: Biological Sciences* 282, no. 1821 (December 22, 2015): 20143085, doi:10.1098/rspb.2014.3085.

4. Keith Block. *Life over Cancer: The Block Center Program for Integrative Cancer Treatment* (New York: Bantam Dell, 2009).

5. Dicken Weatherby and Scott Ferguson, *Blood Chemistry and CBC Analysis: Clinical Laboratory Testing from a Functional Perspective* (Jacksonville, OR: Bear Mountain Publishing, 2002).

6. Alessio Fasano, "Zonulin, Regulation of Tight Junctions, and Autoimmune Diseases," *Annals of the New York Academy of Sciences* 1258, no. 1 (July 2012): 25–33, doi:10.1111/j.1749-6632.2012.06538.x.

7. Marco Skardelly, Franz Paul Armbruster, Jürgen Meixensberger, Heidegard Hilbig, "Expression of Zonulin, C-Kit, Glial Fibrillary Acidic Protein in Human Gliomas," *Translational Oncology* 2, no. 3 (September 2009): 117–20, doi:10.1593/tlo.09115.

8. A. Fasano, "Zonulin and Its Regulation of Intestinal Barrier Function: The Biological Door to Inflammation, Autoimmunity, and Cancer," *Physiological Reviews* 91, no. 1 (January 2011): 151–75, doi:10.1152/physrev.00003.2008.

9. Aristo Vojdani, "Lectins, Agglutinins, and Their Roles in Autoimmune Reactivities," *Alternative Therapies in Health and Medicine* 21, supplement 1 (2015): 46–51, https://www.ncbi.nlm.nih.gov/pubmed/25599185.

10. Margit Brottveit, Ann-Christin R. Beitnes, Stig Tollefsen, Jorunn E. Bratlie, Frode L. Jahnsen, Finn-Eirik Johansen, Ludvig M. Sollid, and Knut E. A. Lundin, "Mucosal Cytokine Response after Short-Term Gluten Challenge in Celiac Disease and Non-Celiac Gluten Sensitivity," *American Journal of Gastroenterology* 108, no. 5 (May 2013): 842–50, doi:10.1038/ajg.2013.91.

11. R. K. Chandra, "Nutrition and the Immune System: An Introduction," *American Journal of Clinical Nutrition* 66, no. 2 (August 1997): 460s–63, https://www.ncbi.nlm.nih.gov/pubmed/9250133.

12. Joseph E. Pizzorno and Michael T. Murray, *Textbook of Natural Medicine* (St. Louis, MO: Churchill Livingstone Elsevier, 2006).

13. Andrew L. Kau, Philip P. Ahern, Nicholas W. Griffin, Andrew L. Goodman, and Jeffrey I. Gordon, "Human Nutrition, the Gut Microbiome, and Immune System," *Nature* 474, no. 7351 (June 15, 2011): 327–36, doi:10.1038/nature10213.

14. John M. Daly, John Reynolds, Robert K. Sigal, Jian Shou, and Michael D. Liberman, "Effect of Dietary Protein and Amino Acids on Immune Function," *Critical Care Medicine* 18, supplement 2 (February 1990): s86–93, https://www.ncbi.nlm.nih.gov/pubmed/2105184.

15. Peng Li, Yu-Long Yin, Defa Li, Sung Woo Kim, and Guoyao Wu, "Amino Acids and Immune Function," *British Journal of Nutrition* 98, no. 2 (August 2007): 237–52, doi:10.1017/S000711450769936X.

16. R. K. Chandra, "Protein-Energy Malnutrition and Immunological Responses," *Journal of Nutrition* 122, supplement 3 (March 1992): 597–600, https://www.ncbi.nlm.nih.gov/pubmed/1542017.

17. Pizzorno and Murray, *Textbook of Natural Medicine*.

18. K. Pino-Lagos, M. J. Benson, and R. J. Noelle, "Retinoic Acid in the Immune System," *Annals of the New York Academy of Sciences* 1143 (November 2008): 170–87, doi:10.1196/annals.1443.017.

19. Katherine Zerdin, Michael L. Rooney, and Joost Vermuë, "The Vitamin C Content of Orange Juice Packed in an Oxygen Scavenger Material," *Food Chemistry* 82, no. 3 (August 2003): 387–95, doi:10.1016/s0308-8146(02)00559-9.

20. Hafeez Ullah Janjua, Munir Akhtar, and Fayyaz Hussain, "Effects of Sugar, Salt and Distilled Water on White Blood Cells and Platelet Cells," *Journal of Tumor* 4, no. 1 (February 2, 2016): 354–58, http://www.ghrnet.org/index.php/JT/article/view/1340.

21. Michael T. Murray, *Encyclopedia of Nutritional Supplements: The Essential Guide for Improving Your Health Naturally* (Rocklin, CA: Prima Health, 1996).

22. E. S. Wintergerst, S. Maggini, and D. H. Hornig, "Contribution of Selected Vitamins and Trace Elements to Immune Function," *Annals of Nutrition and Metabolism* 51, no. 4 (September 2007): 301–23, doi:10.1159/000107673.

23. Cynthia Aranow. "Vitamin D and the Immune System," *Journal of Investigative Medicine* 59, no. 6 (August 2011): 881–86, doi:10.231/JIM.0b013e31821b8755.

24. Johan Moan, Zoya Lagunova, Øyvind Bruland, and Asta Juzeniene, "Seasonal Variations of Cancer Incidence and Prognosis," *Dermato-Endocrinology* 2, no. 2 (April 2010): 55–57, doi:10.4161/derm.2.2.12664.

25. Lisa A. Houghton and Reinhold Vieth, "The Case against Ergocalciferol (Vitamin D$_2$) as a Vitamin Supplement," *American Journal of Clinical Nutrition* 84, no. 4 (October 2006): 694–97, http://ajcn.nutrition.org/content/84/4/694.long.

26. Ruth Sánchez-Martínez, Alberto Zambrano, Ana I. Castillo, and Ana Aranda, "Vitamin D–Dependent Recruitment of Corepressors to Vitamin D / Retinoid X Receptor Heterodimers," *Molecular and Cellular Biology*, 28, no. 11 (March 24, 2008): 3817–29, doi:10.1128/MCB.01909-07.

27. Cedric F. Garland, Frank C. Garland, Edward D. Gorham, Marin Lipkin, Harold Newmark, Sharif B. Mohr, and Michael F. Holick, "The Role of Vitamin D in Cancer Prevention," *American Journal of Public Health* 96, no. 2 (February 2006): 252–61, doi:10.2105/AJPH.2004.045260.

28. Elzbieta Kowalska, Steven A. Narod, Tomasz Huzarski, Stanislaw Zajaczek, Jowita Huzarska, Bohdan Gorski, and Jan Lubinski, "Increased Rates of Chromosome Breakage in BRCA1 Carriers Are Normalized by Oral Selenium Supplementation," *Cancer Epidemiology, Biomarkers and Prevention* 14, no. 5 (May 13, 2005): 1302–6, doi:10.1158/1055-9965.EPI-03-0448.

29. A. H. Shankar and A. S. Prasad, "Zinc and Immune Function: The Biological Basis of Altered Resistance to Infection," *American Journal of Clinical Nutrition* 68, supplement 2 (August 1998): 447s–63, https://www.ncbi.nlm.nih.gov/pubmed/9701160.

30. Janet R. K. Hunt. "Bioavailability of Iron, Zinc, and Other Trace Minerals from Vegetarian Diets," *American Journal of Clinical Nutrition* 78, no. 3 (September 2003): 633s–639, http://ajcn.nutrition.org/content/78/3/633S.full.

31. Mitchell R. McGill, Matthew R. Sharpe, C. David Williams, Mohammad Taha, Steven
    C. Curry, and Hartmut Jaeschke, "The Mechanism Underlying Acetaminophen-Induced
    Hepatotoxicity in Humans and Mice Involves Mitochondrial Damage and Nuclear
    DNA Fragmentation," *Journal of Clinical Investigation* 122, no. 4 (April 2, 2012): 1574–83,
    doi:10.1172/JCI59755.

32. Seema Patel and Arun Goyal, "Recent Developments in Mushrooms as Anti-Cancer Ther-
    apeutics: A Review," *3 Biotech* 2, no. 1 (March 2012): 1–15, doi:10.1007/s13205-011-0036-2.

33. Carolyn J. Torkelson, Erine Sweet, Mark R. Martzen, Masa Sasagawa, Cynthia A.
    Wenner, Juliette Gay, Amy Putiri, and Leanna J. Standish, "Phase 1 Clinical Trial of
    Trametes versicolor in Women with Breast Cancer," *ISRN Oncology* 2012 (May 30, 2012):
    251632, doi:10.5402/2012/251632.

34. Alena G. Guggenheim, Kirsten M. Wright, and Heather L. Zwickey, "Immune Modulation
    from Five Major Mushrooms: Application to Integrative Oncology," *Integrative Medicine* 13,
    no. 1 (February 2014): 32–44, https://www.ncbi.nlm.nih.gov/pmc/articles/PMC4684115.

35. Xiaoshuang Dai, Joy M. Stanilka, Cheryl A. Rowe, Elizabethe A. Esteves, Carmelo
    Nieves, Samuel J. Spaiser, Mary C. Christman, Bobbi Langkamp-Henken, and Susan S.
    Percival, "Consuming *Lentinula edodes* (Shiitake) Mushrooms Daily Improves Human
    Immunity: A Randomized Dietary Intervention in Healthy Young Adults," *Journal of the
    American College of Nutrition* 34, no. 6 (2015): 478–87, doi:10.1080/07315724.2014.950391.

36. Sissi Wachtel-Galor, John Yuen, John A. Buswell, and Iris F. F. Benzie, "*Ganoderma lucidum*
    (Lingzhi or Reishi): A Medicinal Mushroom," chap. 9 in Iris F. F. Benzie and Sissi Wach-
    tel-Galor, eds., *Herbal Medicine: Biomolecular and Clinical Aspects*, 2nd ed. (Boca Raton, FL:
    CRC Press, 2011). Available from https://www.ncbi.nlm.nih.gov/books/NBK92757.

37. Patel and Goyal, "Recent Developments in Mushrooms as Anti-Cancer Therapeutics:
    A Review."

38. Bao-qin Lin and Shao-ping Li, "Cordyceps as an Herbal Drug," chap. 5 in Benzie and
    Wachtel-Galor, eds., *Herbal Medicine: Biomolecular and Clinical Aspects*. Available at
    https://www.ncbi.nlm.nih.gov/books/NBK92758.

39. Qing Li, "Effect of Forest Bathing Trips on Human Immune Function," *Environmental
    Health and Preventive Medicine* 15, no. 1 (January 2010): 9–17, doi:10.1007/s12199-008-0068-3.

40. A. Mooventhan and L. Nivethitha, "Scientific Evidence-Based Effects of Hydrotherapy
    on Various Systems of the Body," *North American Journal of Medical Sciences* 6, no. 5 (May
    2014): 199–209, doi:10.4103/1947-2714.132935.

Chapter 8: The Inflammation-Oxidation Association

1. Subrata Kumar Biswas, "Does the Interdependence between Oxidative Stress and
   Inflammation Explain the Antioxidant Paradox?" *Oxidative Medicine and Cellular Longevity*
   2016, no. 12 (January 2016): 1–9, doi:10.1155/2016/5698931.

2. Udo Erasmus, *Fats That Heal, Fats That Kill: The Complete Guide to Fats, Oils, Cholesterol
   and Human Health* (Burnaby, BC: Alive Books, 1996).

3. Daniel Weber, *Inflammation and the Seven Stochastic Events of Cancer* (Alexandria, NSW:
   Panaxea Publishing, 2010).

4. Mary M. Murphy, Leila M. Barraj, Dena Herman, Xiaoyu Bi, Rachel Cheatham, and
   R. Keith Randolph, "Phytonutrient Intake by Adults in the United States in Relation to

Fruit and Vegetable Consumption," *Journal of the Academy of Nutrition and Dietetics* 112, no. 2 (February 2012): 222–29, doi:10.1016/j.jada.2011.08.044.

5. "Omega-6 Polyunsaturated Fatty Acids and DNA Adducts," *Food and Chemical Toxicology* 35, no. 10–11 (October/November 1997): 1131, doi:10.1016/s0278-6915(97)90098-3.

6. Jian-Hua Yi, Dong Wang, Zhi-Yong Li, Jun Hu, Xiao-Feng Niu, and Xiao-Lin Liu, "C-Reactive Protein as a Prognostic Factor for Human Osteosarcoma: A Meta-Analysis and Literature Review," *PLOS ONE* 9, no. 5 (May 6, 2014): doi:10.1371/journal.pone.0094632.

7. Jill K. Onesti and Denis C. Guttridge, "Inflammation Based Regulation of Cancer Cachexia," *BioMed Research International* 2014 (May 4, 2014): 1–7, doi:10.1155/2014/168407.

8. Norleena P. Gullett, Vera C. Mazurak, Gautam Hebbar, and Thomas R. Ziegler, "Nutritional Interventions for Cancer-Induced Cachexia," *Current Problems in Cancer* 35, no. 2 (March/April 2011): 58–90, doi:10.1016/j.currproblcancer.2011.01.001.

9. Surendra K. Shukla, Teklab Gebregiworgis, Vinee Purohit, Nina V. Chaika, Venugopal Gunda, Prakash Radhakrishnan, Kamiya Mehla, et al., "Metabolic Reprogramming Induced by Ketone Bodies Diminishes Pancreatic Cancer Cachexia," *Cancer and Metabolism* 2, no. 1 (September 1, 2014): 18, doi:10.1186/2049-3002-2-18.

10. David F. Horrobin, "Loss of Delta-6-Sesaturase Activity as a Key Factor in Aging," *Medical Hypotheses* 7, no. 9 (1981): 1211–20, doi:10.1016/0306-9877(81)90064-5; Federica Tosi, Filippo Sartori, Patrizia Guarini, Oliviero Olivieri, and Nicola Martinelli, "Delta-5 and Delta-6 Desaturases: Crucial Enzymes in Polyunsaturated Fatty Acid-Related Pathways with Pleiotropic Influences in Health and Disease," *Advances in Experimental Medicine and Biology* 824 (2014): 61–81, doi:10.1007/978-3-319-07320-0_7.

11. R. A. Kunin, "Snake Oil," *Western Journal of Medicine* 151, no. 2 (August 1989): 208, https://www.ncbi.nlm.nih.gov/pmc/articles/PMC1026931.

12. Paulette Mehta, "TNF-α Inhibitors: Are They Carcinogenic?" *Drug, Healthcare and Patient Safety* 2 (2010): 241–47, doi:10.2147/dhps.s7829.

13. Tzung-Jiun Tsai and Ping-I Hsu, "Low-Dose Aspirin-Induced Upper Gastrointestinal Injury—Epidemiology, Management and Prevention," *Journal of Blood Disorders and Transfusion* 6 (December 26, 2015): 327, doi:10.4172/2155-9864.1000327.

14. Daniel Arango, Kengo Morohashi, Alper Yilmaz, Kouji Kuramochi, Arti Parihar, Bledj Brahimaj, Erich Grotewold, and Andrea I. Doseff, "Molecular Basis for the Action of a Dietary Flavonoid Revealed by the Comprehensive Identification of Apigenin Human Targets," *Proceedings of the National Academy of Sciences* 110, no. 24 (May 2013): e2153–62, doi:10.1073/pnas.1303726110.

15. Saebyeol Jang, Keith W. Kelley, and Rodney W. Johnson, "Luteolin Reduces IL-6 Production in Microglia by Inhibiting JNK Phosphorylation and Activation of AP-1," *Proceedings of the National Academy of Sciences* 105, no. 21 (March 5, 2008): 7534–39, doi:10.1073/pnas.0802865105.

16. Michelle L. Boland, Aparajita H. Chourasia, and Kay F. Macleod, "Mitochondrial Dysfunction in Cancer," *Frontiers in Oncology* 3 (December 2, 2013): 292, doi:10.3389/fonc.2013.00292.

17. Guoyao Wu, Yun-Zhong Fang, Sheng Yang, Joanne R. Lupton, and Nancy D. Turner, "Glutathione Metabolism and Its Implications for Health," *Journal of Nutrition* 134, no. 3 (March 2004): 489–92, https://www.ncbi.nlm.nih.gov/pubmed/14988435.

18. Hu Wang, Tin Khor, Limin Shu, Zheng-Yuan Su, Francisco F. Fuentes, Jong Hun Lee, and Ah-Ng Tony Kong, "Plants vs. Cancer: A Review on Natural Phytochemicals in

Preventing and Treating Cancers and Their Druggability," *Anti-Cancer Agents in Medicinal Chemistry* 12, no. 10 (May 2012): 1281–305, doi:10.2174/187152012803833026.

19. Massimo Fantini, Monica Benvenuto, Laura Masuelli, Giovanni Vanni Frajese, Ilaria Tresoldi, Andrea Modesti, and Roberto Bei, "In Vitro and in Vivo Antitumoral Effects of Combinations of Polyphenols, or Polyphenols and Anticancer Drugs: Perspectives on Cancer Treatment," *International Journal of Molecular Sciences* 16, no. 5 (May 2015): 9236–82, doi:10.3390/ijms16059236.

20. Ching-Chow Chen, Man-Ping Chow, Wei-Chien Huang, Yi-Chu Lin, and Ya-Jen Chang, "Flavonoids Inhibit Tumor Necrosis Factor-α-Induced Up-Regulation of Intercellular Adhesion Molecule-1 (ICAM-1) in Respiratory Epithelial Cells through Activator Protein-1 and Nuclear Factor-κB: Structure-Activity Relationships," *Molecular Pharmacology* 66, no. 3 (October 2004): 683–93, https://www.ncbi.nlm.nih.gov/pubmed/15322261.

21. Xiangsheng Xiao, Dingbo Shi, Liqun Liu, Jingshu Wang, Xiaoming Xie, Tiebang Kang, and Wuguo Deng, "Quercetin Suppresses Cyclooxygenase-2 Expression and Angiogenesis through Inactivation of P300 Signaling," *PLOS ONE* 6, no. 8 (August 8, 2011): e22934, doi:10.1371/journal.pone.0022934; Iris Erlund, Jukka Marniemi, Paula Hakala, G. Alfthan, E. Meririnne, and A. Aro, "Consumption of Black Currants, Lingonberries and Bilberries Increases Serum Quercetin Concentrations," *European Journal of Clinical Nutrition* 57, no. 1 (February 2003): 37–42, doi:10.1038/sj.ejcn.1601513.

22. J. Vlachojannis, F. Magora, and S. Chrubasik, "Willow Species and Aspirin: Different Mechanism of Actions," *Phytotherapy Research* 25, no. 7 (2011): 1102–04, doi:10.1002/ptr.3386.

23. Reason Wilken, Mysore S. Veena, Marilene B. Wang, and Eri S. Srivatsan, "Curcumin: A Review of Anti-Cancer Properties and Therapeutic Activity in Head and Neck Squamous Cell Carcinoma," *Molecular Cancer* 10, no. 1 (February 2011): 12, doi:10.1186/1476-4598-10-12.

24. Mark Barton Frank, Qing Yang, Jeanette Osban, Joseph T. Azzarello, Marcia R. Saban, Ricardo Saban, Richard A. Ashley, et al., "Frankincense Oil Derived from *Boswellia carteri* Induces Tumor Cell Specific Cytotoxicity," *BMC Complementary and Alternative Medicine* 9 (March 18, 2009): 6, doi:10.1186/1472-6882-9-6.

25. John Kallas, *Edible Wild Plants: Wild Foods from Dirt to Plate* (Layton, UT: Gibbs Smith, 2010).

26. S. D. Bhale, Z. Xu, W. Prinyawiwatkul, Joan M. King, and J. S. Godber, "Oregano and Rosemary Extracts Inhibit Oxidation of Long-Chain N-3 Fatty Acids in Menhaden Oil," *Journal of Food Science* 72, no. 9 (December 2007): C504–8, doi:10.1111/j.1750-3841.2007.00569.x.

27. I. Andújar, M. C. Recio, R. M. Giner, and J. L. Ríos, "Cocoa Polyphenols and Their Potential Benefits for Human Health," *Oxidative Medicine and Cellular Longevity* 2012 (October 24, 2012): 1–23, doi:10.1155/2012/906252.

28. Andrea Rosanoff, Connie M. Weaver, and Robert K. Rude, "Suboptimal Magnesium Status in the United States: Are the Health Consequences Underestimated?" *Nutrition Reviews* 70, no. 3 (March 2012): 153–64, doi:10.1111/j.1753-4887.2011.00465.x.

29. Robert Whang, "Magnesium Deficiency: Pathogenesis, Prevalence, and Clinical Implications," *American Journal of Medicine* 82, no. 3A (April 1987): 24–29, doi:10.1016/0002-9343(87)90129-x.

30. James L. Oschman, Gaétan Chevalier, and Richard Brown, "The Effects of Grounding (Earthing) on Inflammation, the Immune Response, Wound Healing, and Prevention and Treatment of Chronic Inflammatory and Autoimmune Diseases," *Journal of Inflammation Research* 8 (March 4, 2015): 83–96, doi:10.2147/jir.s69656.

Chapter 9: Cancer Growth and Spread

1. Christopher I. Li, Janet R. Daling, Mei-Tzu Tang, Kara L. Haugen, Peggy L. Porter, and Kathleen E. Malone, "Use of Antihypertensive Medications and Breast Cancer Risk among Women Aged 55 to 74 Years," *JAMA Internal Medicine* 173, no. 17 (September 23, 2013): 1629–37, https://www.ncbi.nlm.nih.gov/pubmed/23921840.

2. Peter Carmeliet, "Angiogenesis in Health and Disease," *Nature Medicine* 9, no. 6 (June 2003): 653–60, doi:10.1038/nm0603-653.

3. Robert R. Langley and Isaiah J. Fidler, "The Seed and Soil Hypothesis Revisited—The Role of Tumor-Stroma Interactions in Metastasis to Different Organs," *International Journal of Cancer* 128, no. 11 (June 1, 2011): 2527–35, doi:10.1002/ijc.26031.

4. Shalom Madar, Ido Goldstein, and Varda Rotter, "'Cancer Associated Fibroblasts'—More than Meets the Eye," *Trends in Molecular Medicine* 19, no. 8 (August 2013): 447–53, doi:10.1016/j.molmed.2013.05.004.

5. Raghu Kalluri and Michael Zeisberg, "Fibroblasts in Cancer," *Nature Reviews Cancer* 6, no. 5 (May 2006): 392–401, doi:10.1038/nrc1877.

6. Neta Erez, Morgan Truitt, Peter Olson, S. T. Arron, and Douglas Hanahan, "Cancer-Associated Fibroblasts Are Activated in Incipient Neoplasia to Orchestrate Tumor-Promoting Inflammation in an NF-κB-Dependent Manner," *Cancer Cell* 17, no. 2 (February 17, 2010): 135–47, doi:10.1016/j.ccr.2009.12.041.

7. Katsuyuki Miura, Hideaki Nakagawa, Hirotsugu Ueshima, Akira Okayama, Shikeyuki Saitoh, J. David Curb, Beatriz L. Rodriguez, et al., "Dietary Factors Related to Higher Plasma Fibrinogen Levels of Japanese-Americans in Hawaii Compared with Japanese in Japan," *Arteriosclerosis, Thrombosis, and Vascular Biology* 26, no. 7 (July 2006): 1674–79, doi:10.1161/01.atv.0000225701.20965.b9.

8. Zeinab Tahmasebi Birgani, Nazli Gharraee, Angad Malhotra, Clemens A. Van Blitterswijk, and Pamela Habibovic, "Combinatorial Incorporation of Fluoride and Cobalt Ions into Calcium Phosphates to Stimulate Osteogenesis and Angiogenesis," *Biomedical Materials* 11, no. 1 (February 29, 2016): 015020, doi:10.1088/1748-6041/11/1/015020.

9. Daniel J. Goldstein and Jose A. Halperin, "Mast Cell Histamine and Cell Dehydration Thirst," *Nature* 267, no. 5608 (May 19, 1977): 250–52, doi:10.1038/267250a0.

10. Aletta D. Kraneveld, Seil Sagar, Johan Garssen, and Gert Folkerts, "The Two Faces of Mast Cells in Food Allergy and Allergic Asthma: The Possible Concept of Yin Yang," *Biochimica Et Biophysica Acta (BBA)* 1822, no. 1 (January 2012): 93–99, doi:10.1016/j.bbadis.2011.06.013.

11. Liuliang Qin, Dezheng Zhao, Jianfeng Xu, Xianghui Ren, Ernest F. Terwilliger, Sareh Parangi, Jack Lawler, Harold F. Dvorak, and Huiyan Zeng, "The Vascular Permeabilizing Factors Histamine and Serotonin Induce Angiogenesis through TR3/Nur77 and Subsequently Truncate It through Thrombospondin-1," *Blood* 121, no. 11 (March 14, 2013): 2154–164, doi:10.1182/blood-2012-07-443903.

12. Rebekah Beaton, Wendy Pagdin-Friesen, Christa Robertson, Cathy Vigar, Heather Watson, and Susan R. Harris, "Effects of Exercise Intervention on Persons with Metastatic Cancer: A Systematic Review," *Physiotherapy Canada* 61, no. 3 (2009): 141–53, doi:10.3138/physio.61.3.141.

13. Centers for Disease Control and Prevention, "One in Five Adults Meet Overall Physical Activity Guidelines," CDC Newsroom, May 2, 2013, https://www.cdc.gov/media/releases/2013/p0502-physical-activity.html.

14. Steven C. Moore, I-Min Lee, and Elisabete Weiderpass, "Association of Leisure-Time Physical Activity with Risk of 26 Types of Cancer in 1.44 Million Adults," *JAMA Internal Medicine* 176, no. 6 (June 1, 2016): 816–25, doi:10.1001/jamainternmed.2016.1548.

15. Huiqi Xie and Y. James Kang, "Role of Copper in Angiogenesis and Its Medicinal Implications," *Current Medicinal Chemistry* 16, no. 10 (February 2009): 1304–14, doi:10.2174/092986709787846622.

16. Varsha P. Brahmkhatri, Chinmayi Prasanna, and Hanudatta S. Atreya, "Insulin-Like Growth Factor System in Cancer: Novel Targeted Therapies," *BioMed Research International* 2015 (2015): 1–24, doi:10.1155/2015/538019.

17. Tian Lei and Xie Ling, "IGF-1 Promotes the Growth and Metastasis of Hepatocellular Carcinoma via the Inhibition of Proteasome-Mediated Cathepsin B Degradation," *World Journal of Gastroenterology* 21, no. 35 (September 21, 2015): 10137–49, doi:10.3748/wjg.v21.i35.10137.

18. Chia-Wei Cheng, Gregor B. Adams, Laura Perin, Min Wei, Xiaoying Zhou, Ben S. Lam, Stefano Da Sacco, et al., "Prolonged Fasting Reduces IGF-1/PKA to Promote Hematopoietic-Stem-Cell-Based Regeneration and Reverse Immunosuppression," *Cell Stem Cell* 14, no. 6 (June 5, 2014): 810–23, doi:10.1016/j.stem.2014.04.014.

19. Angela M. Poff, Csilla Ari, Thomas N. Seyfried, and Dominic P. D'Agostino, "The Ketogenic Diet and Hyperbaric Oxygen Therapy Prolong Survival in Mice with Systemic Metastatic Cancer," *PLOS ONE* 8, no. 6 (June 5, 2013): e65522, doi:10.1371/journal.pone.0065522.

20. Charlotte Ornstein, "Popular Blood Thinner Causing Deaths, Injuries in Nursing Homes," *Washington Post*, July 13, 2015. Available at https://www.pharmacist.com/popular-blood-thinner-causing-deaths-injuries-nursing-homes.

21. Caiguo Zhang, "Essential Functions of Iron-Requiring Proteins in DNA Replication, Repair and Cell Cycle Control," *Protein and Cell* 5, no. 10 (October 2014): 750–60, doi:10.1007/s13238-014-0083-7.

22. "Micronutrient Deficiencies: Iron Deficiency Anaemia," World Health Organization, accessed September 30, 2016, http://www.who.int/nutrition/topics/ida/en.

23. Louis Harrison and Kimberly Blackwell, "Hypoxia and Anemia: Factors in Decreased Sensitivity to Radiation Therapy and Chemotherapy?" *Oncologist* 9, supplement 5 (November 2004): 31–40, doi:10.1634/theoncologist.9-90005-31.

24. Janet R. Hunt, "Bioavailability of Iron, Zinc, and Other Trace Minerals from Vegetarian Diets," *American Journal of Clinical Nutrition* 78, no. 3 (September 2003): 633s–39, http://ajcn.nutrition.org/content/78/3/633S.full.

25. Adrian R. West, "Mechanisms of Heme Iron Absorption: Current Questions and Controversies," *World Journal of Gastroenterology* 14, no. 26 (July 14, 2008): 4101–10, doi:10.3748/wjg.14.4101.

26. Ahmed A. Alkhateeb and James R. Connor, "The Significance of Ferritin in Cancer: Anti-Oxidation, Inflammation and Tumorigenesis," *Biochimica Et Biophysica Acta (BBA)* 1836, no. 2 (December 2013): 245–54, doi:10.1016/j.bbcan.2013.07.002.

27. L. K. Ferrarelli, "Iron Fuels Glioblastoma Growth," *Science Signaling* 8, no. 400 (October 27, 2015): ec311, doi:10.1126/scisignal.aad7099.

28. Maria José Oliveira, Josef Van Damme, Tineke Lauwaet, Veerle De Corte, Georges De Bruyne, Gerda Verschraegen, et al., "β-Casein-Derived Peptides, Produced by Bacteria, Stimulate Cancer Cell Invasion and Motility," *EMBO Journal* 22, no. 22 (November 17, 2003): 6161–73, doi:10.1093/emboj/cdg586.

29. Gangjun Du, Lingtao Jin, Xiaofen Han, Zihui Song, Hongyan Zhang, and Wei Liang, "Naringenin: A Potential Immunomodulator for Inhibiting Lung Fibrosis and Metastasis," *Cancer Research* 69, no. 7 (April 1, 2009): 3205–12, doi:10.1158/0008-5472.can-08-3393.

30. Hu Wang, Tin Khor, Limin Shu, Zheng-Yuan Su, Francisco F. Fuentes, Jong Hun Lee, and Ah-Ng Tony Kong, "Plants vs. Cancer: A Review on Natural Phytochemicals in Preventing and Treating Cancers and Their Druggability," *Anti-Cancer Agents in Medicinal Chemistry* 12, no. 10 (May 2012): 1281–305, doi:10.2174/187152012803833026.

31. Ke Zu, Lorelei Mucci, Bernard A. Rosner, Steven K. Clinton, Massimo Loda, Meir J. Stampfer, and Edward Giovannucci, "Dietary Lycopene, Angiogenesis, and Prostate Cancer: A Prospective Study in the Prostate-Specific Antigen Era," *Journal of the National Cancer Institute* 106, no. 2 (February 2014): djt430, doi:10.1093/jnci/djt430.

32. Daniel Man-Yuen Sze and Godfrey Chi-Fung Chan, "Effects of Beta-Glucans on Different Immune Cell Populations and Cancers," *Advances in Botanical Research* 62 (December 2012): 179–96, doi:10.1016/b978-0-12-394591-4.00011-8.

33. Jeong-Ki Min, "Capsaicin Inhibits in Vitro and in Vivo Angiogenesis," *Cancer Research* 64, no. 2 (January 2004): 644–51, doi:10.1158/0008-5472.can-03-3250.

34. Jun Lv, Lu Qi, Canqing Yu, Ling Yang, Yu Guo, Yiping Chen, Zheng Bian, et al., "Consumption of Spicy Foods and Total and Cause Specific Mortality: Population Based Cohort Study," *BMJ* 2015 (August 4, 2015): 351, doi:10.1136/bmj.h3942.

35. Slobodan Vukicevic, Vishwas M. Paralkar, and A. H. Reddi, "Extracellular Matrix and Bone Morphogenetic Proteins in Cartilage and Bone Development and Repair," *Advances in Molecular and Cell Biology* 6 (1993): 207–24, doi:10.1016/s1569-2558(08)60203-9.

36. Viktor Chesnokov, Chao Sun, and Keiichi Itakura, "Glucosamine Suppresses Proliferation of Human Prostate Carcinoma DU145 Cells through Inhibition of STAT3 Signaling," *Cancer Cell International* 9, no. 1 (September 10, 2009): 25, doi:10.1186/1475-2867-9-25.

37. Maharjan H. Radha and Nampoothiri P. Laxmipriya, "Evaluation of Biological Properties and Clinical Effectiveness of *Aloe vera*: A Systematic Review," *Journal of Traditional and Complementary Medicine* 5, no. 1 (December 23, 2014): 21–26, doi:10.1016/j.jtcme.2014.10.006.

38. Naghma Khan and Hasan Mukhtar, "Cancer and Metastasis: Prevention and Treatment by Green Tea," *Cancer and Metastasis Reviews* 29, no. 3 (September 2010): 435–45, doi:10.1007/s10555-010-9236-1.

39. Shihong Chen, Zhijun Wang, Ying Huang, Stephen A. O'Barr, Rebecca A. Wong, Steven Yeung, and Moses Sing Sum Chow, "Ginseng and Anticancer Drug Combination to Improve Cancer Chemotherapy: A Critical Review," *Evidence-Based Complementary and Alternative Medicine* 2014 (2014): 1–13, doi:10.1155/2014/168940.

40. Émilie C. Lefort and Jonathan Blay, "Apigenin and Its Impact on Gastrointestinal Cancers," *Molecular Nutrition and Food Research* 57, no. 1 (January 2013): 126–44, doi:10.1002/mnfr.201200424.

Chapter 10: Hungry for Hormone Balance

1. Michael K. Brawer, "Testosterone Replacement in Men with Andropause: An Overview," *Reviews in Urology* 6, supplement 6 (2004): s9–15, http://www.ncbi.nlm.nih.gov/pmc/articles/PMC1472881.

2. Robert H. Carlson, "Targeting Estrogen to Modulate Angiogenesis," *Oncology Times* 29, no. 8 (April 25, 2007): 56, doi:10.1097/01.COT.0000269640.65146.7e.

3. Brian E. Henderson and Heather Spencer Feigelson, "Hormonal Carcinogenesis," *Carcinogenesis* 21, no. 3 (March 1, 2000): 427–33, doi:10.1093/carcin/21.3.427.

4. Medline Plus, "Tamoxifen," US National Library of Medicine, last updated September 1, 2010, accessed August 04, 2016, https://www.nlm.nih.gov/medlineplus/druginfo/meds/a682414.html.

5. Petra Hååg, Jasmin Bektic, Gerog Bartsch, Helmut Klocker, and Iris E. Eder, "Androgen Receptor Down Regulation by Small Interference RNA Induces Cell Growth Inhibition in Androgen Sensitive as well as in Androgen Independent Prostate Cancer Cells," *Journal of Steroid Biochemistry and Molecular Biology* 96, no. 3–4 (August 2005): 251–58, doi:10.1016/j.jsbmb.2005.04.029.

6. Michelle Whirl-Carrillo, Ellen M. McDonagh, J. M. Hebert, Ii Chun Gong, K. Sangkuhl, C. F. Thorn, Russ B. Altman, and T. E. Klein, "Pharmacogenomics Knowledge for Personalized Medicine," *Clinical Pharmacology and Therapeutics* 92, no. 4 (October 2012): 414–17, doi:10.1038/clpt.2012.96.

7. Heather Greenlee, Yu Chen, Geoffrey C. Kabat, Qiao Wang, Muhammad G. Kibriya, Irina Gurvich, Daniel W. Sepkovic, et al., "Variants in Estrogen Metabolism and Biosynthesis Genes and Urinary Estrogen Metabolites in Women with a Family History of Breast Cancer," *Breast Cancer Research and Treatment* 102, no. 1 (March 2007): 111–17, doi:10.1007/s10549-006-9308-7.

8. H. L. Bradlow and M. A. Zeligs, "Diindolylmethane (DIM) Spontaneously Forms from Indole-3-Carbinol (I3C) during Cell Culture Experiments," *In Vivo* 24, no. 4 (July/August 2010): 387–91, https://www.ncbi.nlm.nih.gov/pubmed/20668304.

9. C. C. Capen, "Mechanisms of Chemical Injury of Thyroid Gland," *Progress in Clinical and Biological Research* 387 (February 1994): 173–91.

10. Chandradhar Dwivedi, Wendy J. Heck, Alan A. Downie, Saroj Larroya, and Thomas E. Webb, "Effect of Calcium Glucarate on β-glucuronidase Activity and Glucarate Content of Certain Vegetables and Fruits," *Biochemical Medicine and Metabolic Biology* 43, no. 2 (1990): 83–92, doi:10.1016/0885-4505(90)90012-p.

11. L. D. Cowan, L. Gordis, J. A. Tonascia, and G. S. Jones, "Breast Cancer Incidence in Women with a History of Progesterone Deficiency," *American Journal of Epidemiology* 114, no. 2 (August 1981): 209–17, https://www.ncbi.nlm.nih.gov/pubmed/7304556.

12. Reini W. Bretveld, Chris M. G. Thomas, Paul T. J. Scheepers, Gerhard A. Zielhuis, and Nel Roeleveld, "Pesticide Exposure: The Hormonal Function of the Female Reproductive System Disrupted?" *Reproductive Biology and Endocrinology* 4 (May 31, 2006): 30, doi:10.1186/1477-7827-4-30.

13. Hitomi Takemura, Harue Uchiyama, Takeshi Ohura, Hiroyuki Sakakibara, Ryoko Kuruto, Takashi Amagai, and Kayoko Shimoi, "A Methoxyflavonoid, Chrysoeriol, Selectively Inhibits the Formation of a Carcinogenic Estrogen Metabolite in MCF-7

Breast Cancer Cells," *Journal of Steroid Biochemistry and Molecular Biology* 118, no. 1–2 (January 2010): 70–76, doi:10.1016/j.jsbmb.2009.10.002.

14. Romilly E. Hodges and Deanna M. Minich, "Modulation of Metabolic Detoxification Pathways Using Foods and Food-Derived Components: A Scientific Review with Clinical Application," *Journal of Nutrition and Metabolism* 2015 (2015): 1–23, doi:10.1155/2015/760689.

15. Wendee Holtcamp, "Obesogens: An Environmental Link to Obesity," *Environmental Health Perspectives* 120, no. 2 (February 2012): a62–68, doi:10.1289/ehp.120-a62.

16. Barbara Hammes and Cynthia J. Laitman, "Diethylstilbestrol (DES) Update: Recommendations for the Identification and Management of DES-Exposed Individuals," *Journal of Midwifery and Women's Health* 48, no. 1 (January/February 2003): 19–29, doi:10.1016/s1526-9523(02)00370-7.

17. "EU Tests Confirm Health Risk of Using Growth Hormones," EurActiv, April 23, 2002, http://www.euractiv.com/section/health-consumers/news/eu-tests-confirm-health -risk-of-using-growth-hormones.

18. Renée Johnson, "The US-EU Beef Hormone Dispute," Congressional Research Service, January 14, 2015, https://fas.org/sgp/crs/row/R40449.pdf.

19. Y. Handa, H. Fujita, S. Honma, H. Minakami, and R. Kishi, "Estrogen Concentrations in Beef and Human Hormone-Dependent Cancers," *Annals of Oncology* 20, no. 9 (July 23, 2009): 1610–11, doi:10.1093/annonc/mdp381.

20. V. Beral, D. Bull, R. Doll, T. Key, R. Peto, G. Reeves, E. E. Calle, et al., "Breast Cancer and Hormone Replacement Therapy: Collaborative Reanalysis of Data from 51 Epidemiological Studies of 52,705 Women with Breast Cancer and 108,411 Women without Breast Cancer," *Lancet* 350, no. 9084 (October 11, 1997): 1047–59, doi:10.1016/S0140-6736(97)08233-0.

21. NIH, "WHI Follow Up Study Confirms Health Risks of Long-Term Combination Hormone Therapy Outweigh Benefits for Postmenopausal Women," US National Library of Medicine, March 4, 2008, https://www.nih.gov/news-events/news-releases /whi-follow-study-confirms-health-risks-long-term-combination-hormone-therapy -outweigh-benefits-postmenopausal-women.

22. Jane Higdon, Victoria J. Drake, and David E. Williams, "Indole-3-Carbinol," Micronutrient Information Center, Linus Pauling Institiue,Oregon State University, last updated December 2008, http://lpi.oregonstate.edu/mic/dietary-factors/phytochemicals /indole-3-carbinol; Probo Y. Nugrahedi, Budi Midianarko, Matthijs Dekker, Ruud Vekerk, and Teresa Oliviero, "Retention of Glucosinolates during Fermentation of *Brassica juncea*: A Case Study on Production of *Sayur Asin*," *European Food Research and Technology* 240, no. 3 (March 2015): 559–65, doi:10.1007/s00217-014-2355-0.

23. Neil McKinney, *Naturopathic Oncology: An Encyclopedic Guide for Patients and Physicians* (Richmond, BC: Creative Guy Publishing, 2010).

24. L. Bacciottini, Alberto Falchetti, B. Pampaloni, E. Bartolini, A. Carossino, and M. Brandi, "Phytoestrogens: Food or Drug?" chap. 24 in Andrea R. Genazzani, *Postmenopausal Osteopoersis: Hormones and Other Therapies* (Boca Raton, FL: CRC Press, 2006): 219–31, doi:10.1201/b14631-25.

25. M. J. Glade, "Food, Nutrition, and the Prevention of Cancer: A Global Perspective. American Institue for Cancer Research / World Cancer Research Fund, American Institute for Cancer Research, 1997," *Nutrition* 15, no. 6 (June 1999): 523–26.

26. Joseph E. Pizzorno and Michael T. Murray, *Textbook of Natural Medicine* (St. Louis, MO: Churchill Livingstone Elsevier, 2006).

27. Peter B. Kaufman, James A. Duke, Harry Brielmann, John Boik, and James E. Hoyt, "A Comparative Survey of Leguminous Plants as Sources of the Isoflavones, Genistein and Daidzein: Implications for Human Nutrition and Health," *Journal of Alternative and Complementary Medicine* 3, no. 1 (February 1997): 7–12, doi:10.1089/acm.1997.3.7.

28. Charlotte Atkinson, Katherine M. Newton, Frank Stanczyk, Kim C. Westerlind, Lin Li, and Johanna W. Lampe, "Daidzein-Metabolizing Phenotypes in Relation to Serum Hormones and Sex Hormone Binding Globulin, and Urinary Estrogen Metabolites in Premenopausal Women in the United States," *Cancer Causes and Control* 19, no. 10 (December 2008): 1085–93, doi:10.1007/s10552-008-9172-3.

29. Fen-Jin He and Jin-Qiang Chen, "Consumption of Soybean, Soy Foods, Soy Isoflavones and Breast Cancer Incidence: Differences between Chinese Women and Women in Western Countries and Possible Mechanisms," *Food Science and Human Wellness* 2, no. 3–4 (September–December 2013): 146–61, doi:10.1016/j.fshw.2013.08.002.

30. Lilian U. Thompson, Jian Min Chen, Tong Li, Kathrin Strasser-Weippl, and Paul E. Goss, "Dietary Flaxseed Alters Tumor Biological Markers in Postmenopausal Breast Cancer," *Clinical Cancer Research* 11, no. 10 (May 15, 2005): 3828–35, doi:10.1158/1078-0432.CCR-04-2326.

31. Mitsuo Namiki, "Nutraceutical Functions of Sesame: A Review," *Critical Reviews in Food Science and Nutrition* 47, no. 7 (February 2007): 651–73, doi:10.1080/10408390600919114.

32. Yasuo Imai, Satomi Tsukahara, Sakiyo Asada, and Yoshikazu Sugimoto, "Phytoestrogens/Flavonoids Reverse Breast Cancer Resistance Protein/ABCG2-Mediated Multidrug Resistance," *Cancer Research* 64, no. 12 (June 2004): 4346–52, doi:10.1158/0008-5472.can-04-0078.

33. Emir Bozkurt, Harika Atmaca, Asli Kisim, Selim Uzunoglu, Ruchan Uslu, and Burcak Karaca, "Effects of *Thymus serpyllum* Extract on Cell Proliferation, Apoptosis and Epigenetic Events in Human Breast Cancer Cells," *Nutrition and Cancer* 64, no. 8 (November 19, 2012): 1245–50, doi:10.1080/01635581.2012.719658.

Chapter 11: Stress and Circadian Rhythms

1. "2015 Stress in America Snapshot," American Psychological Association, accessed November 22, 2016, http://www.apa.org/news/press/releases/stress/2015/snapshot.aspx.

2. Myrthala Moreno-Smith, Susan K. Lutgendorf, and Anil K. Sood, "Impact of Stress on Cancer Metastasis," *Future Oncology* 6, no. 12 (December 2010): 1863–81, doi:10.2217/fon.10.142.

3. Bo Christensen, "Melatonin Could Be an Overlooked Treatment for Cancer," *ScienceNordic*, June 1, 2015, http://sciencenordic.com/melatonin-could-be-overlooked-treatment-cancer.

4. Angela Spivey, "Light Pollution: Light at Night and Breast Cancer Risk Worldwide," *Environmental Health Perspectives* 118, no. 12 (December 2010): A525, doi:10.1289/ehp.118-a525.

5. Quentin Fottrell, "55% of American Workers Don't Take All Their Paid Vacation," *MarketWatch*, June 19, 2016, http://www.marketwatch.com/story/55-of-american-workers-dont-take-all-their-paid-vacation-2016-06-15.

6. Torbjørn Elvsåshagen, Linn B. Norbom, Per Ø. Pedersen, Sophia H. Quraishi, Atle Bjørnerud, Ulrik F. Malt, Inge R. Groote, and Lars T. Westlye, "Widespread Changes in White Matter Microstructure after a Day of Waking and Sleep Deprivation," *PLOS ONE* 10, no. 5 (May 28, 2015): e0127351, doi:10.1371/journal.pone.0127351.

7. Sheldon Cohen, Denise Janicki-Deverts, William J. Doyle, Gregory E. Miller, Ellen Frank, Bruce S. Rabin, and Ronald B. Turner, "Chronic Stress, Glucocorticoid Receptor Resistance, Inflammation, and Disease Risk," *Proceedings of the National Academy of Science of the United States of America* 109, no. 16 (April 17, 2012): 5995–99, doi:10.1073 /pnas.1118355109.

8. Lawrence S. Sklar and Hymie Anisman, "Stress and Cancer," *Psychological Bulletin* 89, no. 3 (May 1981): 369–406, doi:10.1037/0033-2909.89.3.369.

9. E. Mavoungou, Marielle K. Bouyou-Akotet, and P. G. Kremsner, "Effects of Prolactin and Cortisol on Natural Killer (NK) Cell Surface Expression and Function of Human Natural Cytotoxicity Receptors (NKp46, NKp44 and NKp30)," *Clinical and Experimental Immunology* 139, no. 2 (March 2005): 287–96, doi:10.1111/j.1365-2249.2004.02686.x.

10. Sefirin Djiogue, Armel Hervé Nwabo Kamdje, Lorella Vecchio, Maulilio John Kipanyula, Mohammed Farahna, Yousef Aldebasi, and Paul Faustin Seke Etet, "Insulin Resistance and Cancer: The Role of Insulin and IGFs," *Endocrine-Related Cancer* 20 no. 1 (February 1, 2013): R1–17, doi:10.1530/ERC-12-0324.

11. Afaf Girgis, Sylvie Lambert, Claire Johnson, Amy Waller, and David Currow, "Physical, Psychosocial, Relationship, and Economic Burden of Caring for People with Cancer: A Review," *Journal of Oncology Practice* 9, no. 4 (July 2013): 197–202, doi:10.1200 /jop.2012.000690.

12. Pesticide Action Network North America, "Apples," What's on My Food?, accessed November 12, 2016, http://www.whatsonmyfood.org/food.jsp?food=AP.

13. Henry McGrath, *Traditional Chinese Medicine Approaches to Cancer: Harmony in the Face of the Tiger* (London: Singing Dragon, 2009).

14. Zhigang Lu, Jingjing Xie, Guojin Wu, Jinhui Shen, Robert Collins, Weina Chen, Xunlei Kang, et al., "Fasting Selectively Blocks Development of Acute Lymphoblastic Leukemia via Leptin-Receptor Upregulation," *Nature Medicine* 23 (December 2016): 79–90, doi:10.1038/nm.4252.

15. Daniel F. Kripke, Robert D. Langer, and Lawrence E. Kline, "Hypnotics' Association with Mortality or Cancer: A Matched Cohort Study," *BMJ Open* 2, no. 1 (February 27, 2012): e00850, doi:10.1136/bmjopen-2012-000850.

16. NIH, "Why Is Sleep Important?" US Department of Health and Human Services, last updated February 22, 2012, https://www.nhlbi.nih.gov/health/health-topics/topics /sdd/why.

17. Lisa Chopin, Carina Walpole, Inge Seim, Peter Cunningham, Rachael Murray, Eliza Whiteside, Peter Josh, and Adrian Herington, "Ghrelin and Cancer," *Molecular and Cellular Endocrinology* 340, no. 1 (June 20, 2011): 65–69, doi:10.1016/j.mce.2011.04.013.

18. "Allergies and Sleep," National Sleep Foundation, accessed November 15, 2016, https:// sleepfoundation.org/sleep-topics/sleep-related-problems/allergic-rhinitis-and-sleep.

19. Erina Nakamura, Ken-ichi Kozaki, Hitoshi Tsuda, Emina Suzuki, Atiphan Pimkhaokham, Gou Yamamoto, Tarou Irie, et al., "Frequent Silencing of a Putative Tumor Suppressor Gene Melatonin Receptor 1 A (MTNR1A) in Oral Squamous-Cell Carcinoma," *Cancer Science* 99, no. 7 (July 2008): 1390–400, doi:10.1111/j.1349-7006.2008.00838.x.

20. T. S. Wiley and Bent Formby, *Lights Out: Sleep, Sugar, and Survival* (New York: Pocket Books, 2000).

21. Antonio Cutando, Antonio López-Valverde, Salvador Arias-Santiago, Joaquin de Vicente Buendia, and Rafael Gómez de Diego, "Role of Melatonin in Cancer Treatment," *Anticancer Research* 32, no. 7 (July 2012): 2747–53.

22. Russel J. Reiter, Du-Xian Tan, Rosa M. Sainz, Juan Carlos Mayo, Silvia Lopez-Burillo, "Melatonin: Reducing the Toxicity and Increasing the Efficacy of Drugs," *Journal of Pharmacy and Pharmacology* 54, no. 10 (November 2002): 1299–321, doi:10.1211/002235702760345374.

23. J. Christian Gillin, "How Long Can Humans Stay Awake?" accessed November 15, 2016, https://www.scientificamerican.com/article/how-long-can-humans-stay.

24. Jennifer A. Mohawk, Carla Beth Green, and Joseph S. Takahashi, "Central and Peripheral Circadian Clocks in Mammals," *Annual Review of Neuroscience* 35, no. 1 (April 2012): 445–62, doi:10.1146/annurev-neuro-060909-153128.

25. Saurabh Sahar and Paolo Sassone-Corsi, "Metabolism and Cancer: The Circadian Clock Connection," *Nature Reviews Cancer* 9, no. 12 (December 2009): 886–96, doi:10.1038/nrc2747.

26. Jens Freese, Daniel J. Pardi, Begoña Ruiz-Núñez, Sebastian Schwarz, Regula Heynck, Robert Renner, Philipp Zimmer, and Helmut Lötzerich, "Back to the Future. Metabolic Effects of a 4-Day Outdoor Trip under Simulated Paleolithic Conditions—New Insights from The Eifel Study," *Journal of Evolution and Health* 1, no. 1 (October 24, 2016): doi:10.15310/2334-3591.1035.

27. Mark P. Mattson, "Hormesis Defined," *Ageing Research Reviews* 7, no. 1 (January 2008): 1–7, doi:10.1016/j.arr.2007.08.007.

28. Mark P. Mattson and Aiwu Cheng, "Neurohormetic Phytochemicals: Low-Dose Toxins That Induce Adaptive Neuronal Stress Responses," *Trends in Neurosciences* 29, no. 11 (November 2006): 632–39, doi:10.1016/j.tins.2006.09.001.

29. Vikneswaran Murugaiyah and Mark P. Mattson, "Neurohormetic Phytochemicals: An Evolutionary-Bioenergetic Perspective," *Neurochemistry International* 89 (October 2015): 271–80, doi:10.1016/j.neuint.2015.03.009.

30. Prasad R. Dandawate, Dharmalingam Subramaniam, Subhash B. Padhye, and Shrikant Anant, "Bitter Melon: A Panacea for Inflammation and Cancer," *Chinese Journal of Natural Medicines* 14, no. 2 (February 2016): 81–100, doi:10.1016/S1875-5364(16)60002-X.

31. Kenneth G. Collins, Gerald F. Fitzgerald, Catherine Stanton, and R. Paul Ross, "Looking Beyond the Terrestrial: The Potential of Seaweed Derived Bioactives to Treat Non-Communicable Diseases," *Marine Drugs* 14, no. 3 (March 18, 2016), doi:10.3390/md14030060.

32. Alexander Panossian, Marina Hambardzumyan, Areg Hovhanissyan, and Georg Wikman, "The Adaptogens Rhodiola and Schizandra Modify the Response to Immobilization Stress in Rabbits by Suppressing the Increase of Phosphorylated Stress-Activated Protein Kinase, Nitric Oxide and Cortisol," *Drug Target Insights* 2 (February 16, 2007): 39–54, http://www.ncbi.nlm.nih.gov/pmc/articles/PMC3155223.

33. Zhongbo Liu, Xuesen Li, Anne R. Simoneau, Mahtab Jafari, and Xiaolin Zi, "Rhodiola Rosea Extracts and Salidroside Decrease the Growth of Bladder Cancer Cell Lines via Inhibition of the mTOR Pathway and Induction of Autophagy," *Molecular Carcinogenesis* 51, no. 3 (March 2012): 257–67, doi:10.1002/mc.20780.

34. Neil McKinney, *Naturopathic Oncology: An Encyclopedic Guide for Patients and Physicians* (Richmond, BC: Creative Guy Publishing, 2016).

35. Tomohiro Shimizu, María P. Torres, Subhankar Chakraborty, Joshua J. Souchek, Satyanarayana Rachagani, Sukhwinder Kaur, Muzafar Macha, et al., "Holy Basil Leaf Extract Decreases Tumorigenicity and Metastasis of Aggressive Human Pancreatic Cancer Cells in Vitro and in Vivo: Potential Role in Therapy," *Cancer Letters* 336, no. 2 (August 19, 2013): 270–80, doi:10.1016/j.canlet.2013.03.017.

36. O. Igarashi, "The Significance of the Issuance of the 5th Revision of the Japanese Standard Tables of Food Components on Study and Research on Vitamins and Diseases," 36th Vitamin Information Center Press Seminar, Tokyo, Japan, 2001.

37. Jo Robinson, *Eating on the Wild Side: The Missing Link to Optimum Health* (New York: Little, Brown and Company, 2013).

Chapter 12: Mental and Emotional Well-Being

1. Michael K. Skinner and Carlos Guerrero-Bosagna, "Environmental Signals and Transgenerational Epigenetics," *Epigenomics* 1, no. 1 (October 2009): 111–117, doi:10.2217/epi.09.11.

2. Thomas Jessy, "Immunity Over Inability: The Spontaneous Regression of Cancer," *Journal of Natural Science, Biology, and Medicine* 2, no. 1 (January 2011): 43–49, doi:10.4103/0976-9668.82318.

3. Jerome Sarris, Alan C. Logan, Tasnime N. Akbaraly, G. Paul Amminger, Vicent Balanzá-Martínez, Marlene P. Freeman, Joseph Hibbeln, et al., "Nutritional Medicine as Mainstream in Psychiatry," *Lancet Psychiatry* 2, no. 3 (March 2015): 271–74, doi:10.1016/S2215-0366(14)00051-0.

4. Pedro Rada, N. M. Avena, and B. G. Hoebel, "Daily Bingeing on Sugar Repeatedly Releases Dopamine in the Accumbens Shell," *Neuroscience* 134, no. 3 (February 2005): 737–44, doi:10.1016/j.neuroscience.2005.04.043.

5. UCSF Benioff Children's Hospital Oakland, "Omega-3 Fatty Acids, Vitamin D May Control Brain Serotonin, Affecting Behavior and Psychiatric Disorders," *ScienceDaily*, February 25, 2015, https://www.sciencedaily.com/releases/2015/02/150225094109.htm.

6. Liang-Jen Wang, Sheng-Yu Lee, Shiou-Lan Chen, Yun-Hsuan Chang, Po See Chen, San-Yuan Huang, Nian-Sheng Tzeng, et al., "A Potential Interaction between COMT and MTHFR Genetic Variants in Han Chinese Patients with Bipolar II Disorder," *Scientific Reports* 5 (March 6, 2015): 8813, doi:10.1038/srep08813.

7. Simon N. Young, "Folate and Depression—A Neglected Problem," *Journal of Psychiatry and Neuroscience* 32, no. 2 (March 2007): 80–82, http://www.ncbi.nlm.nih.gov/pmc/articles/PMC1810582.

8. NIH, "COMT Gene," Genetics Home Reference, January 24, 2017, https://ghr.nlm.nih.gov/gene/COMT.

9. H. J. Baltrusch, W. Stangel, and I. Titze, "Stress, Cancer and Immunity. New Developments in Biopsychosocial and Psychoneuroimmunologic Research," *Acta Neurolgical (Napoli)* 13, no. 4 (August 1991): 315–27, https://ncbi.nlm.nih.gov/labs/articles/1781308.

10. M. A. Visintainer, J. R. Volpicelli, and M. E. P. Seligman, "Tumor Rejection in Rats after Inescapable or Escapable Shock," *Science* 216, no. 4544 (May 1982): 437–39, doi:10.1126/science.7200261.

11. Marilia Carabotti, Annunziata Scirocco, Maria Antonietta Maselli, and Carola Severi, "The Gut-Brain Axis: Interactions between Enteric Microbiota, Central and Enteric

Nervous Systems," *Annals of Gastroenterology* 28, no. 2 (April–June 2015): 203–9, http://www.ncbi.nlm.nih.gov/pmc/articles/PMC4367209.

12. Anastasiya Slyepchenko, Andre F. Carvalho, Danielle S. Cha, Siegfried Kasper, and Roger S. McIntyre, "Gut Emotions—Mechanisms of Action of Probiotics as Novel Therapeutic Targets for Depression and Anxiety Disorders," *CNS and Neurological Disorders Drug Targets* 13, no. 10 (2014): 1770–86.

13. Liya Qin, Xuefei Wu, Michelle L. Block, Yuxin Liu, George R. Breese, Jau-Shyong Hong, Darin J. Knapp, and Fulton T. Crews, "Systemic LPS Causes Chronic Neuroinflammation and Progressive Neurodegeneration," *Glia* 55, no. 5 (April 1, 2007): 453–62, doi:10.1002/glia.20467.

14. A. E. Kalaydjian, W. Eaton, N. Cascella, and A. Fasano, "The Gluten Connection: The Association between Schizophrenia and Celiac Disease," *Acta Psychiatrica Scandinavica* 113, no. 2 (February 2006): 82–90, doi:10.1111/j.1600-0447.2005.00687.x.

15. Richard J. Farrell and Ciarán P. Kelly, "Celiac Sprue," *New England Journal of Medicine* 346, no. 3 (January 17, 2002): 180–88, doi:10.1056/NEJMra010852.

16. Wanyi Tai, Zhijin Chen, and Kun Cheng, "Expression Profile and Functional Activity of Peptide Transporters in Prostate Cancer Cells," *Molecular Pharmaceutics* 10, no. 2 (February 4, 2013): 477–87. doi:10.1021/mp300364k.

17. Sandra Zoghbi, Aurélien Trompette, Jean Claustre, Mahmoud El Homsi, Javier Garzón, Gérard Jourdan, Jean-Yves Scoazec, and Pascale Plaisancié, "β-Casomorphin-7 Regulates the Secretion and Expression of Gastrointestinal Mucins through a μ-Opioid Pathway," *American Journal of Physiology—Gastrointestinal and Liver Physiology* 290, no. 6 (May 10, 2006): G1105–1, doi:10.1152/ajpgi.00455.2005; Katarzyna Gach, Anna Wyrebska, Jakub Fichna, and Anna Janecka, "The Role of Morphine in Regulation of Cancer Cell Growth," *Naunyn-Schmiedeberg's Archives of Pharmacology* 384, no. 3 (September 2011): 221–30, doi:10.1007/s00210-011-0672-4.

18. Flore Depeint, W. Robert Bruce, Nandita Shangari, Rhea Mehta, and Peter J. O'Brien, "Mitochondrial Function and Toxicity: Role of the B Vitamin Family on Mitochondrial Energy Metabolism," *Chemico-Biological Interactions* 163, no. 1–2 (November 2006): 94–112, doi:10.1016/j.cbi.2006.04.014.

19. Edward H. Tobe, "Mitochondrial Dysfunction, Oxidative Stress, and Major Depressive Disorder," *Neuropsychiatric Disease and Treatment* 9 (2013): 567–73, doi:10.2147/NDT.S44282.

20. Pál Pacher, Sándor Bátkai, and George Kunos, "The Endocannabinoid System as an Emerging Target of Pharmacotherapy," *Pharmacological Reviews* 58, no. 3 (September 2006): 389–462, doi:10.1124/pr.58.3.2.

21. Karl W. Hillig and Paul G. Mahlberg, "A Chemotaxonomic Analysis of Cannabinoid Variation in *Cannabis* (Cannabaceae)," *American Journal of Botany* 91, no. 6 (June 2004): 966–75, doi:10.3732/ajb.91.6.966.

22. Lifang Mao, Suizhen Lin, and Jun Lin, "The Effects of Anesthetics on Tumor Progression," *International Journal of Physiology, Pathophysiology and Pharmacology* 5, no. 1 (March 8, 2013): 1–10, http://www.ncbi.nlm.nih.gov/pmc/articles/PMC3601457.

23. Paola Massi, Marta Solinas, Valentina Cinquina, and Daniela Parolaro, "Cannabidiol as Potential Anticancer Drug," *British Journal of Clinical Pharmacology* 75, no. 2 (February 2013): 303–12, doi:10.1111/j.1365-2125.2012.04298.x.

24. D. I. Abrams and M. Guzman, "Cannabis in Cancer Care," *Clinical Pharmacology and Therapeutics* 97, no. 6 (June 2015): 575–86, doi:10.1002/cpt.108.

25. Hong-Fang Ji, Xue-Juan Li, and Hong-Yu Zhang, "Natural Products and Drug Discovery: Can Thousands of Years of Ancient Medical Knowledge Lead Us to New and Powerful Drug Combinations in the Fight against Cancer and Dementia?" *EMBO Reports* 10, no. 3 (March 2009): 194–200, doi:10.1038/embor.2009.12.

26. V. Di Marzo, "The Endocannabinoid System in Obesity and Type 2 Diabetes," *Diabetologia* 51 (June 18, 2008): 1356–67, doi:10.1007/s00125-008-1048-2. Available at http://theroc.us/images/The%20endocannabinoid%20system%20in%20obesity%20and%20type%202%20diabetes.pdf.

Chapter 13: Connecting with the Terrain Ten in the Kitchen

1. William Davis, *Wheat Belly: Lose the Wheat, Lose the Weight, and Find Your Path Back to Health* (Emmaus, PA: Rodale, 2011).

2. James R. Roberts, Catherine J. Karr, Jerome A. Paulson, Alice C. Brock-Utne, Heather Brumber, Carla C. Campbell, Bruce P. Lanphear, et al., "Pesticide Exposure in Children," *Pediatrics* 130, no. 6 (December 2012): e1757–63, doi:10.1542/peds.2012-2757.

3. W. R. Phipps, M. C. Martini, J. W. Lampe, J. L. Slavin, and M. S. Kurzer, "Effect of Flax Seed Ingestion on the Menstrual Cycle," *Journal of Clinical Endocrinology and Metabolism* 77, no. 5 (November 1993): 1215–19, doi:10.1210/jcem.77.5.8077314.

Index

Page numbers followed by *t* refer to tables.

About the Authors

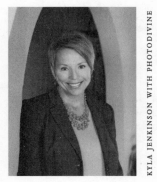

DR. NASHA WINTERS, ND, FABNO, L.AC., DIPL.OM, is the founder, CEO, and visionary of Optimal Terrain Consulting. She has been working in the health care industry for 25 years and is a nationally board certified naturopathic doctor, licensed acupuncturist, practitioner of oriental medicine, and is a fellow of the American Board of Naturopathic Oncology. Initially motivated by a terminal cancer diagnosis 25 years ago, she now lectures all over the world, trains physicians in the application of mistletoe therapy, and consults with researchers on projects involving immune modulation via mistletoe, hyperthermia, and the ketogenic diet. She lives in Durango, Colorado.

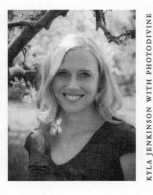

JESS HIGGINS KELLEY, MNT, is the founder of the Oncology Nutrition Therapy Certification Program at the Nutrition Therapy Institute in Denver, Colorado. She also is the founder and CEO of the metabolic nutrition consulting, education, and research enterprise Remission Nutrition. With an undergraduate degree in journalism, Jess has written health and nutrition articles for local and national publications and is the former managing editor of *Edible Southwest Colorado* magazine. She lives in Mid Coast Maine.

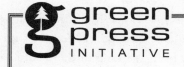

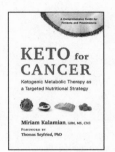
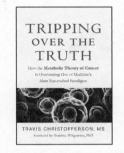
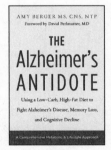
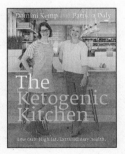
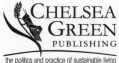

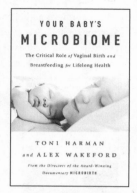
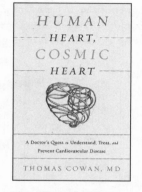
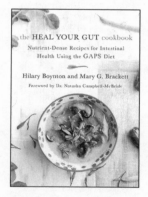
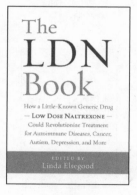
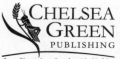